M

Soul-Full Eating

A *(Delicious!)* Path to Higher Consciousness

*"The greatest pleasure comes
from being in sync with
what resonates with our Souls."*

~ Maureen Whitehouse

Soul-Full Eating

A *(Delicious!)* Path to Higher Consciousness

Maureen Whitehouse

AXIOM PUBLISHING
HOLLYWOOD, FL

Published by Axiom Publishing, Post Office Box 682, Hollywood, FL 33022 U.S.A.
Orders@ExperienceAxiom.com | www.ExperienceAxiom.com

Publisher's Cataloging-in-Publication
(Provided by Quality Books, Inc.)

    Whitehouse, Maureen.
      Soul-Full eating : a (delicious) path to higher
    consciousness / by Maureen Whitehouse. -- 1st ed.
      p. cm.
      Includes index.
      LCCN 2006907116
      ISBN-13: 978-0-9745869-6-0 (print ed.)
      ISBN-10: 0-9745869-6-X (print ed.)

      1. Nutrition. 2. Spiritual life. 3. Health.
    I. Title.

    RA784.W58 2006   613.2
                          QBI06-600325

DISCLAIMER: This book is for informational and educational purposes only. The material in this book is not meant to replace medical advice. Please consult with a physician or other qualified health care professional if you have questions about your health.

Never change any treatment or medication without consulting a physician or other qualified health professional. The author and Axiom Publishing shall have neither liability nor responsibility to any person or entity with respect to any damage, loss, consequences or injury related to information including recommendations, products and services contained in this book.

Book Design by Dotti Albertine / Jessica Trussell

Unattributed quotations are by Maureen Whitehouse.

This book is dedicated to
My Beloved One
Whose Fullness I taste every day
In all of my life
With all of my life.
I am deeply in your Grace.

ACKNOWLEDGMENTS

Before I began writing books, I used to read these acknowledgment pages with curiosity wondering how it was that the author found so many people to work with and to thank for getting their book to print. After all, I thought, what is there to it? Don't you just sit down with a pad of paper or a computer in front of you and write? Isn't it all just between you and the page? Oh was I ever mistaken!

Now that I've worked on several book projects, I see that there are far too many elements and interactions with people that go into the creation of a book to even begin to recount all of them. So thank you to anyone I missed in my list below. I am grateful for your help too!

This book is my first of many books to be published—I know that. In this way, I see it as a "firstborn." And writing it made me recall a remark a friend made to me when I was carrying my first child: "They say you make all of your mistakes on the first one." I'd like to thank all of the following beautiful Souls for being there for me and not only "cleaning up my many mistakes" as I wrote *Soul-Full Eating*, but also helping to transform this project into a beautiful, helpful, inspiring message that hopefully can help heal our planet. I love you all…

First, Heather—my bright, beautiful talented daughter—who helped me get the very first words of this book on a page back when we still thought it was just a chapter in another book I'm writing called *True Beauty*. You are a gifted writer.

Next Fritz, Maeve and Chauncey for eating all of my meals for all of those years, but mostly for being such powerful living breathing examples of absolutely unconditional love in my life.

Theresa Nardi, my sista—you know how much I love you. Thank you, just for being YOU so brilliantly, and for being so much FUN!

For Robin Quinn, I thank you not only for your unsurpassed editing skills but for your extremely encouraging, genuinely enthusiastic and effervescent persona. I feel blessed to have met and worked so closely with you. I look forward to collaborating on many more future projects together.

Linda Collie, for your "eagle eye" copy editing and invaluable input, many, many thanks.

Saeedeh Naderi, your artistic talents are surpassed only by your ability to be *the most* self-less, loving, caring and supportive friend. Thank you for designing such an exquisite cover and elegant inside illustrations for this book. Ya Allah Salam!

For Your Supreme Light, my dear friend Ani St. Germaine, you know I am always grateful.

Peter Cervoni, chef extraordinaire, for your helpful information and continual encouragement.

Aaron Vanderpool, for your inspiring presence. You shine so bright.

For Josh's Organic Garden—I Thank God!

Deborah Lazar, your organizational skills and computer expertise contributed greatly to the ease of the formatting process.

Dotti Albertine and Jessica Trussell, words are so much more poignant when arranged with Soul in mind. Thank you for adding your beautiful, spacious style to the formatting of *Soul-Full Eating*.

And last but not least, to Mom and Dad, two beautiful Twin-Souls who always encouraged me to Be Who I Am as they've watched me embrace and walk "the road less traveled by" for many, many years. I love you both.

Just Sit There

Just sit there right now.
Don't do a thing.
Just rest.

For your separation from God
Is the hardest work in this world.

Let me bring you trays of food
And something that you like to drink.

You can use my soft words
As a cushion
For your
Head.

~ Hafiz, Persian Poet (ca.1320-1389)

"Love is All there is.
You live that you may learn to love.
You love that you may learn to live.
There is no other lesson.
Your Soul knows this.
Your Soul is empty of all else.
Hence, your Soul is always full,
Of Love."

CONTENTS

FOREWORD

"Great book!" the photographer says as he hands my portfolio back to me. "You'd be perfect for this job. I hope we get a chance to work together." Smiling, I thank him, but think, "How many times have I heard that before?"

Out on the street, a man lies in a doorway on a pile of grimy clothes. Extending his rumpled Dunkin' Donuts coffee cup to me, he says, "Ma'am, got any spare change?" I shake my head, fingering the only two quarters in my pocket, my subway fare, wishing I did have extra money to give. It's noon, and I've been beating the streets since 10 a.m. With three appointments behind me, I have four more to go, each one on near opposite sides of the city. I know, as usual, that I'll be hoofing my way around Manhattan for hours, trying my utmost to look not only good, but "perfect." Today I'm attempting it in suffocating 95 degree heat.

I pat down my frizzling hair as I look at my reflection in a shop window and then proceed down the street. I imagine I'm in a sauna, paying for this luxury, as I feel a drop of sweat run down my cheek. I walk further up the block and spy a church. I feel instantaneous relief as my hand touches the long brass handles, cool as icicles, and pull open the door.

An instant rush of still, fragranced air greets me and lures me into the darkened sanctum. There I sit in the candle-lit silence, and let out a deep, full sigh. I go into my own little world, far, far away from the streets of New York. I begin envisioning myself the picture of success—to me that means being a globe-trotting, sleek top model, the only thing fat about me being my bank account. I picture that account as full as my modeling portfolio is of magazine spreads and covers of me.

About ten minutes later, the clink, clink of some coins in the poor box snaps me out of my reverie. Standing up, I grab my portfolio, heave my shoulder bag into position, and once again head out into the street, leaving the church behind.

Moments later, I pass a construction crew on lunch break.

"Hey honey. How ya doin'? What'cha got there? A modeling portfolio? Can I see? Got any pictures of those legs?"

I ignore them. Like ants, the construction workers are everywhere, on nearly every block of the city there's another steel-raftered hole from which they emerge in droves. Thankfully I'm about to arrive at my next appointment. I dodge in the doorway, take the elevator to the top floor, and head for a typical photographer's loft that has a job in full swing.

Seated on chairs behind the camera are several ad agency reps and an art director. Two assistants are setting the lights as the photographer chats with his studio manager. The models, all in various stages of being prepped and camera readied, are positioned around a full wall-sized mirror, which is surrounded by white-hot light bulbs. A makeup artist applies foundation, taken from his massive case, to the women's faces, with deft strokes, a la Renoir painting a portrait. The hairstylist lacquers a chignon. The stylist steam-irons a silk dress.

As I walk towards the photographer, I pass a buffet table, which runs nearly the entire length of the studio. It has been cursorily picked over. Involuntarily, my mouth waters like one of Pavlov's dogs. The photographer notices me and he tramples through the ordered confusion to extend a warm smile and then his hand for my book. We exchange small talk as he thumbs through it appreciatively. As he closes the book, I hear for the fourth time that day, "You're great. I'd love to work with you."

I smile, murmur my thanks, and while walking out I find myself tempted to grab a roll as I pass by the lunch spread. But I refrain, knowing next week I could be here again—hopefully getting paid to smile in front of the camera. So in anticipation of a someday, once again I starve myself today…

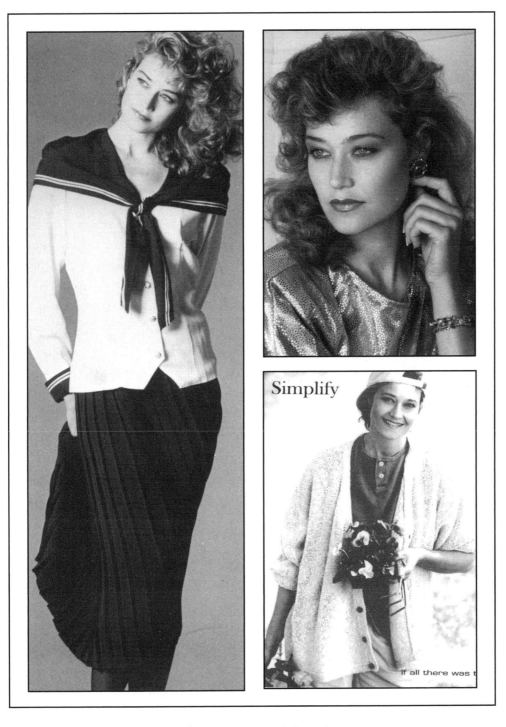

Pictures of me in my modeling daze...

That's a snapshot from my glamorous life as a fashion model. A girl-next-door type, I was particularly well-known for being able to sell anything that normally would never make it past my big, white-toothed smile, and into my stomach, such as savory snacks and sweet indulgences. I held McDonald's burgers and fries, various supermarket whipped-cream-laden bakery goods, synthetically contrived breakfast cereals, and even the biggest no-no of all—cigarettes!

Why? Well, I can't say I didn't know any better than to be such a vital cog in the "do what the beautiful people do" driven wheel of consumption—I did. In fact, I made it my daily practice not to get sucked into this consumption myself as I put on my high-heels to wade each day in the muck of commercial advertising. Maybe I can chalk it up to selfishness—the money was so good— or the need for excitement—I never knew where I'd be from one day to the next. Fame and fortune lingered just around each and every corner. Or maybe I had just bought into the fast-held American Dreamer's belief that somewhere out there I could find something fulfilling if I just tried it all.

I didn't find it. That is, not until somewhat by default, after so many years of taking refuge in churches and metaphysical bookstores between go-sees and auditions, I finally found my Soul and realized "it" never was *out there*. IT is *in here*. This is the same for each and every one of us, whether we are the person acting in the commercials or the one sitting in an Easy Boy watching them. You will never know satisfaction until you go deep—past all superficiality, trends and material-driven hungers—to something infinitely more pleasurable… to the unveiling of *your Soul*.

I've written this book so that you can devour something that is not filled with empty calories, but with juicy, golden nuggets of wisdom and truth. Take your time to savor each and every page, put what resonates with you to good use, and then pass on the pleasure you've found from it to others.

In Soul Territory, the only way to keep something that you truly love is to give it away.

*"Eat with love
what's grown with love,
prepared with love,
and served with love."*

Basic Principle of *Soul-Full Eating*

"I find it is easy
to give a plate of rice to a hungry person,
to furnish a bed to a person who has no bed,
but to console or to remove
the bitterness of anger and loneliness
that comes from being Spiritually deprived,
that takes a long time."

~Mother Theresa of Calcutta

INTRODUCTION

"I had been feeding my body's hunger for approval but not feeding my Soul..."

I grew up in a typical middle-class American household, eating some variation of meat and potatoes almost every night for dinner. When I was in high school, my brother Michael brought home some very basic health food. It was nothing too avant-garde, just something like honey, granola bars, fresh ground nutbutter and whole-wheat bread. Even so, my mother quickly banished it to the back corner of the pantry, far away from our "normal" food, which was more of the Kraft Macaroni and Cheese, Wise Potato Chips, and Jif Peanut Butter variety. After leaving home for college, I progressed to supping on dining-hall food—need I say more!—and then eating in a similar manner as I had at home when I moved off campus into a rented house where I lived with several roommates.

But, little by little, I began to be exposed to whole foods during my first two years in college. Then, during my junior year, my brother and I visited some cousins who lived in Hawaii. For nearly a month, we camped on the beach and ate food picked directly from vines and trees, or purchased at a nearby health-food store. At the store, I was introduced to Paavo Airola's classic book, *How to Get Well*, which gave me a glimmer of understanding about the relationship between diet and health.

It was also at about this time that Ralph Nader came to speak at my college. In vivid detail, he exposed the makings and ingredients of hot dogs. After this, my stomach did flips at just the thought of consuming one. I was an Animal Science major and the visit from Nader—on top of a school field-trip to a slaughterhouse, plus the experience of one too many dissections—had me making a firm vow to give up eating meat for life.

By the time I began modeling in New York City after college, I was a full-fledged vegetarian and well aware of the benefits of a healthy diet. My imperative to keep in shape guided me towards attaining a virtual Masters Degree in nutrition and holistic health. If anything was written about food, nutrition or health, I devoured it.

Yet, now, instead of having a nutritious meal for the pure enjoyment of it, eating became more of an obsession, an experience that was almost always tinged with guilt. I had to keep that perfect figure in order to be marketable, or worth anything in anyone's eyes. Although eating well was a wonderful focus, my motivation was completely outside of myself.

It wasn't until years later that I realized I had been feeding my body's hunger for approval but not feeding my *Soul*, and that my struggle with food was largely because I was living a surface existence and expecting it to somehow feel deeply fulfilling—an irreconcilable difference. Little did I know how vital it would be for me to make this connection.

Even though I was basically unconscious about the Spiritual symbolism behind eating and food back in my modeling days, I was aware of some things. Like most people, I knew that food—like air and water—is vital to support life and serves a primary physiological human need. But later on I learned the key to mastering an effortless, healthy relationship with food (or anything else for that matter). I saw that the most important connection for us all to make is with the *Spiritually* nutritive quality of life, which is every bit as important as the physiological—if not more so. I saw that carrying out typically mundane actions, such as eating, with a **Soul-Full**, sacred intention is liberating, and it allowed me to realize, *"I am not just a body! I am an Eternal Being."* Ingesting food with this perspective fills us with Spirit, tapping a wider, higher, deeper experience which makes eating supremely satisfying. In other words, *it is not only* **what** *we eat that's important, but also* **how**, *and with what perspective, we eat it.*

This book is aimed at giving clear, concise information about a way of eating that will best foster your own Soul-Full connection. First "digest" it, then adjust the approach considering your own lifestyle, habits, likes and dislikes. You alone can determine how to put the book's suggestions into practice for your optimum benefit. Only you know the path that is right *for you.* And I will stress this. *You do know! No one else does.* By being in touch with your Soul, by truly being aware, you can know yourself and how best to proceed.

One more thing… above all else recommended in these pages… love yourself.

If you begin to notice where Self-love is present—or not—in the entire process of eating, then the changes will come quite naturally. Soon you'll begin to become realigned with your Soul's internally set guidelines for peace and perfection. You will become that which is love. Then you will automatically begin to resonate with, and eat, only that which is healthy and whole.

CHAPTER ONE

Soul Food

Nourishing Yourself from the Inside Out

"Eating well becomes another way that we demonstrate self-love, a greater connection to our Soul."

ONE FUNDAMENTAL MISPERCEPTION that taints our world also forms the basis of most every diet that's ever been conceived—that we are *only* our bodies. As we now know, a human being is so much more than just a physical form. We are also Souls having what is meant to be the delightfully blessed experience of wearing a body for a time.

If we look at ourselves in this way, an entirely new world of perception opens up to us, including the way that we view diet. We realize that pleasure comes from being in sync with what resonates in our Souls, not necessarily from doing what we think gratifies our physical bodies. From this perspective, eating well—"dieting" if you will—becomes only one part of a greater connection to our true Selves. It becomes another way for us to nourish our connection with who we truly are, a way in which we demonstrate Self-Love.

So many diets don't work because they only acknowledge the most superficial aspects of us. For instance, look at the issue of maintaining an ideal

*"We are new
every day."*

~ Irene Claremont
De Castillego

weight. Our bodies gain excess weight because they are ideal indicators of our environment—both internal and external. Whatever is hidden internally cannot stay hidden for long—it will be projected outward from within us. In other words, the thoughts we think affect us physically. Excess weight is our heavy, un-happy thoughts about ourselves, or our uneasy lives, projected outward. Its presence is just a signal that we are out of connection with ourselves, or out of sync with life the way it was meant to be lived. The primary way to maintain an ideal weight is by honoring your Self and getting in sync with your Soul. Fall in love with your life and see what happens next!

THE IDEA BEHIND SOUL-FULL EATING

If we honor and connect to our Soul-Self, we can take an entirely different approach to diet—one with *no deprivation*. We can eat anything we want, any time we want, as long as it is indeed furthering our connection to our Divinity. That's the catch. Which foods actually compliment our Divinity and advance our connection to our Souls and which do not? That answer is simple... *The most nourishing food is that which is consciously grown, lovingly selected and prepared, and mindfully eaten.*

- CONSCIOUSLY GROWN refers to food produced in harmony with the greater environment—the greater Soul found in all of creation. When food is grown in this way, with a deeper connection and reverence for nature, it intrinsically connects us to "the bigger picture." To me, being conscious means acting in a way that demonstrates that you fully understand all of the consequences of your actions. You are aware that the way you talk, act, think and carry out your daily affairs affects yourself and others. So, when we eat food grown consciously, we more easily feel ourselves to be an intimate part of the circle of life. Consciously grown foods include those that are grown without artificial substances such as hormones, chemicals, pesticides and the use of genetic engineering. Without such false interferences, these foods maximize the benefits of sunlight, thus allowing us to receive the greatest energy exchange possible. They contain vital earth-energy and this is transferred to us.

- LOVINGLY SELECTED FOODS are those we choose that compliment our own unique, individual needs, as well as the foods that we know we will savor, such as those that are fresh and locally grown. Choosing to eat only foods that we truly love and are attracted to with all of our five senses automatically eliminates foods that we tend to eat on the run or just to fill our stomachs. Eating foods we take care to select fosters a greater sense of Self-recognition and Self-reverence.

- CAREFULLY PREPARED FOODS are made in ways that release their vitality. These dishes can be simple or elegant, but they are created and served in a manner that magnifies the food's nutritional value—in an environment that feels balanced, nurturing and healthful—i.e.: full of love! Those qualities are then imbued energetically into the food.

- CONSUMING FOOD MINDFULLY means eating with awareness and gratitude for all the effort and positive energy that has been focused in order to provide the bounty about to be enjoyed. Paying attention to not only what is on our plate—but how it got there and also how we eat it—is a powerful way to practice the art of true presence.

WHY "SIMPLE" CAN BE DIFFICULT

Eat with love only that which has been grown, prepared and served with love. It sounds simple. Well, the truth *is* always simple, but then we humans add the complications. And it seems that we are expert at complicating our world. Particularly in recent years, many of our "advances" have brought us far from recognition of the perfect balance, simplicity and innate order in ourselves and in all things. The development and proliferation of *chemical additives and preservatives, processed and fast food* have affected us in numerous ways—and not for the better. Industrial methods take the life out of food and then manufacturers add synthetic "flavor" and "zest" back into it. Sadly, our once vital, Light-filled, natural food-supply is now upstaged by the vast supply of altered, highly processed foods.

Because of this, maintaining a balanced, loving relationship with food has become difficult. We have gotten so far from the original path of simplicity that we now need guidance to carry out one of our most natural functions—eating. But eating food isn't meant to be an obstacle to surmount, a chore, or a situation of fear; it's meant to be an enjoyable part of life. It should also be the most natural and innate part of existence. The reason it is not, for so many, is that we have learned to dishonor life, and in turn the feelings of our bodies, the vehicles of our Souls. This, however, is learned behavior.

Think back to a day many years ago when you sat in an elementary school classroom, knowing that you had to go to the bathroom but instead opted to wait until "the proper time." Our "civilized" societies have institutionalized life, have made us conform even our most basic needs into what "fits" in. It has been physically ingrained in us that our own individual comfort levels can be taught to us, appropriately met, and even dictated to us, from sources outside of ourselves. That's why it seems nearly impossible these days to rely on ourselves to make choices that easily promote contentment and well-being. The only way to get back to an effortless, joyful experience with food is to deliberately make the act of eating sacred, entirely personal, and honoring of one's deepest needs.

SOMETHING TO CHEW ON

Spend five minutes meditating on or writing about the following questions. When you were young, were you given praise for finishing every last bite on your plate? Were you ever coerced into eating even after you felt full by being told about the starving children in other parts of the world or about how others suffered and sacrificed to provide you with your meal? If so, then it's likely that guilt has been coloring your world when it comes to eating—guilt for not eating enough, or guilt for eating too much. We are all born with an internal comfort-seeking mechanism—the Soul—The "Voice" of sanity. However, for many of us, it's been layered over, smothered and silenced by the guilt inherent in our fear-based conditioning.

SOUL-FULL EXERCISE #1

Just for one day, do only what you genuinely love to do. Can you do that? Lucky you, if you don't have to put a hold on everything and completely rearrange your entire life to do this. That means you are already being True to your Soul!

But if you do have to do a bit of finagling of time and space in order to allow your authentic-self to emerge, that's still fine. Why? Because now you can see that you really do deserve to love yourself more. Once you do this once, there may be no turning back!

Eating what you really don't love, without love, is just one small symptom of a greater picture of denying your brilliance and self-worth.

"True contentment is the power of getting out of any situation all that there is in it. It is arduous and it is rare."

~ G.K. Chesterton

CHAPTER TWO

Transition Time

"The curious paradox is that when I accept myself just as I am, then I can change."
  ~ Carl Rogers

IT IS VITALLY IMPORTANT that you love yourself as you give up old habits, tastes, textures and affinities. Remember that you are transitioning to a whole relationship with food, the ultimate objective of this approach to diet. There is no room for guilt in this process. Recognize that this is a new way of looking at food, relating to it, and allowing it to become you. Most transitions with this degree of impact do not happen overnight. But as the Spiritual text, *A Course in Miracles*, teaches, "The miracle minimizes the need for time." And the ultimate miracle is recognizing that you are not a body, but an unlimited Spirit, whose essence is as timeless as love itself. So once you align with a Soul-Full perspective, how long it takes to drop pounds or establish a healthier lifestyle becomes less important and simply part-and-parcel of following the urge to release yourself to a more fulfilling and peacefully oriented identity. While whole grains may not initially sound as enticing as a glazed donut, each time you make a healthy food choice you will both strengthen your body *and* your subtle Spiritual sensitivities. You will weaken your palate's habitual cravings and allow your Soul to come to the fore.

*"To change,
a person must
face the dragon
of his appetites
with another dragon,
the life energy
of the Soul."*

~ Jalaluddin Rumi

Until you feel entirely aligned with your Soul, take it as slowly and gradually as you must—patience is key. Staying in sync with whatever makes you feel most connected and happiest with yourself is the only imperative here. It's what's inside you—not outside—that we are focusing on. Hence the #1 Rule—*No Guilt*.

LOVE VS. GUILT

Eating with guilt is not eating with love. In fact, guilt (self-judgment) and love cannot occupy the same place at the same time. Why is it then that in our abundant society, guilt often goes hand-in-hand with eating? Perhaps it is in part that, unlike in more underdeveloped cultures, the variety of foods we have access to as Americans is astounding. This could be viewed as both a blessing and a curse. Blessed with bounty, those who don't make aware choices—and also relish and give thanks for them—often abuse themselves with food.

For women especially, guilt often plays a major role in the process of eating. We frequently experience some elusive emotion about ourselves that we can't put our finger on, one that we feel a continual need to squash and silence. This turns out to be guilt, not for anything in particular, other than just for being alive! Meanwhile, guilt is more toxic than any unhealthy food could ever be.

Often it's the guilt that pushes us toward the double-dip hot fudge sundae. We eat, or don't eat, in hopes of being able to control what seems so hopelessly out of control in our lives. At other times, we eat to de-sensitize ourselves in a shallow world that keeps us always looking for something satisfying. Still other times we unconsciously "bulk up" to protect ourselves from being seen in a purely superficial way. Yet only love and a Soul-Full connection can satiate our real needs. Diet after diet, it's not difficult to see that it's our illusory needs, our over-identification with the body and the guilt inherent in that perspective, that hang on much more tenaciously than the fat.

So, to reiterate, the most important rule here is to *love yourself entirely*, while remembering you are not limited to a body mind-set when you align with a Soul-Full perspective. Center your intention on loving and being present while you choose, prepare and eat food. When you do this, everything else will seem clear and fall into place.

THOUGHTS ON THE TRANSITION

As you cultivate a healthy relationship with food, begin by *loving* the fact that you live in a society that allows you such an abundance of food choices. Think of the variety available to gift yourself with, and the plethora of ways in which you can connect yourself to the Soul of life. Cultivate genuine gratitude for yourself and for your plenty. Give thanks for what you have. Then, as you choose, honor your choices fully while you transition to Light-filled foods. Now if you happen to choose a piece of Devil's Food Cake, eat it with awareness. A little treat now and then needn't plummet you into the depths of hell. If you really watch yourself eat it, you'll be able to discern what about the experience brings you joy, satisfaction and fullness—or conversely pain, sadness and feelings of self-defeat. By bringing this food into your experience, are you promoting a healthy relationship with life?

If you really enjoy this indulgence while being mindful, you will feel satisfied and satiated afterwards. If, on the other hand, you feel that this was not a great food choice, you can fully feel why. Watching yourself mindfully with love will allow you to see almost immediately what effects any type of food has on your body. Does it promote cravings, mood-swings, hyperactivity or sensitivity? Based on these mindful realizations, the next time you eat, you can make a more informed, self-honoring, conscious decision about what you desire to put into your mouth and body.

Initially while transforming your diet, you may feel as though you are off somewhere in left field and far from the mainstream of life. And that's no surprise, since about 90% of the money that Americans spend on food is used to buy processed, canned, frozen or dehydrated products. If you're eating wholesome foods in a mindful manner, you may not appear to be "normal" to others. Now another rule of mastery will come in handy.

Rule #2: *No Judgment*—of yourself or of others. Now is the time to live, and let live. Don't try to convert others, no matter how zealous you feel. That's a sure way to sabotage yourself. If you feel any judgment about another's lifestyle, you are just avoiding experiencing even greater Self-love. Notice that you can't realize your own advances while focusing on someone else's failures. If you feel inclined to change or convert others to your new way of being, get back into your own business. Your determination to be an authentic, living breathing example of one who lives Soul-Fully will speak volumes. Allow others to watch your new relationship to food without feeling the need to make any excuses for being "different." Wait until someone asks you, *with sincere interest*, for information about your new lifestyle before you speak about it. This is kind to both you and others.

Think back to a time (possibly very recently) when you didn't know that there was a more satisfying way of relating to food. A time when you felt you loved inhaling nachos and cheese at midnight in front of the TV without tasting them, infinitely more than you loved the idea of having a Soul-Full relationship with food. Fully get in touch with that way of thinking. What did it take to consider changing? Now know that change is just as scary to others as it is to you. Most of us make any excuse in the book to avoid changing. So be easy on yourself and other people while you take this courageous step in your life. And remember, actions always speak louder than words.

A basic reason to be gentle with yourself as you transition is that it may take a while for you to adapt physically. Our taste buds develop mostly within the early years of childhood. Therefore, tastes and food preferences are acquired as we are growing up. If we were fed large amounts of sugary and greasy fast-foods as children, we will continue to have an affinity for this as we grow older—that is, until we consciously "reprogram" ourselves. As you change your eating habits, I think you'll find that you begin to prefer simple, whole foods—as opposed to highly flavored, processed foods. *Your tastes can change*.

You may also find that you not only crave the tastes and textures of certain foods, but that you may even experience some physical withdrawal symptoms.

Watch for this particularly if your diet has included highly processed foods such as sugary baked goods (yeast and sugar), coffee and soda (caffeine), diet soft-drinks (artificial flavors, colors and sweeteners), and packaged goods with a long shelf-life (preservatives).

INTUITION VS. CRAVINGS

"One change leaves the way open for the introduction of others."

~ Niccolo Machiavelli

This book is not meant to tell you what to eat or how to eat it; it is merely meant as a source of information to supplement what your Innate Wisdom already knows about your nutritional needs. Because that's just it—you do know what you need, better than anyone else ever could. Each of us is programmed to instinctually hunger for foods that will contribute to our health and vitality. The trick is getting past cultural programming and learning to listen to your true needs. The information given in this book is meant to help block out all the societal white noise surrounding diet and nutrition, assist you in letting go of poor programming, and allow you to intuit what approach to eating will really work for you.

In our world, we are so accustomed to being told what we want, what we need, and what is good for us, that many of us have forgotten that the best gauge of our own bodily nutrition needs is our very own authentic tastes and hungers. Do you ever have cravings for particular foods without knowing why? Have you noticed that sometimes you may want a salad, while on another day a bowl of soup or burger seems more appealing? While in the humidity of Florida I am often satisfied with fruit, but when I visit relatives in Boston I often crave foods that are more substantial. This is because my body knows that it needs heartier foods and more protein in a colder climate.

You may be thinking, "I crave chocolate chip cookies and ice cream, but my body can't possibly need that!" The truth is that in our modern day culture, it is easy for our intuition to be skewed. On one hand, we are constantly barraged with advertisements selling us sweet, processed commercial foods. On the other hand, our society's obsession with body image and fad diets tells us that actually wanting any of these things is wrong. In addition, many of these foods contain addictive substances, such as sugar and caffeine. No wonder we are confused! But even with "junk-food" cravings, our bodies are tying to tell us something. A craving for fried chicken could be your intuition's signal that you need some protein. Do you really crave the potato chips or could it be the salt that comes with them? Sugar and salt cravings often signal mineral or vitamin deficiencies.

Whenever you are shopping for food, perusing a restaurant menu, or staring into your refrigerator deciding on a meal, pause to ask your deeper intuitive Self what you really feel like eating. Not what you think you *should* be eating, but what *you* feel that you need. Once you have an idea, ask your Self why you think you want this. Is it a craving influenced by advertising or the advice of others? Is it triggered by an attachment to "comfort foods" that help you to cover up feelings of pain or inadequacy? Once you are able to clear such outside noise or internalized bad programming (which gets easier with practice), you will eventually be able to identify which nutrients your Inner Wisdom is telling you that you need. Use the information given in this book to help discern what this Voice is telling you—to make conscious eating choices. By consuming what *your* body needs, you will feel more satisfied after each meal.

MAKING ADDITIONS, SUBSTITUTIONS, AND CHANGES WITH MODERATION

Ayurveda (one of the ancient eating approaches from India that is discussed in greater depth in Chapter 29) approaches healing and lifestyle changes in a gradual, positive way, rather than through deprivation, rigidity or "slash-and-burn" removal. Starting dietary changes by cutting out huge quantities of things that you previously enjoyed will, in most cases, not be very effective. Most likely you will resent the diet and may struggle with your own willpower and feelings of guilt. In addition, quitting addictive substances such as sugar and caffeine can bring along withdrawal symptoms. It is much more effective to *be certain your body is receiving the proper nutrients it needs **before** you start removing foods.*

Here are some ways to more easily transition to a healthy diet, and they will be discussed in greater detail throughout the book:

- **First—Begin with healthy additions** without depriving yourself of anything you currently enjoy.

- **Second—Substitute healthy alternatives for less desirable food choices**, such as mineral-rich sweeteners instead of sugar; homemade soups instead of canned ones; fresh cooked grains and vegetables instead of processed meals; and high-quality meats and fish instead of conventional supermarket meats.

- **Third—Eliminate some unhealthy foods and addictions.** This will be a lot easier if you have already made some of the above changes and are feeling their benefits.

- **Fourth—Avoid extremism.** The 19th century German naturopath Heinrich Lahmann stated: "It's not what you eat on Sunday that matters; it's what you eat the other six days." His practice was to prepare feasts of "stimulating" foods that were off the menu for the patients in his spa one day a week. Once in a while, it's fine to overindulge on foods you truly love if your typical approach to eating is moderation. Our physiology can handle feasting as long as it is not every day. And most people's psyches demand it occasionally.

MORE TIPS FOR TRANSITIONING:

1. In a culture that promotes the "Super-size," you may feel slighted at first when comparing truly healthy portion sizes to the norm. To prevent them from looking meager, use smaller plates and arrange foods on them creatively, attractively and, of course, lovingly. A plate of fresh vegetables or fruits in an assortment of colors representative of nearly every hue of the spectrum fills us up with light—affecting not only our body, but our mind, and enhancing our connection to Spirit as well. Eating this way enlivens us and our senses.

2. If you feel the urge to eat but realize you aren't hungry, nurture your body in other tangible ways—such as with deep breathing, relaxation exercises and meditation.

3. Get plenty of rest, fresh air and sunshine.

4. Drink lots of fresh water. It will help rid your body of toxins and also keep you feeling more full and satisfied while you are transitioning. If you feel that your body is releasing too many toxins too quickly, you can slow down the detoxifying process a bit by drinking fresh vegetable and fruit juices instead of water.

5. Finally, if you feel physical food-withdrawal symptoms of any kind, relax and be joyous in knowing that programmed into each of us is *self-healing*. Symptoms such as skin eruptions, headaches, slight nausea and a thickly coated tongue are quite normal. You are just healing and your body is detoxifying. Just as our skin rejuvenates when we are cut, our entire bodies are designed—from the cellular level to vital organs—to be self-healing. And the vital ingredient that each of our cells thrive on, and which heals us most assuredly, is *love*.

This Is How a Human Being Can Change

There's a worm addicted to eating grape leaves.
Suddenly he wakes up,
call it grace, whatever,
something wakes him,
and he's no longer a worm.
He's the entire vineyard,
and the orchard too,
the fruit, the trunks,
a growing wisdom and joy
that doesn't need
to devour.

~ Jalaluddin Rumi

SOMETHING TO CHEW ON

In the Hindu Spiritual tradition, our physical bodies are considered to be just one part of us. This tradition proposes that we also have mental, emotional, vital and Spiritual bodies—all of which exhibit their own qualities. You'll find that your physical body will feel less deprived as you transition to any new way of eating if you are satisfying the "hunger" of your other four bodies in some way.

For example, your vital body can be fed with rest or a daily brisk walk. Your emotional body could find satisfaction in journaling or writing an old friend. Your mental body could enjoy finding out more about a topic in this book that you find interesting by exploring some of the resources listed. Your Soul can be nurtured by taking time out to reflect or by simply noticing how great it feels to just "Be" with it all.

In addition, know that any activity that you bring your full attention and presence to nurtures all five of your bodies simultaneously and will always add the greatest sense of joy and fulfillment to your life. This aligning with all five of your bodies simultaneously will also help remind you that you are so much more than what you typically believe yourself to be and help you to release yourself from the dream of self-limitation.

SOUL-FULL EXERCISE #2

Have someone take a photo of you today—just as you are. And then sit down and write a short one-day autobiography. Here's your first sentence: *"This is who I am today—physically, mentally, emotionally, vitally and Spiritually."* Then describe in detail—objectively and nonjudgmentally—the present state of each of your bodies (physical, mental, emotional, vital and Spiritual). Next, write on the same paper: *"This is who I am loving myself into being in one week, one month, three months, six months and one year."* Illustrate on that page the most healthy, happy, vibrant, radiant picture of yourself that you can imagine—*and more.*

When the photo that you've taken of yourself is developed, put it together with this paper and save them in a "sacred" place. You can go back and look at them at the above intervals—taking a new picture of yourself to put in your box each time you look. Don't be surprised if—just by beginning to pay attention to all five of your bodies, even without *trying* to change one thing in your diet—you start to become the person you'd most love to be. And remember, in Reality you are not limited to even one body, let alone 5! You are a Soul—having a "fun" but impossible dream that you could ever be confined in any way, shape or form.

The 10 Key Concepts

"The Sun is simply bright. It does not correct anyone. Because it shines, the whole world is full of light. Transforming yourself is a means of giving light to the whole world."
~ Ramana Maharshi

EVEN IF YOU DECIDED to never count another calorie, read another food label, or assess another plate of food for its possible vitamin and mineral content, you could feel well-nourished, balanced, energized and able to live your life's purpose. How? Just by following the guidelines given in this section of the book.

I consider some of the concepts contained in this section to hold the key to having an effortless relationship with not only food, but also all other important aspects of your life. Implementing the information in these chapters will remind you of what's most important to you, restore your sanity, and reacquaint you with the essence and fullness of life. The overall message?... whenever you are not wholly joyous, it is because you have reacted with a lack of love.

Only love makes us feel full and complete. Eating with love will afford you a fullness beyond anything else you've ever experienced. Eating with love reminds us of Spirit. While you read this section, make a conscious effort to let go of all previous labels you may have had about yourself, eating, and your relationship to food. Step up to the plate with an open heart. Love yourself. *And remember: Simplicity is stuffed with pleasure!*

CHAPTER THREE

Be Mind-Full

"A baby tasting a certain food for the first time, if left alone, literally consumes it with every sense."

IN THE WORLD OF TV COMMERCIALS, they call it "the bite and smile," and in my day as a commercial actor, I learned to be masterful at it. *As the camera zooms in, the actor eyes the food in rapt anticipation, sniffing the air and sighing at its delectable aroma. Then she reverently picks it up and takes a slow, sumptuous mouthful. Her eyes close as her tastebuds take in the full effect of the heavenly cuisine. Only then does she slowly chew and swallow, before flashing to the camera a satisfied smile that drips with delight.*

Sure the food on commercial sets is intensely prepped and perfected (so much so, in fact, that the slang name for it, befittingly, is the "hero"), and certainly the actors are skilled in the dramatization of these simple moments of enjoying food. Still, the "bite and smile" is a great example of how food is meant to be eaten. Our food is supposed to be appreciated, and eating intended to be a delightful experience.

Imagine how much more satisfied we would be if we took in our food with a greater awareness of our senses—smelling the food's aroma, noticing how it is arranged on our plate, feeling its texture as we put a forkful into our mouth and again as we swallow it down. This would make the experience of dining much more satisfying and pleasurable, and also bring us more fully into the moment.

EXPERIENCING DEEP MINDFULNESS

The mystic side of me is drawn to the intimate exploration of the world's many Spiritual traditions. Mainly this is because I realize Spirit as the largest part of who I am. However, I also feel it's important to live, first-hand, anything that I relate to others about spirituality, or anything else for that matter, before I dare claim any authority to teach it. So while I was studying various forms of meditation, I attended a week-long silent meditation retreat with Thich Nhat Hahn, a Buddhist monk, and his disciples. At the very core of Nhat Hahn's Spiritual philosophy is mindfulness—i.e., purposefully being present with the moment you are in. We practiced this approach all day, every day, and although eating was considered to be a less significant part of the retreat, the power of being mindful became most blatantly apparent to me at mealtime. Throughout the retreat, food was very intentionally consumed in a mindful, reverent manner, as though eating was itself a sacred meditation.

Here is a snapshot of our typical meal... The fresh, organic food was served buffet style. Each person got in line at the sumptuous smorgasbord and, before taking any food, blessed their plate and utensils. We blessed ourselves, followed by blessing the kitchen staff for preparing such a lovely feast, and finally we blessed the variety of food that was in front of us. As we made selections, the monks reminded us that each plate of food holds the entire universe within it because the food has been grown in the earth with the aid of the air, sun and water—all these elements can be found in the food that we eat.

After gathering their food, each person then went to a table where we stood silently waiting for everyone to choose a seat. When all of the seats

"Be very still an instant. Come without all thought of what you ever learned before, and put aside all images you made. The old will fall away before the new without opposition or intent."

~ A Course in Miracles

at the table had been selected, each person silently looked at the others standing with them, and honored those gathered with bows. It was wisely pointed out that if one doesn't honor and recognize the others who dine with them, they are not honoring the space that they are in, and therefore are not being entirely present. It was a wonderful, almost royal, thing to then sit down and eat the whole universe with other people, and realize that this was what we were doing while we were doing it.

Each person was encouraged to consciously chew every bite 50 times. Doing this, I often realized how little I really needed of the food that I had taken from the buffet. (Needless to say, portion-sizes dwindled significantly as the week progressed, yet people always left each meal feeling very contented and satisfied.) During the meal, at some unpredictable and unannounced point, a monk would sound a mindfulness gong to keep diners aware of precisely how present they were being. Each time that happened, all are asked to stop, put down their forks, and sit quietly, becoming acutely aware of what we were doing, even more than we had been previously. At this point, we would simply sit back and notice things such as whether or not we were chewing 50 times or what else was happening inside and outside of ourselves that we hadn't noticed before. After a while, the gong would sound once more and we'd resume eating. The whole thing was such a beautiful, fulfilling process. After experiencing it, I couldn't imagine ever eating again in the same old unconscious, irreverent way.

The process of eating happens every day, yet so often we miss the opportunity to become aware, to be present, and to be Soul-Fully connected in those moments. And as a result we often fail to notice the miracles that are taking place around us. It's a beautiful experience to live so mindfully, to be plummeted so deeply within yourself, that there is nothing to feel but gratitude for what surrounds you.

> *"There are things you do because they feel right*
> *and they may make no sense and they may make*
> *no money and it may be the real reason we are here:*
> *to love each other and to eat each other's cooking*
> *and say it was good."*
> ~ Brian Andreas (Storypeople)

A STUDY IN CONTRASTS

A few weeks after I returned home from the retreat with Thich Nhat Hahn, I accompanied my then-husband to a corporate banquet for his work. Long tables were draped with thick white tablecloths. A buffet stood in the center of the room including metal platters filled with grilled vegetables or creamy Fettuccini Alfredo. A chef wearing a tall white paper-hat carved thin slices of roast beef. Steam rose out of a basket filled with warm rolls which one of the waiters had just placed on the buffet table, while a salad of iceberg lettuce and carrot shavings stood nearby. I watched as business people and their spouses rushed about the room. They greeted others and shook hands between moments of filling their plates, then hurried back to their tables. Seated, they shoved forkfuls into their mouths amidst small talk and laughter.

On one side of this room was the dessert table, overflowing with all manner of gooey, creamy and sugar-laden "delights"—the kind I'd drooled over so many times in the past. But this time, my eye was drawn to a large platter in the middle of the table filled with fresh fruit. Among the juicy squares of pineapple and melon sat a gorgeous, ripe strawberry. I'd spotted it from across the banquet hall and I knew from my experience at the retreat that that one strawberry could satisfy my appetite for the entire evening.

So I put the strawberry right in the center of a dessert plate and returned to my table. In the past, I might have felt silly or made up some excuse to the others for my "odd" preference. But this time, I just filled my senses entirely with the sight and scent of the bright red treat. If any of the others noticed me while I took each Soul-Full bite and *genuinely* smiled, I never noticed them. Gone were the days of performing for the camera. At that moment, everything else fell away and I was in heaven.

A MIND-FULLNESS EXERCISE

I begin the "diet" section of my *True Beauty* workshops without saying a word. Instead, I hand each of the participants three raisins. Then I tell them to imagine that they have never seen such a food before. They are to experience them anew, or as Zen Buddhists call it, with a "beginner's mind."

You can get three raisins now, and try this yourself while reading. Here's how I take the women through the exercise...

Taking the first raisin, begin to examine it carefully—touch it, feel it, roll it in the palm of your hand. How does it feel, smell and look? Then lick the raisin; how does it taste? When you have fully considered this, put it in your mouth, but don't chew it. Let it sit there, allowing your tongue to explore it. Notice what your tongue does—how it reacts to this "object." Now roll it all around your mouth with your tongue. Be aware of your tongue as well as of the raisin. Notice any new observations or realizations about this object. Now allow your teeth to touch it and slowly begin to chew. Try to consciously chew it until you no longer can, until it turns completely to liquid. Then, and only then, swallow it.

Now, take the second raisin. Explore it in the same way—very deeply, slowly and consciously. Note how this experience differs, and how it is the same, as the first.

Finally, take the third raisin and do the same—proceeding even more slowly and mindfully. Try to find anything in or about the raisin you may have missed the other two times, remembering that no matter how similar these objects appear to be, they are all unique and have some differentiating qualities about them.

After this "raisin meditation," I ask the women to comment on their experiences. Here are some of their responses:

"I never knew you could hear a raisin!"
"I usually eat these by the handful and barely taste one."
"Raisins have belly-buttons!"

I am always amazed to find that each time a group does this, someone, somehow, comes up with something entirely new about raisins. This is usually inspired by a flash of insight, or a reckoning about something they have been missing in their own lives on many levels. The women have made comments such as:

"While you fear missing a meal, you aren't fully aware of the meals you do eat."

~ Dan Millman

"I realized I could learn to like and actually savor something I thought I had no affinity or liking for."

Or, *"I tasted a medley of flavors when before this I had labeled raisins as having only one taste."*

All of these insights can be metaphors for how we live, how closely our relationship with food mirrors our relationship with life. What did you discover if you did the exercise as you read through it?

SOMETHING TO CHEW ON

The ultimate act of transcendence is to become one with someone or something. Just as brilliant actors become the character they portray, drawing us into the scene with them completely, we can be that absorbed in the everyday graces—such as the act of eating—in our own lives.

The next time you sit down for a meal, imagine yourself experiencing the sensory feast that a baby experiences while tasting a food they love for the first time. If left alone, they will literally become their food, consuming it with every sense. Food to a baby is a source of communion, in which they become fully satisfied, long before what they consume reaches the belly.

That may be the extreme, but you get the idea. See how it feels to resist eating unless you can make it a full-bodied experience for yourself—no matter where you are or what you're eating.

SOUL-FULL EXERCISE #3

If you haven't already, try the above Mind-Fullness Exercise with the raisins. It is derived from a popular exercise designed by mind/body medicine researcher, Jon Kabat-Zinn, Ph.D., of the University of Massachusetts Medical School.

By the way, if you hate raisins, all the better; do the Mind-Fullness Exercise anyway. And while you're experiencing the raisin with your every sense, ask yourself why you find those taste sensations distasteful. You may find that it's not the taste or texture of the raisin at all!

For many of us, food preferences are formed early based on a certain experience we've had with the food. I know I haven't been able to eat custard for a long time now. This used to be one of my favorite foods when I was young. That is, until the day I got a stomach virus after eating a big helping of it. Now my stomach does turns and I get an instant headache just thinking of eating it. So while doing the raisin exercise, you may discover a repressed memory.

If you don't dislike raisins, think of another food you've avoided since childhood, and try the Mind-Fullness Exercise with a very small portion of that too. See if you can discern whether it's the food's taste, or the feeling or memory that eating it elicits in you, that turns you off.

In the introduction of her book, *The Power of the Mind to Heal*, cellular biologist Joan Borysenko included a story about her Uncle Dick who hated cheese. One day at a family gathering, he wolfed down two huge pieces of cheesecake smothered in strawberries—thoroughly enjoying every morsel. About an hour later, Joan's mother commented that she was surprised he'd eaten the cheesecake. As soon as she told him what the "delicious dessert" he'd eaten was, the uncle "turned green and threw up all over the living room rug."

Your reaction to a certain food could very well be the result of being on the receiving end of a scolding or punishment for not eating that item as a child. At such a moment, your brain makes an emotional connection between the yucky item you are chewing and not feeling free to make an independent choice. This situation is then infused in the subconscious so that years later you find that item gives you terrible indigestion, for instance. It may not be the food item that you are adamant to avoid at all costs, but the fused memory of having no choice. You may have forgotten all about the situation that caused your distaste for the food, but your subconscious hasn't. A pattern has then been set and this food item is the trigger.

This type of realization translates to your other experiences in life. How many things might you be avoiding and finding distasteful based on your past experience of them? I have a friend who says he hates Boston because he had a bad experience with an ex-girlfriend there. He's missing out on experiencing the delights of an entire city that's filled with millions of people and offers thousands of potential experiences based on emotions that get triggered at just the mention of the name "Boston." The good news is that your biocomputer can be reset once you take a look at why you dislike anything—and the perfect method is by forgiving the past, and becoming conscious and mindful in the present.

So get out that list of foods you've been avoiding and try having a mindful taste test. You never know what juicy piece of information you may unearth about yourself. It could open up a whole new world for you.

CHAPTER FOUR

Buy Locally/ Grow Your Own

"It's difficult to think anything but pleasant thoughts while eating a homegrown tomato."
~ Louis Grizzard

PARTICULARLY IN DEVELOPED, INDUSTRIAL NATIONS—such as Great Britain and the United States—food appears to be traveling farther and farther to get to the table. Why is this? While there are many reasons, one is particularly significant for those of us who cherish the wide-open spaces—we are developing prime growing-land.

The term, *food miles*, is food-systems professional vernacular for the distance a food travels from where it is grown to where it is ultimately purchased by consumers. Today the average food mile for *locally grown produce* is about 56 miles. In contrast, according to an Iowa State University study, the typical *conventionally grown* food mile is an ever-widening 1,494 miles—nearly 27 times farther. That's a lot of shipping and handling!

And we're not just talking about getting pineapples to New Jersey or kiwi fruit to Ohio; this study was done on fruits and vegetables typically grown in any region. So, for example, the local food mile distances reported in the study

"Shipping is a terrible thing to do to vegetables; they probably get jet-lagged, just like people."

~ Elizabeth Berry

ranged from 20 miles for broccoli and sweet corn to 75 for potatoes, whereas the conventional food mile distances ranged from 311 miles for pumpkins to 1,838 miles for carrots. The study also found that conventional-source broccoli traveled more than 90 times farther than the locally grown variety. Conventional-source carrots, garlic, sweet corn, onion and spinach all traveled at least 50 times farther than their locally grown counterparts.

One reason to pay attention to where your food comes from is that the number of food miles any food travels affects the product's freshness, quality and taste. I believe a person hasn't truly lived until they've tasted a food that still feels warmed by the sun. In my family, one person would watch over the pot of water boiling on the stove while another would run out to the garden and pick the corn. So we were able to eat the corn on the cob within minutes of prying it from the stalk! My favorite "meal" this year was an enormous organic peach I devoured while still standing on the ladder leaning up against the tree I'd just picked it from!

It's wonderful to eat with a sense of connection in mind. Eating foods grown in our own gardens or from local farmers allows us to experience a more tangible bond with the larger whole. It also gives us greater recognition of the divine network that brings food to our table. Seek out farmer's markets, which are proliferating now, especially in big cities, and whenever possible be sure to support local farmers who use high-quality farming techniques.

Most towns and cities at least have farm stands and weekend farmer's markets during growing seasons. If you haven't yet been to one, it's an experience worth the effort and the ultimate sensory experience.

There are many advantages to buying from local farms. Not only is the produce fresh, but you will know exactly where it came from—it's not far from the farm to your table. If you have any questions about pesticides or preparation, you can ask the farmers personally. Knowing what you are eating and how it is grown connects you to the whole, which is always a full-filling experience.

SOUL-LINKING FROM A DISTANCE

All of this is not to say that eating a mango can't fulfill you if you live in Connecticut, where mangos don't grow. But to further highlight a Soul-Full connection, when you eat the mango, be appreciative of the chain of events and people involved in the miracle process that brings food from so far away to your table. This can fulfill you as well as connect you to California, Bali or wherever the food is from. Recognizing the privilege of being able to take part in this commonplace marvel will also help make you feel satisfied and whole.

I received the following note from a woman who attended one of my mindfulness workshops several years ago: *"A few days after I returned home from your workshop, my five-year-old daughter had two of her friends over to play. It was about 11 a.m. when they said to me, 'We're staaaaaaaarvin!' so I gave each of them a banana.*

"About a half-hour later, I found all three bananas lying on the nightstand in my daughter's room, barely eaten. It was at just that moment I remembered your lesson in mindfulness and connectivity. So I called all three girls into the room, and I asked them if they'd like me to tell them a story called The Life of a Banana. Their eyes widened as they chorused a resounding 'Yes please!' and scampered to sit at my feet.

"I began, 'Once upon a time, there was a banana tree on a tropical island, far, far away from Massachusetts (where we live). The banana tree took many, many years of rooting itself deeply into the ground, reaching its leaves towards the sun, and soaking in the tropical rain showers to grow a perfect bunch of bananas. One morning, a banana farmer got up very early in the morning to harvest his banana crop. He kissed his wife good-bye and walked into his banana grove to meet the other workers. There he found a beautiful bunch of perfect, almost ripened bananas...' " You get the idea. I told them exactly how the bananas they'd barely eaten that morning got all the way from a tropical island and into their hands.

"The girls were enthralled. When I was done, my daughter was the first to say, 'I'm hungry,' and to jump up to grab her banana. The others followed. This time I smiled as I watched them relish every single bite."

Food can spark the realization of how privileged we are to live in a day and age when the entire world is accessible and available to us for our enjoyment. Even if we don't personally know the grower in South America, we are Soul-Fully linked by a common appreciation.

GETTING TO KNOW YOU...

Back when I lived in New Hampshire, I made it a point to be on a first-name basis with everyone who worked at the local farm stand I used to frequent near my home. They could see my appreciation for their work and my love of their produce, so they'd always reserve the freshest pick for me.

Talk to everyone at your local farm stand—staff and customer alike. You'll get all kinds of great tips about things like how to pick the very best cantaloupe (I was told that you smell for a sweet aroma, squeeze it looking for a soft firmness, and thump it, looking for a "hollow" sound) or how to pick a great ear of corn without peeling back the husk (you ask!!). You'll find people eager to share tips like their grandmother's "secrets" and prize-winning recipes for strawberry rhubarb pie and strawberry jam. It's not difficult to find people who *love* their food at farm stands.

If you ever find yourself feeling over-worked, over-tired or stressed, try stopping by a local farm market with the deliberate intention to reconnect to the basics. Use all of your senses to breathe in every sight, smell, taste, touch and sound. You'll find it comforting to every part of your being.

Since moving to Florida, I demonstrated the power of intention by manifesting through prayer one of the most amazing organic farmer's markets on the East Coast every Sunday right next door! The staff at Josh's Organic Garden are my second family. The only way I could find food any more fresh, or pure, is if I were to grow it myself—which just so happens to be another wonderful option.

BEING YOUR OWN FARMER

Last year, at the age of 80, my father decided to grow his first vegetable garden. He lights up like a kid when speaking about it, and literally glows when he displays his harvest. I know my father's decision to plant vegetables is a direct result of his feasting on beefy red organic heirloom tomatoes and organic basil salads from my next-door organic market when he and my mother visited me last winter. The taste of those salads stayed with my father until spring, when he could plant his own prize-worthy crop.

By the way, my parents don't have a backyard of their own; they live in a condo community. My father heads off each morning, with his next-door neighbor, to a communal plot of land that his condo association owns. For a small annual fee, many cities and communities offer similar plots of land, with access to running water for those interested in growing vegetables and flowers. If you live in an apartment, or don't have access to a growing space by your home, inquire at your city or town hall to see if they have such "victory gardens." The experience of tending the soil, and watching the sun and earth meet to support life right along with you, can be both a grounding and expansive experience. It's also a great way to meet and spend time with like-minded people.

You can also grow tomatoes and many herbs—such as chives, thyme and parsley—in containers or pots on decks or balconies, even if just for the fun of it. I adore fresh herbs, so I always have a small kitchen container garden of some kind growing in my home. Even if all I do is sniff them from time to time, just knowing they are there for that alone is nourishing to me.

It's easy to see that this kind of "food loving" encourages our overall health and well-being. The closer I am to the soil, the more Soul-Full and grounded I feel in every area of my life—whether it's digging in it to weed or plant vegetables, flowers and herbs, or washing the dirt off a just-picked carrot, potato or chive.

"You shall eat the fruit of the labor of your hands. You shall be happy, and it will be well with you."

~ Psalms 128:2

CONSIDER A CSA

If you don't like to garden, there is another option that may be available to you, and it can still offer this same tangible feeling of connectivity. You can join a CSA—a Community Sponsored (or Supported) Agriculture program.

A CSA is essentially a partnership between the grower and the consumer. The CSA farmer estimates the growing capacity of his land—the number of people it can feed for a season. Then each consumer pays a lump sum in advance of the growing season to purchase one of those "shares" of the harvest for the length of the growing season. There are organic CSAs and also many other kinds, so be sure if you decide to join one that it reflects your unique lifestyle, tastes and values. Some require people to pick up produce at the farm itself, others have satellite pickups—in the nearest city, for example. Some CSAs even have work involvements, such as picking, washing, loading or unloading the produce on market day. For some, this work is mandatory and, for others, there is a reduction in share cost with a work commitment. The cost of the membership varies as does the size of the share. Some CSAs let you pay as you go, as opposed to paying the full fee up front. Often single people can buy in with a half-share as opposed to a full share for small families. Some even take food stamps. So shop around for one that fits your needs and budget.

This is certainly a wonderful way to eat fresh whole food, but it does require a commitment. If you sign on, you do need to show up and commit to at least getting your food or arrange to have another person pick it up for you—more opportunities for Soul-linking!

OTHER WHOLE FOOD OPTIONS

While I'm an advocate of locally grown produce, I fully understand the need for moving beyond the local proximity to find produce in some cases. That's partially because I lived in New Hampshire for 16+ long winters before moving to Florida.

"When I think of how far the onion has traveled just to enter my stew today, I could kneel and praise all small forgotten miracles."

~ Naomi Shihab Nye

When the seasons don't cooperate, you have no farmer's markets and farm stands close by, or you cannot grow your own produce, choose to shop in supermarkets, specialty stores and health food stores that sell quality food. By requesting that the stores stock specific items, it becomes easier to see which ones will support your convictions to eat consciously. Even supermarkets are open to doing this.

I've convinced local supermarkets to stock hormone-free and organic dairy products as well as a good variety of organically grown produce. When I didn't feel like my voice alone was enough, I asked friends from my baby-sitting coop—or other parents in my neighborhood and at my children's schools—to sign a letter requesting certain items. Don't be afraid to be a visionary, or a bit "ahead of your time." When I first started doing this, not one supermarket in my area (a large suburb of Boston) stocked organic milk. Now look in the dairy section in your local supermarket. Chances are pretty good you'll see not only organic milk, but many other organic dairy products. Start by filling out suggestion cards or asking store managers how to get their store to stock items you know you'll purchase regularly.

It works. This is a consumer-driven economy. Companies do listen when we make our voices loud enough and they do their utmost to deliver. This is evidenced by the recent emergence and success of the large supermarket-sized health food stores, such as Whole Foods and Wild Oats, in many major cities. What a far cry these chains are from the little mom and pop health food stores that were the only places to find healthy selections for so long.

If, however, you happen to live in a remote area and none of the above alternatives are available to you, there is another wonderful and viable option—start a food cooperative. I know people who've pooled their interest and began purchasing organic produce from large suppliers who will deliver all manner of organic fare to them at a drop-off point once a week. Not only is this very convenient and cost effective, but it's a great way to meet like-minded friends.

And, finally, let's not leave out the Internet. I have several friends who sell their unique and hard-to-find organic products, such as raw chocolate, on the Web. Do a search for organic products or organic produce, and you'll be absolutely amazed at the whole new world you'll open up for yourself.

TOP 7 REASONS TO BUY LOCALLY

1. **Freshness**
    On average, produce travels 1,500 miles from the grower to your plate. When you buy your produce fresh from the field, you reduce the distance from the farm to your dinner table and lessen transportation costs and environmental impact.

2. **Flavor**
    Foods that are allowed to ripen longer on the vine and tree taste much better! This is more of a possibility when longer travel times aren't a factor.

3. **Connection with the seasons**
    Buying locally offers you a full experience of seasonal and regional flavors, and a wider range of unique and heirloom varieties.

4. **Interaction with community growers**
    Putting a face behind the product gives you a tangible connection to the farmers. It also allows you to ask questions and learn many subtleties, hints and suggestions for handling and preparing your produce.

5. **Support of local jobs**
    When you buy locally, you give back to your community. It helps create and save jobs, and because the wholesaler is often eliminated, it provides the farmers with a living wage. With direct sales, the growers receive full price for their product.

6. **Support of responsible land development**
    Small local farmers value and care for the land and preserve the beauty of open spaces.

7. **Support of independent farmers**
   Independent farmers have the power to make decisions about how to treat their own land. They are personally concerned with the sustainability of the quality of life in their community.

HOW TO FIND LOCAL GROWERS

To find farmer's markets, farm stands and CSAs in your area, you can utilize the following resources:

- **Local Harvest**—A national search engine of local food sources.
  www.localharvest.org

- **Alternative Farming Systems Information Center**—The USDA's comprehensive listing of CSA farms.
  www.nal.usda.gov/afsic/csa/csastate.htm

- **Farmer's Markets**—An alphabetical directory maintained by the USDA of farmer's markets (organized by state).
  www.ams.usda.gov/farmersmarkets/map.htm

- **Robyn Van En Center for CSA Resources**—Provides support for sustainable agricultural initiatives and has a search engine for locating CSAs.
  www.csacenter.org

- **Just Foods in New York City**—Connects low-income people with CSA growers who will work on a sliding scale.
  www.justfood.org

- **The International Co-operative Alliance**—The home of the ICA, which is a base for all co-op activity worldwide.
  www.coop.org

- **COOP Directory Service**—Provides information about finding and starting a co-op.
  www.coopdirectory.org

- Plus, here are two great websites for finding local markets near you.
  www.seasonalchef.com
  www.localharvest.org

SOMETHING TO CHEW ON

Do you live outside of a city, in a suburb or in a smaller community, and want to keep urban sprawl at bay? If so, know that when you buy local produce you give those with the space—farmland, pastures, etc.—an economic reason for staying underdeveloped. Buying that bunch of carrots from your local farm stand can actually help preserve the beauty of open spaces.

SOUL-FULL EXERCISE #4

Using some of the above resources, find out where you can find locally grown produce in your area. Make use of these contacts. If you're reading this book in the dead of winter and live in a region with pronounced seasons, think ahead and plan for warmer days. If helpful, contact and visit those farmers who are accessible in the off-season to make arrangements.

CHAPTER FIVE

Choose Organic Foods

"These fruits and vegetables may not look flawless, but one taste tells the whole story. The imperfections are the perfections in organics. That's the beautiful thing... "
~ Neil Ims, organic grower

I FIRST LOOKED FOR ORGANIC FOODS with a vengeance when I moved back to the States from Germany when my daughter Heather was just about one year old. We had been living in Berlin, and as in most German cities, people there tended to shop for their fresh produce at the local markets almost every day, buying small amounts of groceries instead of a week's worth. Before that I'd lived in New York City, where people pretty much followed the same trend. But now I not only had my eye on fresh food, I wanted THE BEST food for my family—and to me that meant *organic*.

Heather's 21 now. Back when she was an infant, it was slim pickings for organics, so at times I had to be a very ingenious shopper. There were no health food supermarket chains, and I usually had to shop each week at four or five small health food stores that were sprinkled around my area of New Hampshire. Today my local supermarket in Southeast Florida has more organic items on their shelves and in their produce section than I could find in all of those New

"We think
we may be
entering a
culinary
golden age.
We make a
prediction:
More and more
natural foods
will become avail-
able, and they will
be better and
better, especially
as educated
consumers
demand more."

~ The Moosewood
Collective,
authors of
The Moosewood
Cookbook

Hampshire health food stores combined. Now I eat primarily organic foods, and since I have an organic market right next door, it's very easy for me to find fresh organic produce there. I also find additional organic products at the local supermarket, at nearby *Whole Foods* or *Wild Oats*, and even online.

In Boston, where I often visit, there are even services that will deliver organic produce right to your door, just as there are in many other major cities. No matter where you live, it's easier to find organic produce today. So there's no time like the present to determine which foods you eat that can be purchased as organic. You'll find a big difference with the addition of organic foods into your life—not just taste-wise, but health-wise. More on this later in the chapter.

OUR BASIC CHOICES

There are many methods of farming practiced today, but they can all be grouped into basically two types—*conventional* and *organic*.

We call large scale factory-farming "conventional," and the long enduring, simple, aggregate approach to agriculture "organic." It's interesting that organic farming methods are often labeled as alternative when you consider that people have been farming for thousands of years and only recently—since World War II—began using pesticides and other "scientific" approaches to farming. The widespread use of chemical fertilizers, synthetic pesticides, industrial mass-production techniques, and process shortcuts were instituted as output maximizers, ideal for making large profits, and they are all characteristic of modern-day conventional farming. While the organic approach is much simpler than this, organic food is now the fastest growing sector of US agriculture due to consumer demand. That is because even though organic products often cost more than conventional foods, many consumers believe they are a better value. It's clear that by eating organically grown foods, we can avoid the negative aspects of conventional farming techniques.

WHAT "ORGANIC" MEANS

Below are several reasons sited by NOFA—The Northeast Organic Farming Association—as to why organic farming methods are superior to conventional methods.

- **No pesticides**

  Organic standards prohibit the use of synthetic pesticides, exposure to which has been linked to a number of serious human diseases. The conventional approach allows such pesticides.

- **No genetic engineering**

  Organic standards prohibit the use of genetically modified organisms (GMOs) for feed and livestock, although the US government has allowed and even encouraged the development and release of many GMOs into our environment and food system.

- **No growth hormones**

  Organically grown foods cannot be grown with the presence of growth hormones. These substances are used to increase the size and rate of growth in animals raised for meat and to stimulate the production of animal products, such as milk. The US government permits the wide-scale use of such hormones in conventional livestock operations.

- **No antibiotics**

  Although the US government allows the routine use of antibiotics in livestock operations, organic standards prohibit this. In the overcrowded, conventional factory-farm, animals are *routinely fed* subtherapeutic levels of antibiotics to promote growth and prevent disease. Antibiotics can only be administered to an organic animal when the animal is sick and needs treatment, in which case such animals may no longer be marketed as organic.

- **No irradiation**
Organic standards prohibit the use of ionizing radiation to preserve food. Again, the government policy permits irradiation of both produce and meat. Irradiation is used to extend shelf life and to kill microbes, which may spoil food and cause human illness. But this may also impact the enzymes, vitamins and the healthfulness of food. Opponents of irradiation suggest cleaning up feedlots and industrial food-processing operations as an alternative way of protecting the public from disease.

- **No sludge**
The conventional farming approach routinely uses sewage sludge, as well as dioxins and other chemicals, to fertilize their crops, despite concerns about contamination by high levels of heavy minerals. Organic farmers use only naturally based fertilizers to provide needed nutrients to plants, such as composted manure, crop residues, cover crops, and rock powders.

- **No animal cannibalism**
Although this practice has been associated with outbreaks such as "Mad Cow Disease" in Europe, our government standards allow rendered animal products to be fed to cattle, sheep, and other herbivores as a protein supplement. Organic standards specifically prohibit such practices.

- **Healthy soil and water**
A program of soil building, which protects the soil from erosion and water pollution, is adhered to in organic farming. Organic farmers believe that healthy soil promotes vigorous soil life that

in turn breaks down minerals and makes a complex meal of nutrients available to plants. The synthetic fertilizers used in conventional farming deliver only the three primary nutrients needed for plant growth, but leave out the many diverse macronutrients that lead to plant vigor and health.

- **Free range**
  Organically raised animals generally must be allowed access to range or pasture, as organic standards prohibit confinement or feedlot-style livestock operations. This promotes animal health and well-being as well as contributes to maintaining large areas of open land in otherwise developing communities.

- **Humane conditions**
  Finally, organic standards require that animals be treated humanely. This is spelled out in specific detail in the form of housing requirements for space, ventilation, and manure accumulation, as well as access to appropriate pasture or range, healthcare, food and water, treatment of the young, etc. The organic approach is based on the belief that ethical agriculture must produce thriving plant and animal products to ensure a healthy cycle of life.

The pesticides, irradiation and genetic engineering used in conventional farming are virtually undetectable to our senses, but nonetheless they affect our food. Therefore it is hard to build a case in favor of conventional techniques which are not based on the above principles. When we ingest conventionally farmed foods, they influence our bodies in many ways. Pesticides are poisons, and though some of them can be washed or peeled off, others are systemic—that is, they've become part of the very fiber of our food. Chemical fertilizers not only leave damaging chemical traces in our food, but in our soil and water as well—impacting large sections of our ecosystem.

"Most organic farmers encourage complex relationships between crop roots, soil microbes and minerals— relationships that become wholly disrupted by chemical additives."

~ Dan Barber, from *The New York Times*

It can generally be said that organic farmers are in the business of farming because they love it. Farming is in their Soul, as the organic farming approach is quite often a very complex process requiring the farmer to express an enormous amount of commitment. These farmers must not only meet standards which are much more stringent than those imposed on conventional farmers, but their methods are subject to intense scrutiny in order to stay certified. Though regulations are strictly imposed in most states, it is often found that the farmers hold themselves to a higher standard and ethic than that enforced by regulators.

BUY ORGANIC FOR THE HEALTH OF IT

A very significant reason to buy organically grown foods is that they are more nutritious and better for us than their processed or synthetic counterparts. Since organic farming prohibits routine pesticide and herbicide use, chemical residues are rarely found. In contrast, non-organic food is likely to be contaminated with residues that often occur in potentially dangerous combinations. It is also believed that the micronutrient deficiencies found in so many people today have their roots in the mineral depletion of soils by intensive agriculture. While plants extract a wide range of minerals from the soil, artificial fertilizers replace only a few principal minerals. This means a clear long-term decline in the trace mineral content of fruit and vegetables.

Pesticide exposure is also suspect for contributing to the alarming rise in allergies as well as other illnesses and maladies such as various cancers, neurological disorders, disruption of the endocrine system, and immune system suppression. Research has also suggested that pesticide exposure affects male reproductive function.

Children, in particular, may stand to benefit from eating organic foods. In one recent study, covered in the journal *Environmental Health Perspectives*, scientists monitored preschool children in Seattle, Washington to assess their exposure to pesticides in their diet. The total dimethyl metabolite chemical concentration was approximately six times higher for children with conventional diets than those with organic diets. This suggests that consumption of organic fruits, vegetables and juice can reduce children's exposure levels from above to below the US Environmental Protection Agency's guidelines, thereby shifting exposures from a range of uncertain risk to a range of negligible risk. The study concluded that consumption of organic produce could be a relatively simple way for parents to reduce children's exposure to OP (organophosphorus) pesticides. Additionally, organic food production bans the use of artificial food additives such as hydrogenated fats, phosphoric acid, aspartame and monosodium glutamate, which have been linked to health problems as diverse as heart disease, osteoporosis, migraines and hyperactivity.

Study after study shows that organic crops on average contain significantly higher mineral levels, more nutrients such as vitamin C, and significantly fewer nitrates (a toxic compound). They also provide higher phytonutrient plant compounds which can help prevent cancer. A review of 41 studies and 1240 comparisons covered by *The Journal of Alternative and Complementary Medicine* found statistically significant differences in the nutrient content of organic and conventional crops. In addition, here's information based on a particular study done at Rutgers University, which also compared the nutritive qualities of organically and conventionally grown vegetables.

"Organic products are the fastest growing area of the food industry, increasing 20 to 25 percent every year."
~ Daniel W. Lotter

ORGANIC VS. CONVENTIONAL PRODUCE

A comparative analysis of the nutrient content of organic and non-organic food from the Firman Bear Report, Rutgers University. The shaded rows are organic produce, unshaded rows are conventional produce.

Crop	Calcium	Magnesium	Potassium	Sodium	Thiamine	Iron	Copper
Snap Beans Organic	40.5	60	99.7	8.6	60	227	69
Snap Beans Conventional	15.5	14.8	29.1	<1	2	10	3
Cabbage Organic	60	43.6	148.3	20.4	13	94	48
CABBAGE Conventional	17.5	15.6	53.7	<1	2	20	<1
Lettuce Organic	71	49.3	175.5	12.2	169	516	60
Lettuce Conventional	16	13.1	53.7	<1	1	9	3
Tomatoes Organic	23	59.2	148	6.5	68	1938	53
Tomatoes Conventional	4.5	4.5	58.6	<1	1	1	<1
Spinach Organic	96	203.9	257	69.5	117	1584	32
Spinach Conventional	47.5	46.9	84	<1	1	19	<1

* Firman Bear Report, Rutgers University, all numbers represent Milliequivalents per 100 grams, dry weight.

Become an informed, active consumer. Don't just take what is handed to you, organic or conventional, unless you feel it is grown with consciousness, harvested at the right time, and handled with care. Inquire about how and where your food is grown. When shopping in supermarkets, read the labels that identify where the produce is grown. And use all of your five senses (as well as your Soul sense!) when choosing fruits and vegetables. You'll see that once you practice this kind of presence, it becomes easier and easier to discern what *feels* the best for you to buy and consume. Gift yourself and your loved ones each time you sit down to a meal by holding to high standards of quality. By this approach, you not only honor and love yourself, but you do the entire world a favor. Act locally to change things globally.

SOMETHING TO CHEW ON

Objectively and nonjudgmentally look at your own diet for a moment. How much of your daily fare is organically grown? Maybe you have options to find and buy organic foods that you haven't explored yet. Remember, you can increase your nutrient intake just by switching to organic, even without changing anything else about your diet at all.

SOUL-FULL EXERCISE #5

Do a taste test. Find two identical pieces of fresh produce—one conventionally grown and one organically grown. Then use all of your five senses to decide which one *feels* best to you in every way. As you do this, keep this in mind…

The Copenhagen Zoo began feeding their chimpanzees organic fruit in an effort to become more ecological. Lo and behold! The chimps were able to easily tell the difference between the organic and regular fruit. The zookeeper, Neils Melchiorsen, told the Danish magazine, *Ecological Agriculture*, "… the tapirs and chimpanzees are choosing organically grown bananas over the others… It seems they instinctively tell the difference and their choice is not at all random." When the zookeeper left only conventional bananas, the monkeys peeled them before eating, but ate the organic ones peel and all!

CHAPTER SIX

Avoid Mind-Less Fast Food

"Fast food is neither produced, nor prepared, in a mindful or loving fashion."

I WAS OUT WALKING MY DOG Chauncey one crisp, fall morning, along the empty side streets and busier roads of my neighborhood in Southern New Hampshire. Looking down at the curb, I noticed that mixed in with the red and orange autumn leaves were Styrofoam packages, milkshake cups, paper Big-Mac wrappers, empty Kentucky Fried Chicken tubs, and other colorful fast food waste. I realized that on my two-mile walk through this typical suburban, seemingly pristine neighborhood, I could have easily filled a large 30-gallon trash bag with the refuse. Later on that same day, I did go back to collect it. I also realized then that these were all wrappers and packaging of dead food, the food which is served in mass quantities by the fast food industry. The opposite of Soul-Full food, fast food promotes unconsciousness about our true needs.

When we stuff ourselves with fat-laden, greasy ground beef and synthetic white flour buns, we are not respecting our bodies. And so it is only natural that

"Americans now spend more money on fast food than on higher education, personal computers, computer software, or new cars."

~ Eric Schlosser, author of *Fast Food Nation*

our dishonored bodies will take this dishonoring further to the next "natural" step of disrespecting the environment. The food that had been contained by those packages and wrappers, which were now lying largely empty by the roadside, deadens the senses and the mind. It disconnects us from feelings of wholeness and from that which honors our world. Despite its numbing effects, Americans spent more than $110 billion on fast food in 2000. In fact, a new fast food restaurant opens somewhere in the world every two hours.

The negative effects resulting from the current trend of producing and eating the synthetic food served in millions of fast food restaurants are far-reaching. In his book, *Fast Food Nation*, Eric Schlosser illustrates the impact that the fast food industry has had on America. He states, "On any given day in the United States, about one-quarter of the adult population visits a fast food restaurant. During a relatively brief period of time, the fast food industry has helped to transform not only the American diet, but also our landscape, economy, workforce and popular culture."

He goes on to give two astonishing examples of the impact of the popularity of fast food. First, a survey of American children found that 96% could identify Ronald McDonald; the only fictional character with a higher degree of recognition was Santa Claus! But even more flabbergasting is that they also found the golden arches are now more widely recognized than the Christian cross!

Moving beyond the US, I've noticed fast food's influence as I have traveled extensively and lived in many other countries. As any traveler knows, fast food is not prevalent in just America; today we live in a fast food world.

I am not relating this information to put a guilt trip on fast food lovers. I am writing it to remind all of you that eating should be a joyful and enriching experience—one which connects us to our Source. Our food is meant to nourish and enliven all of our senses, not deaden us to our world, or to our feeling of connection with ourselves and one another.

Most fast food is neither produced, nor prepared, in a mindful or loving fashion. On the contrary, its methods can seem quite mind-less and un-loving—towards the environment, the animals and plants that provide the nutrients, the workers who help to produce the food at various stages along the way, and towards you, the consumer, who eats the finished product.

Much of the reason that the fast food industry now occupies such an important position in our society is due to the fact that most families have two wage-earners. The effect on our eating habits has been debilitating. According to author Eric Schlosser, three quarters of the money used to buy food in America a generation ago was spent to prepare home-cooked meals. Today, roughly half of the money is spent at restaurants and mostly at fast food restaurants.

We're a society on the go. And it's due to this and the larger social and economic trends that the fast food industry is thriving. It may appear that fast food is inexpensive, but Schlosser says the low cost of a fast food burger or fries does not reflect its real cost. It's sobering to realize that the only reason the fast food profits have been possible is because of the huge losses they have imposed on the rest of society. The annual cost of obesity alone is now twice as large as the fast food industry's total revenues.

Whether our lives are busy or not, it's time for us to get mindful in this area that so greatly affects our health and the future of our world in so many ways. As consumers, we hold the reins. When we act consciously, we can greatly affect change for the better. Here are some ways to positively influence the changes that occur in this industry:

1. By far, the most effective and evident action is to stop buying fast food that is grown, prepared and served without love.

2. Speak to your children about food. The fast food industry is not only making its way into our nation's school cafeterias, but classrooms as well, via advertisers. There are pizza-party awards for reading books, discount coupons offered in back-to-school packets, and sponsorships given to motivational speakers who sport the well-known company logos.

3. Seek out and buy food from manufacturers who produce nutritious food, refuse to pollute the environment, treat their employees with respect, and support worthy causes.

4. Realize that this industry was created to serve you and it is therefore dependent on the consumer. Voice your disapproval if you notice unethical practices.

5. Ask for tougher food-safety laws and more thorough food-inspection systems to be implemented.

SOMETHING TO CHEW ON

The word "fast" has become synonymous with progress. However, the fast food industry is one very blatant example of where the thrust towards high-speed living is causing many people to become out of step with their Soul.

History has proven that anything that does not promote peace—which is a deep, indwelling experience and a natural expression of the Soul—cannot be long sustained. The most blatant example of this is war, which is synonymous with instantaneous destruction. Given the fact that the fast food industry is sustained by a short-term benefit mentality of instant gratification consumerism, are these restaurants destined to become the world's next dinosaurs?

Yes, the only things that are enduring are those that are sustained by and with peace—a natural expression of the Soul. This is true for institutions as well as for people. Centenarians have one thing in common, an ability to maintain a peaceful persona, which enables them to outlive many people they love—even their children. Perhaps fast food was conceived with the intention to promote a more peaceful, convenient way of life. However, unless the current approach of disregarding the Soul takes a change towards a more conscious and connected approach, its future is questionable. Word is spreading of its ill effects in books like Schlosser's and movies like *Super Size Me*.

SOUL-FULL EXERCISE #6

Next time you find yourself drawn to eating fast food, pay attention to your frame of mind. What is it that you have been doing and why are you doing it? Are you under stress? Have you been trying to accomplish too much? Are you acting out of obligation? Are you tired or confused? Does the activity or action you were involved in truly nourish you?

To a Soul, there are no superficial concepts such as "convenient," "in a rush," or "on the run." Your Soul abides in a deeper, more still and peaceful place within you.

Food choices can be illustrative of the many empty ways we spend our time and seek fulfillment, striving for the approval of others and therefore missing the opportunity to experience greater depth in our lives.

"You can find your way across the country using burger joints, the way a navigator uses the stars."

~ Charles Kuralt

CHAPTER SEVEN

Practice Soul-Full Food Preparation

"Preparing food is at once child's play and adult joy...and done with care, it is an act of love."
~ Craig Claiborne

THERE CAME A POINT in my Spiritual journey when I kept hearing the same idea over and over. It was that if I am experiencing unrest in my life, it is merely misperception. A vast amount of what I was learning dealt with the concept that I could transform any seemingly gloomy situation by showing up to it whole and happy. If, however, I was feeling "less than" able to rise to the occasion, I could feel resentful and jilted by life.

This whole notion really galled me at first. I had so little awareness that I could be the one tainting my perception and causing myself such a great deal of pain. I really had a hard time accepting the idea. That's probably because at this time in my life, I was heavily into blaming others and outside situations for all of my discomforts and angst.

At this time, we were just beginning to practice the art of mindfulness in my meditation class. Our assignment for one particular week was to consciously watch ourselves and how we were living our lives. As a means to this end, the instructor handed out a heart sticker to each student. She said, "Take this home and put it in a place where you feel it will best remind you to be mindful."

"Simple enough," I thought. "I know exactly where to put mine."

When I got home, I stuck the heart right at eye level above the stove in my kitchen. This was because on most nights I sat at our dinner table feeling more like the dishrag I'd been using to mop up spills on the floor all day than a jovial dinner companion. So I took the brave step of choosing to be mindful and present at the spot where I prepared the evening meal.

At first, the heart was a great reminder to me to be present and I happily hummed along chopping vegetables, boiling water and the like. But it wasn't too long before I found myself caught up in my old mindset. I just couldn't lie about this whole dinner thing, which was for me the biggest symbol of my victimhood in life. I started banging around pots and pans on the stove, as I found myself thinking, "I'm trapped. I'll be stuck here the rest of my life, playing slave-maid to a bunch of ingrates. Why did I break my butt for all those years trying to get somewhere in a career?!—For this!? My life stinks. Blah, blah, blah… " I went on and on, further perpetuating the self-abuse.

This was not an easy time in my life. I was trying so hard and felt I was totally missing the mark. However, I could no longer deny the pain I was causing myself.

It was at this point that I felt the need to take a serious look at changing my behavior.

The next time I sat in meditation, I simply prayed, "I don't know. I don't know how to fix this one… Please, please, give me an answer." It was then that I heard from deep within myself, from my Soul:

You are worthy. Not sad, stupid, guilty, weak or pathetic—simply worthy. In My sight, which is the only true sight there is, you are Perfection. You are Perfection so worthy of my all abiding Love that I weep when you refuse it and instead congeal with these painful convoluted thoughts. And as you experience this thinking, you believe it is the truth.

How can you really be anything but whole if I so dictate?

You will accept your worthiness, your very Oneness—of that I am sure. Choose to accept it now, and be at home in a peace-filled oasis of Truth that proclaims to once deafened ears your perfection, your worthiness, your Oneness, in peace with Me.

I had to admit my own self-loathing and sense of unworthiness were the very things that were keeping me from experiencing not only a happy, carefree family life, but my connection to the rest of life as well. My giving to my family had been done from a place of self-sacrifice. Somehow I'd come to believe that giving myself away would make me worthy enough to be loved.

Soon I could finally grasp that all of my angst had little to do with my duties as a wife and mother, but with the way I perceived my role in life. This understanding came while considering the ways of Mother Theresa. I had sought out her background because what I most often found myself inwardly screaming each time I watched myself fail so miserably at being present was "I am not Mother Theresa!"

The reason Mother Theresa could find boundless energy to tend to the needs of others nearly unceasingly, and well into old age, was because it gifted her—*immediately.* When Mother Theresa went into a hospital ward filled with dying people, she saw all people as God giving her an opportunity to Love and connect with the Divine. When you Love in such a manner, the instant you give you receive tenfold. You are giving yourself total permission to Be God attending to God. This is how Mother Theresa loved and lived.

After that realization, I made dinner in quite a different manner. My family became free to help me in my kitchen, the very place which used to imprison us all. They found it easier to be included because I stopped fanatically picking at them, lording over their every move, or analyzing their every mistake. I finally knew I was worthy of Love and happiness, and so were they. Does God ever deserve anything less?

After these revelations, any time I'd spy that heart—which remained on the top of the stove until the day we moved from that home—I'd smile.

IMBUING FOOD WITH THE INGREDIENTS OF LIGHT AND LOVE

The antithesis of adding negative emotion to the food you prepare is to consciously saturate it with love. I've practiced Reiki, and I have many friends who are Reiki Masters—that is, they are healers who work with the body's subtle energy fields. It's a common practice in Reiki circles to "turn on" the healing energy of the hands while preparing food.

The ability to add an energetic charge to a meal is not a talent reserved for Reiki practitioners alone—anyone can do it! In fact, most of the world's best chefs do this naturally, their passion for their work and the artistic medium of food turns them on. So their love flows to the food each time they approach the preparation of a meal. If you choose to prepare food with this in mind, you can add the extra ingredient to any meal which can make it taste heavenly.

Just as a beautiful work of art is created though the constant interaction between artist and canvas, a Soul-Full meal is the result of the cook's attention, care and contact with the food. You will find that as you practice this approach to food preparation, you'll gain a heightened sensitivity for the field of energy of the food. Your state of consciousness will expand. You'll begin to feel the life force as it flows from you to the food and vice versa.

So you can see how important it is to act with a mindful presence while you are preparing food—not only for yourself, but for the others you serve. Food is most nourishing to the Soul when prepared with love and care—when it's well cleaned and carefully handled. Cooking can actually be regarded as an act of self-expression and creativity. How many times do we afford ourselves the luxury of performing this everyday task in that way?

THE ART OF MINDFUL FOOD PREPARATION

In many traditional cultures and in some less "advanced" ones today, the women gather together to make the food as a community. It is not only a creative act, in which each woman contributes to the final masterpiece, but also a time for social interaction—for *connection*. We've gotten so far from that.

Today, it is not uncommon to open up a frozen dinner, pop it in the microwave, and then throw it on the table so that we can just get on to the next thing.

Cooking and eating are a huge part of our lives. To miss these minutes and hours of our day because we are not honoring such activities—seeing them instead as merely a means to an end—seems a shame. There can be beauty in food preparation, particularly if we view and approach it with loving attention. Savoring the process as if it were itself the main event allows something as simple as an aroma alone to elevate your consciousness. It's centering to hear crisp vegetables crack under the knife, euphoric to breathe in deeply the aroma of fresh picked herbs, and tantalizing to inhale the scent of sizzling onions while watching simple ingredients transform into a luscious *pièce de résistance*—no matter how simple it may be. The time taken to cook with love and creativity is time spent in communion with your Soul. And how vibrant is the food we eat—when we begin to assimilate that vigor simply by noticing the delectable tastes, textures and colors contained within it.

> "We all cook together around a fire. Our yearning music builds. We share our tools and instruments and plates. We are companions on this earth."
>
> ~ Hafiz

COMMUNION THROUGH COOKING

At best, food preparation becomes an inclusive act, uniting people with a common focus and drawing them together. A woman in one of my workshops related her experience of just how fulfilling, and uniting, food preparation can be: *"My mother-in-law and my brother were both visiting for ten days. It was so nice to be in the kitchen with them. Just going down to the farm, buying fresh fruits and vegetables, and bringing them home to chop together brought that experience to new heights. I realized then that the preparation process is as important as the event of sitting down to eat. One night, my mother-in-law and I spent a really long time preparing a special meal for my husband because she wanted to make something that would remind him of his childhood. We had gotten all of these fresh vegetables. We must have sounded crazy to the rest of the family once we sat down to eat, because after every few bites we commented on how wonderful the food was. We went back and forth saying, 'Can you believe the squash?' and 'I know, I can't get over this!' We were enjoying it so much that eventually everyone else joined in."*

Often, today, the whole process of meal preparation—from start to finish—doesn't feel fulfilling to us because we don't think of it as something that everyone can join and share in. Yet with the intention, we can make every dinner into a family "Thanksgiving" meal. Children, family, friends—whoever happens to be eating with you—can help with the preparation. Washing and chopping vegetables for a salad, picking herbs from the garden, stirring a pot of spaghetti or just boiling water—there are many ways for others to help out. And someone who is an active participant in the food preparation often enjoys the food much more, having that sense of connection with what they consume.

"Small but stellar moments occur even when cooking the simplest things."

~ Deborah Madison, author of *Vegetarian Cooking for Everyone*

ABOUT KITCHEN EQUIPMENT

After making the effort to buy healthy, organic food, it is wise to give some consideration to the tools that are used in the preparation process. It's most advantageous to use only stainless steel, glass or cast-iron cookware. This can be expensive, but it will last a lifetime. Plus, food cooked in cast-iron pans can actually be enriched with natural iron from the pot. Aluminum cookware and utensils should never be used because they can leave residues of highly toxic aluminum in the foods they come in contact with. There have been numerous studies that link aluminum to Alzheimer's Disease.

Teflon-coated pans are a no-no, due to concerns about toxic emissions released at high temperatures. The Environmental Working Group has been a leading force on the issues related to such non-stick cookware. According to the *Townsend Letter*, studies have found that 95% of Americans have detectable levels of Teflon-related chemicals in their blood. At the time of this writing, the Environmental Protection Agency (EPA) was taking action to eliminate the use of certain perflourochemicals in Teflon, other non-stick cookware and stain-resistance coatings. Their goal is to eliminate sources of exposure by 2015. And in May 2006, the 3M Corporation (which makes Scotchgard) announced that it will stop producing perfluorochemicals. Meanwhile, *MotherJones.com* reports that based on internal company documents which were obtained, it believes that 3M and Dupont (manufacturer of Teflon) "have suspected for decades" that the chemicals "pose serious health hazards." Note that these chemicals are also found in a grease-resistance coating which has been used for many microwavable containers, such as popcorn bags, as well as fast food containers and pizza boxes.

Take care when using pottery and ceramics to cook and hold food. Some glazes can contain cadmium and lead. Pottery and ceramics that are imported from Mexico, Spain, Italy and China are the most likely to have this. Also, do not use antiques or collectibles to hold or serve food or beverages. The manufacturing standards in the past were not as high as they are today, and these items may contain lead and other poisonous elements.

Whenever possible and practical, store things in glass.

Also consider storing fresh produce and herbs in *Evert-Fresh Green Bags*. These bags absorb and remove the natural gasses that are released from fruits and vegetables during the natural ripening process that occurs after harvest. They are reusable and keep produce just-picked fresh for weeks! (*Evert-Fresh Green Bags: website, www.Evert-fresh.com; Tel, 979-885-0340.*)

In addition, I usually wrap items such as school lunches in waxed paper or unbleached parchment paper to avoid the contact of my food with the aluminum in foil or the petrochemicals in plastic wrap. Attach a piece of tape to secure it, or use an outer layer of tin foil or plastic wrap to keep it closed.

COOKING GUIDELINES/TIPS

Nutrition-wise, raw is usually best. However, when cooking vegetables, steaming is preferred to boiling or frying. Steamed vegetables retain more of their vitamins, minerals and flavor. The crispier the vegetables are when steamed, the more nutritious they are.

Remember to wash your hands prior to preparing food, using a good natural soap, such as Dr. Bronners, and rinse well. You can also use a nail brush to clean under your fingernails. Then get your hands into the food as much as possible and, while you do, feel yourself activating the energy of the food as you infuse it with your presence and love.

Unless you plan on eating salad greens immediately, they should be torn instead of cut during preparation. Otherwise, they will begin to oxidize (go brown) while stored because of the exposure to the metal.

Ceramic cutlery, once used almost exclusively by chefs, is now becoming more widely available and also a preference for many—although it is still quite expensive. According to Chef Peter Cervoni of Angelica's Kitchen in New York City, "It is super hard and holds its edge a lot longer than stainless steel." Because of costs, stainless steel cutlery is still the mainstream preference as well as a very good and viable option.

Wooden or bamboo cutting boards are both great surfaces to cut on, and according to Cervoni, one reason they're better than glass is that the glass dulls the knives faster. Bamboo is not only an extremely hard surface to cut on; it comes from a beautiful, fast-growing tree, which is a highly sustainable resource. Also, if you do use wooden or bamboo cutting-boards, be sure to have two of them—one for meat, poultry and fish and one for fruits and vegetables. Always wash them thoroughly with natural soap and water after using them. To prevent the cutting boards from drying, use a high-quality walnut oil to treat them periodically.

Use fresh herbs and spices in your foods whenever possible; they not only add flavor but life and additional energy to food. As you add these fresh ingredients, let them touch every one of your senses by allowing yourself to engage in their textures and aromas. Later, notice how they add to the distinct creation and flavor of your meal.

Vow today to make every meal a work of art, fit for a queen or king—something that speaks of your immanent awareness of your own self-worth!

Going to the Kitchen

The kitchen is alchemical,
a place where we cook—actually
and Spiritually. We come to it
for nourishment and ease.
We come to it as to a center—

The heart of the house,
the heart of the dwelling.
In the kitchen we are one,
linked by hunger—
actual Spiritual hunger.

We go to the kitchen to be
nourished and revealed.
It is a holy place.

~ Gunilla Norris in *Becoming Bread*

Have you ever been to a trendy restaurant and despite the rave reviews felt that something about your meal was just a bit "off"? There may be a very good reason for that. I'm just as experienced in the restaurant industry as I am in the world of high-fashion. I literally grew up in the business, securing my first job as a busgirl in a busy New York restaurant when I was just 14. And just like with the modeling industry, the world of high-end gastronomy has its "dark side." Behind the scenes of most any establishment with a well-noted reputation, there can be immense pressure for the chefs and staff to perform in what is already a pressure-ridden industry. While initially many chefs often consider themselves lucky to have the opportunity to blissfully express their creative talents freely, often their euphoria succumbs to the hectic, nerve-racking pace and constant demand to perform that comes along with the reputation. Add this to the typical drama which goes on behind the perpetually swinging kitchen doors of any busy restaurant and you have the ingredients for a meal that can demand much more energy from you when you eat it than it can possibly offer to you in the exchange.

Be discriminating.

Whether it's a five-star establishment or a pizza parlor, choose a place to eat based on how you personally feel about the atmosphere and energy at least as much as its notoriety.

Prepare yourself a meal that is filled with Love—from start to finish. Use whole, fresh, vital foods, and while creating the meal, get in touch with how it feels to love the process as much as the "destination." Eat as much as you like once it's ready. Savor every moment, every sensation that flows through your five senses until you swallow the very last bite. Feel what it means to feel truly FULL in every sense of the word. When you feel you've relished the experience long enough, gently and objectively observe how this meal compares with your former approach to eating.

CHAPTER EIGHT

Less Is More

"The more you eat, the less flavor. The less you eat, the more flavor."
~ Chinese Proverb

I ONCE HEARD A STORY about the yogi, Paramahansa Yogananda, from the time when he first arrived in America in the 1920s as one of the initial representatives of Far East spirituality. Yogananda was drawing large audiences, and not just because he had shoulder-length hair and wore ochre-colored robes. This Spiritual leader also had an unusual way of demonstrating the great strength he possessed as a result of his yoga practice. After taking the stage, he would call for several large male volunteers from the audience, and ask them to lean on his belly. Then, with a single flex of his stomach, Yogananda would send them tumbling, just like dominoes, cross the stage.

How did he cultivate such power? By focusing his breath on his power center. In the Taoist Spiritual tradition and in Qi Gong, this area where you can access your power is called the *tan tien*—or as I prefer to call it, the Soul's Fire. It is located around the navel area. This is where you experience "willpower" or a lack of it. The ideal state is to experience a free flow of energy through this part of your body. That would be the liberating experience of living your free will as a human being who is entirely connected to your Divine potential.

THE "THICK AROUND THE MIDDLE" SYNDROME

> "Happiness is
> a way station
> between too
> much and
> too little."
>
> ~ Channing Pollock

Realizing that we each have the potential to experience this source of power certainly puts a different spin on the common experience of being "a bit thick around the middle." You can now objectively view the widely acceptable "pot belly" syndrome which is so prevalent in our comfort-driven world in an entirely different way. Excess weight around the middle is a symptom of a much greater dis-ease than being over-weight or obese. Overeating is a symptom of denying who we truly are, as we try to fill the insatiable hole we feel whenever approaching a relationship to ourselves from the outside-in instead of from the inside-out. It is the most common way people block internal messages and deny the beauty inherent in the present moment as well as their creativity, passion and Soul-Full essence. It is here, in this power center of ourselves, that we align with the Divine or not—that is our free will— to choose a Divine connection, or not. If we choose to do anything with a "fire in our belly," it is usually Divine action. The world seems to miraculously comply and formidable obstacles crumble. There is no stopping us.

Yet, there cannot be any "fire in the belly" if you have layers and layers of dormant energy—fat—covering it. If you happen to have a "spare tire" and you are reading this, don't feel embarrassed or defensive. Instead, see this information as a wakeup call to your true potential and all of the power lying dormant at your core that you have forgotten how to access.

Cultivating a love for the feeling of a "Greater Emptiness" in your belly will help you unearth your passion and purpose as well as powerful Divine support here on earth. Now you can feel "emptiness" in a whole new way— it is not a feeling of deprivation as you may have previously been thinking. Instead, it is a wider open receptacle from which your inner command— your all-mighty Self—can build and emerge. When considering losing weight around the middle, you can now consider the effort as a very convenient way to access the mightiness you hold within that has been hidden from you and the world. (See Chapter 26, "Breathe Deep," for more information on tan tien deep-belly breathing. It's a method you can use to access the energy in this power center.)

THE GOOD NEWS AND THE BAD NEWS

In America, we have a consumer-driven society. Even when you are entirely unaware of it, you are being barraged with "consumer-ese" input. As a result of this, many people in the US have an insatiable appetite for purchasing consumer goods. That means no amount of material consumption can possibly satisfy them. This, in my view, is both the good news and the bad.

It's bad if you forget that you didn't come to this earth to be satisfied. Rather, you came here to know your power to overcome all of your limited beliefs. Your Soul's purpose and greatest desire is to know yourself as free—and one of the final steps to adopting this free identity is to know yourself as a fully autonomous, ever-evolving, creative human-being propelled by unique tastes and desires. To go along with "the crowd" by investing your time, energy and money on the trend-of-the-day, while hoping to feel any sense of ultimate satisfaction, is futile. This will always feel unfulfilling because you are not going for what is right for you as an individually evolving Soul. Any satisfaction you could ever experience from this motivation and perspective would be fleeting at best.

On the other hand, the fact that you now know material consumption can never satisfy you is good news—*if* you decide that now is the time for you to get off this wheel and begin marching to a different drummer. But know that if you choose to do that, by the very nature of the choice, you'll soon feel compelled to focus more deliberately on your own individual and unique desires and less on the mind-numbing media and its pick-of-the-day trends. This will leave you free to choose a more conscious, discerning and discriminating path—one in which you can, for instance, tune out, turn off, or turn down the volume on commercials and other media and take the time to know yourself.

If you begin to spend such deliberate time with yourself—10 minutes here and there, one morning, one whole day, etc.—you'll no doubt discover something that the "emptier" crowd knows. You are not a human "doing," you are a human "being"—and the being part of you is your Soul. By honoring your "gut" knowing and cultivating a deep connection, you'll enhance your personal presence and power from the inside out.

SYSTEMATICALLY UNDER-EATING

Let's focus now on the food aspect of consumption. How do you cultivate self-control in this arena? Well, there is a practice honored in many monasteries associated with various Spiritual traditions—*stop eating before you are full.* Spiritual eaters know that you must leave room for the essence of food to be infused with the essence of your Soul. If you do this, you'll experience a natural commingling of your human side—the concrete part of you that chews and digests food—and your being side—your Soul—which is very fulfilling. You cannot know this same fullness when stuffed to the gills.

To adopt this practice, it can be helpful to become aware of healthy portion sizes of the foods you eat. This can be a real eye-opener! Our stomachs can really only comfortably accommodate two fistfuls of food, without having to expand, like a balloon, to accommodate more. To get an idea of healthy portion sizes, look at the labels on food packages. Also, try this—put about two fistfuls of food onto a plate and see how much it is. The amount will be less than most restaurant-sized portions are today. In order to compete with one another, restaurants serve food on platters instead of plates. "All you can eat" is a standard lure and portion sizes have become part of the way food is sold to us. We are trained as consumers to want bigger portions and fuller stomachs. It's so easy to forget that *less is more*. An over-stuffed belly will most definitely make you identify with a body and not the lighter aspects of your Soul.

As stated earlier, in "Tips for Transitioning," one way to enhance the appeal of smaller portion sizes is to creatively arrange the food on smaller plates, while paying particular attention to the variety, color and assortment of foods you choose. When we eat such a meal, comprised of fresh quality fruits or vegetables representative of nearly every hue of the spectrum, it insures that we feel fulfilled in body, mind and Spirit. Eating thoughtfully and colorfully enlivens us and our senses.

THE "MORE MECHANISM"

Another advantage of systematically under-eating is that you will find yourself to be better in touch with what I call the *"more mechanism."* This is the inner-gauge we all have that signals when we are full. If you have ignored this feeling barometer for a while, chances are that your more mechanism gauge is set very high. As a result, you may eat much larger amounts than are healthy for you without feeling full.

Even if you don't typically overeat, chances are that you've overindulged at times—like on Thanksgiving, for instance. Of course, there you're not alone. If our more mechanisms could be serviced by a technician like washing machines or cars are, nearly every American would need a service tune-up for their more mechanism after Thanksgiving! Instead, that day just seems to set the tone for the rest of the holidays in which it is seen as typical and quite often expected that you overeat.

Interestingly, in your body, your more mechanism works very much in the same way endorphins do when they kick in after an experienced runner hits the zone. While the skilled runner feels entirely "done" with running at some point and would much rather stop than continue, they know from experience that they should just push on a little longer. The result? They'll hit a stage where it feels as though they could just run forever. Well, your more mechanism is just like that, only the antithesis of the experience really; whereas the runner is typically letting go of the body-oriented limitation, an overeater is anchoring themselves to it more and more with each and every bite.

But if you are overeating once you hit a certain full point, you can't tell whether you are hungry or filled to capacity. What would normally be a very uncomfortable state becomes comfortable, since you've become comfortably numb!

> *"The hardest thing is to take less when you can get more."*
>
> ~ Kim Hubbard

*"Who
covets more
is evermore
a slave"*

~ Robert Herrick

To reset your more mechanism, begin to eat while mindfully paying attention to the precise moment when you first feel full. When you do feel it, put down your fork or spoon immediately and thank your body for letting you know your own optimum satiation point. Then if at first while trying to change, you decide to pick up your fork and start eating again, ignoring your more mechanism, that's perfectly alright! Just noticing that you do have such inner intelligence is enough. Eventually you'll find yourself listening to it more and more. Another powerful and very effective way to reset your more mechanism is through fasting. (See Chapter 34, "Getting on the Fast Track," for more information.)

Many people feel as though they've been left out of paradise somehow, that they are uncared for by God. But we are never dropped by the Divine. It's just that so many people focus outwardly for answers, instead of looking within, to their Soul.

If you've been overindulging and find yourself overweight or unhealthy because of it, you just haven't been paying attention to the unceasing and unconditionally loving Small Still Voice that is inside of you. Tune in and ask that Small Still Voice, and the more mechanism, for guidance. Once you find that voice of fullness and follow it, you will never feel dropped by God again.

SOMETHING TO CHEW ON

Do you watch television commercials? If so, ask yourself why and then notice some things about them. First, notice what is being presented to you—see how food products tease and tantalize. The commercials are designed to appeal, but to never overload your senses. Then notice that the consumers on TV always seem to look and feel delightfully satisfied, or in a state of hungry anticipation, but they are never overindulged—unless it's a commercial for antacids! You won't often see an overstuffed plate on a television advertisement either. Typically portion sizes are small and delicately alluring. For instance, a bag of chips may be held, but only one bite of one chip per person will ever be shown. A similar approach is used for even a mealtime feast. The plates will all be perfectly filled to entice—and highlighted by everyone's vivacious enthusiasm—but they won't be stacked enough to "stuff" each eater.

Pay attention to this. Most likely you've never noticed it before, and there's a good reason. While you're watching shows that carry you along in the plot, you are under a form of hypnosis, and this is the very reason why advertisers pay such big bucks to flaunt their goods in front of your very susceptible eyes for 30 seconds between segments. Don't be surprised if out of nowhere, while you're viewing a commercial, you find yourself feeling a little hungry as you watch a group of teens romp about snacking on a shared bag of nacho chips or *need* to have a bowl of ice cream after you see that well performed "bite and smile." It all looks so fun and inviting—so alive, while you sit there observing. You're not given the impression that you'll feel stuffed and uncomfortable after eating this food. And feeling like you're missing out on the fun can seem mighty empty and certainly not like you're experiencing the most fulfilling way to live. So you eat to at least fill yourself up with something.

SOUL-FULL EXERCISE #8

Watching television is just one of the many ways people "numb-out" and distance themselves from their inner feelings. Still, it is an excellent place to become more mindful in your life and to practice self-control in order to tap your willpower more tangibly.

Next time you are watching TV, make it a point to do so with a deliberate presence. See if you feel pulled into wanting to purchase or consume anything that may not necessarily enhance your life. It's very easy for advertisers and marketers to manipulate the collective consciousness via the airwaves. That's because the primary experience of most television viewers as they watch—although very few people are aware of this—is that of becoming connected to others. Not only do you, as a viewer, feel linked with the performers you see on the screen, but you also feel joined with all of the other unseen viewers as well. But the satisfaction gained by this type of inactive participation with the world is always short-lived and ultimately very unsatisfying to a powerful, interactive, expansive and expressive Soul.

However, in the short-term, while you are viewing, you don't even have to leave your living room to feel part of the collective whole, and isn't that what everyone longs for on a deep level—*connectivity*? That's the only "fullness" we notice missing in our lives. Consuming more and having more "stuff" is not the answer. Adding more things to your life and "more layers" to your body will only make you feel more separate and less powerful to live the unique and individual life you were born to live.

So as you watch TV, try getting up when a commercial comes on. Stretch and drink a glass of water during the break instead of numbly "consuming" the ad. Or stand up and deliberately deep breathe for the duration.

You'll find more information about the Soul-connecting experience of drinking water in Chapter 24, "Do Drink the Water," and deep Soul-Full breathing in Chapter 26, "Breathe Deep."

CHAPTER NINE

Recognize Your Blessings

"Wherever there is a human being, there is an opportunity for a kindness."
~ Marcus Annaeus Seneca

AMERICANS HAVE THE LUXURY of a wide-range of food choices—something that less advanced cultures often don't experience. Away from the cities, in areas of many third-world countries, people basically live off the land and therefore eat what they can harvest. Mother Earth is not just a metaphor to these people. They know the earth as the feminine nurturing aspect of God—the Goddess feeding her children.

If we were all to honor the Truth, we'd understand that when one person on earth hungers, starves, or has "less than" feelings, the rest of us feel the same—if not on the surface, then deep within. Therefore it's only natural that so many of us have "can't quite put my finger on what they are" elusive guilt feelings when we overindulge with food. Again, I don't say this to put further guilt on the process of eating; there is far too much of that already. I say this to promote gratitude, inner connectedness and presence. To liberate ourselves from guilt, we can cultivate an appreciation of our bounty—a sense of knowing that we are blessed, and a state of being aware of the grace that comes from having so many choices.

MAKING THE CONNECTION

I was at a talk given by Andrew Cohen, a wonderful Spiritual teacher and a friend of mine. He was speaking about Liberation and Enlightenment. During his talk, Andrew mentioned the poverty he had just witnessed on a trip to India. He said, "Most of us have no idea how fortunate we are. We don't see how the rest of the world lives. It would be very good for us to witness this."

Shortly after that comment, a woman raised her hand and said with a bit of an edge to her voice, "I want to stick to the subject here. I don't want to get sidetracked speaking about what is happening halfway around the world. I have enough problems in my own immediate life to think about without getting sucked into thinking about that. I want to know what I can personally do right here, right now, to be free."

Sidestepping a confrontation, Andrew was very gracious with her, and he began to give the woman some Spiritual pointers, all very wonderful. I raised my hand next, feeling the need to add to what he had related to her. I said to the woman, "I hope you don't mind me commenting on what you said previously. It's been my experience that the very reason so many people are in so much pain is the lack of connectivity we feel. We are all so self-ishly living in our own little world, trying to be free of the pain of that self-imposed isolation. When we do this, we can miss the fact that those people 'way on the other side of the world' are our saviors. Because if we can truly connect with them, we recognize we are One, we've broken our boundaries, and then miraculously we'll find ourselves set free."

Selfishness, or isolated thinking, is a very unfulfilling state to be in. It will always keep us looking for something to fill the void and the pang of separation that we feel. Some people who seem to need food all of the time, who are continually grazing, are very unaware of this. These people don't

"Always be a little kinder than necessary."

~ Sir James M. Barrie

realize that they are only reaching for the food to satiate the empty feeling inside that's caused by feelings of separation. No amount of food will ever appease that type of hunger.

Think of it this way—thoughts can be either *thought-full* or *thought-less*. You'll know which of the two are taking up space in your mind by the way you feel—full or lacking.

There is an easy way to get an instantaneous bellyfull of satisfaction. As I stated in the previous chapter, our solar plexus, which lies at the center of us, just below the rib cage, is our body's own individual power center. It's where we radiate love, and can pull the miraculous energy of ourselves from within us to push it out towards the rest of the world. "I, me, mine"—selfish (thought-less)—thoughts create an inward movement of energy and ultimately a "black hole" type sinking feeling. Whereas, Universal or "We" (thought-full) thoughts create just the opposite—free, expansive, radiant and full feelings. When we "feed other's Souls" by connecting with them in caring ways, we automatically feel more power-**full**. And if not, we feel power-**less**.

SOMETHING TO CHEW ON

It's natural when contemplating a situation as huge as world hunger to think, "I'm only one person. Any gesture I make doesn't even put a dent in the situation." That's the ego's thought-less way of thinking, and it will keep you feeling small-minded and insignificant. But consider this, any little bit of giving helps *you* to know the Greatness of your Soul. That's one of the powerful opportunities for connectivity our impoverished brothers and sisters offer to us.

Here are some facts from the *Bread for the World Institute* that will help you to see how every "little bit" really can make a great difference…

- Today our world houses 6.47 billion people. In 2005, statistics showed that 852 million people across the world are hungry, up from 842 million a year earlier. That's a jump of 10 million people—most of whom are children.

- Every day, more than 16,000 children die from hunger-related causes—one child every five seconds.

- In essence, hunger is the most extreme form of poverty, where individuals or families cannot afford to meet their most basic need for food. Hunger manifests itself in many ways other than starvation and famine. Most poor people who battle hunger deal with chronic undernourishment and vitamin or mineral deficiencies, which result in stunted growth, weakness and heightened susceptibility to illness.

- Countries in which a large portion of the population battles hunger daily are usually poor and often lack the social safety-nets we enjoy, such as soup kitchens, food stamps, and job-training programs. When a family that lives in a poor country cannot grow enough food or earn enough money to buy food, there is nowhere to turn for help.

- In the developing world, more than 1.2 billion people currently live below the international poverty-line, earning less than $1 per day. Among this group of poor people, many have problems obtaining adequate, nutritious food for themselves and their families. As a result, 815 million people in the developing world are undernourished. They consume less than the minimum amount of calories essential for sound health and growth. Undernourishment negatively affects people's health, productivity, sense of hope and overall well-being. Economically, the constant securing of food consumes valuable time and the energy of poor people, allowing less time for work and earning income. Socially, the lack of food erodes relationships and feeds shame so that those most in need of support are often least able to call on it.

In addition, below are a collection of food "myths" that, according to the organization *Food First*, are the reasons there is such widespread world hunger today—even though we live on such an abundant planet. To find out more, visit: *www.foodfirst.org*.

Myth 1—There is not enough food to go around.

Reality—There is, in fact, enough meat, fish, grains and produce to provide every human being on the planet 4.3 pounds of food a day—that's enough to make most people fat. But many people are too poor to purchase the foods grown right in their own regions and so it is exported.

Myth 2—Famine is a result of natural causes.

Reality—Human causes are increasingly responsible for making people vulnerable to nature's variances. Millions continually live on the brink of disaster, and natural disasters become the final push over the edge. In the eyes of Food First, the real disaster is that many of the world's societies are apparently run by economies that fail to offer opportunity to all and that place private-profit over compassion.

Myth 3—Overpopulation causes hunger.

Reality—For every densely populated and hungry country, there are others where abundant food resources coexist with hunger. It is the underlying iniquities that deprive people, especially poor women, of economic opportunity and security.

Myth 4—Environmental concerns cause less food to be grown.

Reality—Efforts to feed the hungry are not causing the environmental crisis. Environmentally sound agriculture alternatives are often more productive than environmentally destructive ones.

"You have not lived a perfect day unless you have done something for someone who will never be able to repay you."

~ Ruth Smeltzer

Myth 5—Growing more food can alleviate world hunger.

Reality—Due to the Green Revolution, millions of tons more grain is harvested each year; however this has not alleviated hunger largely because this approach fails to alter the distribution of economic power that determines who can buy the additional food. Other concerns related to this increase in production are that the long-term capacity of the soil may be degraded and that there are ill effects—both to the consumer and to the environment—due to the genetic alteration of the seeds.

Myth 6—Larger farms are the answer to hunger.

Reality—Today large landowners are some of the most inefficient growers, while small farmers typically achieve four to five times greater output per acre. This is due, in part, to the more sustainable, integrated production systems that small farmers use. Also, although large landowners have most of the best land for growing, they leave much of it idle, so redistribution of land is one viable option, as in the land reform seen in countries such as Zimbabwe, China and Taiwan, where markedly increased production was experienced after redistribution. A World Bank study of Northeast Brazil estimated that output could be raised an astounding 80% through redistributing farmland to smaller holdings in that country.

Myth 7—The free market alone can end hunger.

Reality—Although a free market policy is a step in the right direction, any overly dogmatic approach ultimately does more harm than good and pits those who are pro-market against governments and vice-versa. A true, long-lasting solution is a combination of both the market and government that allocates resources and distributes goods. It's important to realize that the market's marvelous efficiencies can only work to alleviate hunger when the purchasing power is widely dispersed. And perhaps most important of all is focusing on promoting not just the market but the consumers themselves— by offering genuine tax credit and land reforms to disperse buying power

"Eating is the most essential act of every living creature. And in virtually every human culture, growing, eating and sharing food has a Spiritual dimension too."

~ Anna Lappe and Bryant Terry, authors of *Grub*

toward the poor—and moving away from the current tendency towards privatization and deregulation.

Myth 8—Free trade is the answer.

Reality—There still needs to be many reforms in the current free-trade promotion formula. Currently Third World countries exports have been booming while hunger has continued unabated or even worsened in recent years. The majority of people are still too poor to buy the foods grown on their own country's soil. Not surprisingly, those who control productive resources still direct production towards more lucrative markets abroad.

Myth 9—More aid from the US government will help.

Reality—Unless we focus on empowering the poor and hungry to help themselves, we are doing little more than perpetuating the problem. The answer is not to shore up the very forces that work against the poorest people. For instance, it is not helpful to give money to governments that repress their people by promoting exports or by providing the armaments that repressive governments use to stay in power. Despite the images we see of weak and suffering poor people, it is a fact that people will feed themselves if given the opportunity to do so. It would be more helpful to focus on removing obstacles to such self-sufficiency. Our foreign aid budget would be better spent on unconditional debt relief, since it is the foreign-debt burden that forces many Third World countries to cut back on the essential education and anti-poverty programs and basic health care.

Myth 10—There must be poor to benefit the rich.

Reality—Although low wages both abroad and in inner cities may mean cheaper bananas, computers, t-shirts and fast food for many Americans, it also causes us to pay heavily for the hunger and poverty it creates in the lives of others. The low wages paid to workers in Third World countries cause US corporations to seek cheaper labor abroad, thus adversely affecting the job availability, wages and working conditions for many Americans. It is important to finally see what is becoming so evident—we are One! In a global economy, the advances that American workers have attained in employment benefits, wage levels, and working conditions are protected only when working people all over the world are freed from economic desperation. If we choose to educate ourselves about the commonalities that many privileged Americans share with both the poor in Third World countries and at home, we will naturally become more compassionate without sliding into pity. By working to support the poor in freeing themselves from economic oppression, we free ourselves.

Myth 11—My lone voice doesn't matter.

Reality—Although to you, your opinion may seem insignificant in the grand scheme of things, your individual choices do matter. When you buy locally grown, organic foods, avoid GMOs, and/or make other conscious consumer decisions, and then share your opinions and reasons for doing so with others, you benefit the whole of humankind. Remember, a bonfire can be lit with just one match!

SOUL FULL EXERCISE #9

If you feel concerned or upset in any way about issues concerning world hunger, it's your time to do something about it. But don't do this to be benevolent or altruistic for someone else—do this for yourself. You'll see that once you get out of your own "little world" and begin to cultivate a more universal mindset, you will not feel any better until you take some action to make a difference. As Mahatma Gandhi once said, *"You must be the change you wish to see in the world."*

There are a lot of ways for you to feel your power by thinking in globally connected ways while taking action right where you are. Here are some organizations and websites that can help you get started…

The Institute for Food and Development Policy/Food First

I found this website particularly interesting because the Institute does not just solicit donations—it also works for social change. Their position is that there is plenty of food being produced on the planet, however a scarcity mentality and the skewed distribution of economic power keep it from getting into hungry mouths. Their mission is to shape how people think by analyzing the root causes of global hunger, poverty, and ecological degradation. Their goal is also to develop solutions in partnership with movements working for social change.

www.foodfirst.org

Bread for the World Institute

Bread for the World's 55,000 members contact their senators and representatives about legislation that affects hungry people in the United States and worldwide. They do not provide direct relief or development assistance. Rather, the organization's focus is on using the power that people have as citizens in a democracy to support policies that address the root causes of hunger and poverty.

www.bread.org

Feed the Children

Feed the Children is an international, non-profit relief organization that delivers food, medicine, clothing and other necessities to individuals, children and families who lack these essentials due to famine, war, poverty or natural disaster. It is one of the world's largest private organizations dedicated to feeding hungry people.

www.FeedTheChildren.org

Christian Children's Fund

The Christian Children's Fund organization operates under the belief that children have the right to experience life with as much joy and hope as possible. Donations made go to a specific child with whom the donor can correspond, thus creating a tangible bond between them.

www.christianchildrensfund.org

"It's time we turn the 'you are what you eat' truism on its head: I am, in effect, what you eat; you are what I eat. It's time to awaken to a diet of interdependence."

~ Anna Lappe and Bryant Terry, authors of *Grub*

Heifer International

Heifer International is a wonderful organization that promotes strong communities, sustainability, environmental protection and peace. It currently supports projects in more than 50 countries, including the United States. Their goal is to create sustainable small-scale farm enterprises to improve nutrition and supplement incomes. Local community groups conceive and manage Heifer International projects, empowering people to solve their own problems and equipping the next generation to face challenges successfully.

www.heifer.org

CHAPTER TEN

Weigh Your Thoughts

"As ye sow, so shall ye reap."
~ Galatians 6:7

THE MOST POWERFUL WAY to affect your outer world is to be mindful of your inner world. Your mind is like a field into which you can plant any seed and it will grow. That is why it is of utmost importance that you notice what kinds of thoughts you consistently think and then weigh them to see if they are life-enhancing or in fact diminishing of your quality of life. As you nurture seed-thoughts of compassion, joy, accomplishment, acceptance and love, those things will appear in your life abundantly. Conversely, if you choose to plant a briar patch of negative, doubtful and fearful thoughts, they too will grow. Choose wisely. And remember, not only your present experience, but your destiny is shaped by the thoughts you think each day.

Relating this to food, what are you thinking as you fill your grocery cart or pick vegetables or fruit from your garden? The process of eating mindfully starts at the gathering stage. When you begin to deliberately pay attention to what your thoughts are about what you eat, those times when you are choosing food should be included. Here's an example.

One of the very first stories I told to illustrate how dramatically I had changed after my discovery of a Soul-Full way of living was about grocery shopping. I chose to speak about this because, strangely enough, I found that I was filling up with bliss most unexpectedly, not in churches, but in the supermarket!

Walking into the produce section of the supermarket one day, I spied a large, full display of cherries in the center of the aisle. They were in season, and as I reached up to rip a plastic bag off of a nearby roll, I admired the cherries lying invitingly before me. Most were plump and dark red.

In the past, I used to speed through the store, quickly grabbing produce and items off the shelves. I just tried to get the food-shopping chore over with so I could get to the next obligation on my long "to do" list. Before, bagging cherries would have been done in one fell swoop—bag open, fist-full of cherries shoved in.

Not this time! I picked the cherries up and, one by one, began touching, smelling and examining them before dropping the fruit into my bag. After a moment, I looked up from the bin to see a woman and two men standing in a circle around the display, filling their bags as well.

I said aloud, "This is funny. We're like orchard workers all picking side by side." They laughed and we continued selecting cherries.

Then I was inspired to share a childhood story at the supermarket with strangers! "We used to have a cherry tree in my backyard when I was a little girl. My friends and I never ate the cherries; we just had fights with them. One year, about two dozen of my cousins came over for a summer barbecue and we waged a huge cherry war. Just as it was really getting going, my grandmother ran out of the house yelling, 'Don't throw those cherries. That's food!' We yelled back, 'Awe come on Nan, this tree's rotten. We never eat them. They're no good.' She disarmed us all the same. A few weeks later, that tree was completely full of red, ripe delicious cherries for the first time ever."

"Watch your thoughts; they become your words. Watch your words; they become actions. Watch your actions; they become habits. Watch your habits; they become character. Watch your character; it becomes your destiny."

~ Frank Outlaw

When I looked up from my bag, now filled with cherries, the men and the woman were smiling at me. The woman started to relate her favorite recipe for cherry pie and one of the men described his favorite dessert, which was flaming cherries jubilee. After that, I walked through the aisles joyfully astonished at how simple it is to find heaven and angels on earth. The supermarket and all the food in it were nearly the same as ever. The only thing that had changed since the time when I hated food shopping was me!

How would these cherries taste to me when I shared them later with my family? Would the pleasant memories of both my shopping experience and my childhood influence my appreciation of the food I had bought? *Of course.*

"Everything you see is a result of your thoughts. There is no exception to this fact."

~ A Course in Miracles

A PRIVILEGED ABUNDANCE

What many of us take for granted, others may experience as life-changing—food shopping included. I remember hearing a story about a Russian man who came to the US for the first time during the period when travel from his country to other nations was still restricted. During his visit, he was taken to a supermarket in order to observe the opulence to be found in America. The man was very unimpressed and in response to his hosts' comments, he said, "I've heard of this being done in Russia too. Everything from all of the stores is put in one place to impress foreign dignitaries and such." So he was taken to another store, and another, and still another, only to find the very same variety and amount of goods being sold. Finally he was convinced, and incredulous at what he saw to be the norm, the man broke down and cried.

We are privileged to enjoy such abundance. If you want to practice connection with your own heart and others, try going food-shopping. Supermarkets can be sacred places, if you go with a grateful heart. And think of the opportunity for Soul connection—many more people go to the grocery store each week than to churches, temples or mosques!

SOMETHING TO CHEW ON

We are continually making decisions and faced with options in our lives. Grocery shopping is one very tangible experience of this. How do you make your choices while food shopping? Do you choose items based solely on price or are you filling your cart with "bliss" by buying items you know help sustain and support our planet? Are your purchases based primarily on convenience? Or do you buy foods you know make you and those you love feel most whole and balanced? Everything we do speaks of who we believe ourselves to be.

SOUL-FULL EXERCISE #10

Any supermarket employee who works the checkout will tell you that most shoppers consider themselves stressed by the whole process of shopping for their consumables. It's just one more obligation added to a long list of others. If that's how you often feel, why not allow your next trip to the supermarket to be a "Zen" experience by feeling your connectivity to it all—row by row, item by item, encounter by blessed encounter.

When you are choosing an item, pause for just a moment to consider the orchestration that took place to get that specific product into your hands. Inquire about items, or read labels, not just to find out their ingredients, but also to discover the orientation and even the mission statement of the companies whose products you choose most consistently. Greet the store's staff when you encounter them in the aisles, see them stocking shelves, or stand across from them at the registers.

I discovered one of the most amazing people I've ever met while chatting with Aaron, an employee at Whole Foods, as he packed my grocery bags. What started out as a casual conversation deeply touched me, because Aaron told me he'd just left New Orleans after his home was flooded during Hurricane Katrina. He had lost practically everything and his house would have to be destroyed. I would never have guessed that; he had such a profound sense of peace about him, and treated me and the items I'd purchased with such caring attention. Then I realized that Aaron had gotten "it"—the realization that life's not about "things," it's about a deeper connection to the everyday blessings.

Take time to connect with store workers and fellow shoppers with a genuine smile or kind word. You'll never know what treasures these seemingly insignificant encounters can hold until you do. Just be present, and you'll notice just as I have—*what you give, you receive.*

CHAPTER ELEVEN

Eat What You Want

"He who distinguishes the true savor of his food can never be a glutton; he who does not cannot be otherwise."
~ Henry David Thoreau

I WAS ON THE SET OF A PHOTO SHOOT in New York City with one of the top super-models at that time. When we broke for lunch, a sumptuous catered buffet was laid out before us. We sat down, and one of the ad agency reps remarked, "Looks great, but I guess you models won't be eating much." The other model, who was as slim as a beanpole, piped right up, "Oh, I can eat anything I want." To this, the wide-eyed agency rep quickly replied, "Geeze, you must not want much."

The model did eat everything she wanted and the ad agency rep was right—it wasn't much. But she did seem to enjoy savoring every bite.

I also modeled in Paris. There, it wasn't just the models, but most people who exhibited this same basic eating philosophy. According to my Parisian friends, they feel it's possible to eat anything *in moderation.* Apparently, they'd learned this approach to eating early on and continued to practice it all their lives.

"Happiness is a bowl of cherries and a book of poetry under a shade tree."

~ Astrid Alauda

Parisians often enjoy lavish meals, which typically contain several small courses. The foods they eat are of high quality, as it's the norm in Paris to shop at small, local markets and buy only produce that's in season and packed with flavor. They may enjoy a few ounces of baked fish rather than half a pound. And they've discovered that one small piece of high-quality chocolate is much more satisfying than a mile-high piece of Double Fudge Cake. In other words, it's all about maintaining a balance. If they happen to over-indulge, they simply choose to eat less at the next meal or get more exercise. So a dessert at lunch might mean eating a lighter dinner or taking the dog for an extra-long walk that night. They typically don't skip meals or replace them with prepackaged diet bars. They don't avoid fats and sugars at all costs, or even count calories. Instead, they focus on eating in a way that ensures the greatest possible appreciation and enjoyment of food, emphasizing quality over quantity and slowing down to mindfully savor meals instead of eating on the run or while otherwise distracted.

Although the French are known world-wide for their passionate love affair with food and the culinary arts, their slim physiques show the effectiveness of this mindset. And more importantly, this approach to eating cultivates balance. It adds more color and flavor to life—enhancing one's existence and promoting a sense of deep satisfaction and fullness. So next time you sit down to eat, remember *less is more*. Instead of a huge plate of mediocre food, you may want to try savoring several flavorful small courses.

A FINAL NOTE

We can all eat "anything we want" once we begin to pay attention to our body's signals and feelings. If you work toward eating only when you are hungry and stopping when you are full, you'll notice that much of the time when you do overeat you really don't want what it is that you're eating at all. Extra helpings, even of the most delicious food, lose their flavor once you've eaten one bite too many. When we truly want to feel good, we will eat only foods that make us feel and (as a result!) look good.

SOMETHING TO CHEW ON

When I was a little girl, I loved babies, so I used to watch mommies and daddies with their little ones all of the time. From these experiences, I vividly got the strong message that it was very important to make a baby eat—a lot!—sometimes even until they spit it back up at you! I remember hearing exclamations like, "He's such a good eater!" and "Look at those cheeks, how beautiful. I see you have no problem getting her to eat!" I also recall seeing parents use distraction techniques, such as flying a paper airplane by their baby's face just as they shoved that extra-important spoonful of cereal into her mouth, even though she had previously refused it. Television was another good distraction. You could shovel spoonful after spoonful of previously unwanted food into a baby if you sat them in front of a mesmerizing kiddie show.

We've all been programmed by our childhood experiences, most of which we don't even remember. So don't be surprised if you've found that it's a pattern for you to want more food, even when you're completely full, and you don't have a clue as to why.

It really doesn't matter why, or what happened to you in your past—that's not the point I'm making. Everyone's always doing the best they can, based on their own life experiences. Just realize that now, in the present, you can change the patterns that don't suit you by paying attention to your feelings and respecting them. *Honoring your deeper feelings is the key to your every success!*

"Nothing in excess."

~ Solon

SOUL-FULL EXERCISE #11

Next time you're reaching for something to eat, ask yourself, "Why am I eating now? Am I hungry?" If you are hungry—great! Go ahead and thoroughly enjoy your food. But while you are enjoying it, try being Soul-Fully present with yourself. For instance, notice how delicious the first bite tastes when you are hungry. Then, as you eat, notice when you begin to feel satisfied. Does the food still taste as delicious to you now? Keep on eating while noticing your feelings. When you begin to feel very full, notice the subtleties of what this is like and whether the food still tastes as delicious as it did with that first bite.

If you pay attention to your feelings while you are eating, instead of gulping down food as you are being distracted by something else, you'll notice that you actually enjoy food much more but often eat less!

"Moderation is the key to lasting enjoyment."

~Hosea Ballou

CHAPTER TWELVE

Amazing Grace

Tap Into the Power of Prayer

"We love our bread, we love our butter, but most of all, we love each other."
~ My family meal prayer

I'VE BEEN TO INDIA several times, and I've eaten my share of meals in places that in the States would be considered downright gross. I've paused between bites to watch a family of cockroaches, each one "the size of me fist," parade across the kitchen floor. In one less-than-appetizing place, I watched as a flock of crows had a pool party in the vat of rice left to soak in the courtyard—a vat just like the one used to make the Vegetable Briyani I'd just eaten! Yet I have never experienced any stomach upsets in India—not even one. I firmly believe that's because before I partake in a meal, any time or any place, I always bless my food. I don't feel it's what I say so much as how and why I say it.

The way I see it, everything is either love or fear. Wherever love is present, no sickness or dis-ease can prevail. Love, or the Soul's light, is of the highest, purest vibration. So I pause and center myself on my Soul before consuming anything I eat. Next I feel the essence coming from the food to be sure it is of the highest quality possible and if it is, I simply give thanks. If it's not, I add my Soul's light to it—in other words, I bless it.

As I've paused to put my hands over my food in some eating establishments, not only in India but most any place in the world, I could literally feel the state of mind of those preparing the food. Some food that looks wonderful can feel formidable. Don't let looks fool you! As I've said, even in Five Star restaurants, the energy of the food can be gut-wrenching if there is lots of ego or anger in the kitchen. If I find that's the situation, I not only bless my food, but the kitchen help as well!

Many people don't travel as much as I do and so they know the quality and origin of their food and exactly how it's prepared. In that case, blessing food before eating it takes on a bit of a different intent—one of feeling a sense of gratitude—the very best "seasoning" of all. How delicious a home-cooked meal can taste when you've given thanks not only for the food, but for the one who has prepared it.

Think about your own life and how you can bring more grace into your experiences at meal-time. If you truly want yourself and your loved ones to get the most out of every meal, remember that centering on the Soul is an essential, oft overlooked element of a well-balanced diet. Prayer before meals is a wonderful way of getting ourselves into the moment, and consciously expressing gratefulness for what we are about to receive. It is the perfect beginning to a mindful eating experience. By prefacing our meal with prayer, we acknowledge the higher purpose for which our actions are intended. This ensures that they represent more than the mechanical motion of putting food in our mouths, chewing and swallowing.

FOOD AND SACRED TRADITIONS

It's no coincidence that in most Spiritual traditions, important rituals center on the preparation of food. Any tradition worth its weight in salt couldn't help but notice the powerful opportunity for deeper connection that sharing a meal naturally provides. The Catholic miracle of the consecration of bread and wine, the Jewish celebration of Seder, and the cooking of *Prasad*—consecrated food—at many Hindu ceremonies all center on food preparation as part of the sacred feast of joining in communion. Traditions throughout the world see the sharing of food as symbolic of a deeper, more Spiritual mingling of Souls. Breaking bread together is a privilege—one to be honored and acknowledged.

The originators of these traditions realized that mealtime is sacred and food is a very powerful symbol conducive to centering on the trinity of our body, mind and Spirit as one. Mealtime is a time for gathering and community, and for being aware of the Divine.

PRAYER AT OUR TABLES

I remember going to church with my family on Sunday mornings when I was a child and feeling a sense of connection with them. However, that feeling of communion was nowhere near as powerful as the one I felt later in the afternoon when my grandparents joined us for Sunday dinner and my grandfather said the blessing before the meal. By this time, my taste buds tingled and my mouth watered—tickled for hours by the delectable aromas wafting from the kitchen. Finally it was time to feast! But first, we all gathered around the dining-room table and said our prayer, which we called the "Grace before the meal." This was such an appropriate name for it, as that moment was when I always felt closest to Grace. It wasn't an obscure concept to me then. It was as tangible as the steaming mashed potatoes I'd soon be piling high on my plate.

Prayer doesn't necessarily have to be a religious act, or the recitation of a formalized doctrine. Its best purpose is just putting us in a frame of mind in which we are totally dedicated to being present and grateful for what we have. It is equally powerful to bless your food in the fellowship of others or simply in your own company.

Below are examples of prayers related to mealtimes from various traditions. Perhaps you've heard some of them.

- This prayer is from the **Christian** tradition, but can be made relevant and accessible to any faith by realizing that Christ is the essence of perfection, or holiness, or Godliness within us all.

  Bless us oh Lord, and these thy gifts,
  Which we are about to receive from thy bounty,
  through Christ, our Lord.
  　　　Amen.

- Here's a prayer from the **Buddhist** tradition.

  This food is the gift of the whole Universe—the earth, the sky, and much hard work.
  May we eat in mindfulness, so as to be worthy to receive it.
  May we transform our unskillful states of mind, and learn to eat with moderation.
  May we take only foods that nourish us and prevent illness.
  We accept this food to realize the path of understanding and love.

- This prayer comes from the **Hindu** tradition.

  God, bless this food so that it brings vitality and energy to fulfill thy mission and serve humanity.
  God, bless this food so that we remain aware of Thee within and without.
  God, bless this food so that we love all and exclude none.
  Bless those who have provided this food, who have prepared this food, and who eat this food.
  Bless all, my Lord.
  　　　Amen.

- The following prayer, from a Western Sect of the **Muslim Sufi** order, is sung to many different tunes before meals.

Oh Thou, the Sustainer of our body, hearts and Souls,
Bless all that we receive in thankfulness.

- This meal prayer is part of the **Hebrew/Jewish** tradition. It is a prayer said over bread.

Ba-ruch a-ta, A-do-nai, E-lo-hei-nu, me-lech ha-o-lam, ha-motsi le-chem min ha-a-rets.

   This means:
We praise you, God, Ruler of the Universe, who brings forth bread from the earth.

- And the prayer over wine is:

Ba-ruch a-ta, A-do-nai, E-lo-hei-nu, me-lech ha-o-lam, bo-rei pe-ri ha-ga-fen.

   This means:
We praise you, God, Ruler of the Universe, and Creator of the fruit of the vine.

- Here's a **Talmudic** blessing of food. The Talmud is an authoritative body that's also part of the Jewish tradition.

Blessed be He who created this object. How beautiful it is.

"Gratitude is the memory of the heart."

~ Massieu

- This meal prayer comes from the **Baha'i** religion.

   He is God!
   Thou seest us, O my God, gathered around this table,
   praising Thy bounty, with our gaze set upon Thy kingdom,
   O Lord, send down upon us Thy heavenly food
   and confer upon us thy blessing.
   Thou art verily the Bestower, the Merciful, the Compassionate.

- The following is a **Celtic** Prayer, which I found in *The Open Gate* by David Adam.

   Be gentle when you touch bread.
   Let it not lie, uncared for,
   Unwanted.
   So often bread is taken for granted.
   There is such beauty in bread—
   Beauty of surf and soil.
   Beauty of patient toil.
   Wind and rain have caressed it.
   Christ often blessed it.
   Be gentle when you touch bread.

- This **Native American** blessing is said by a server as the food is placed in front of the person dining.

   Spirit partake.

- Here is a prayer my family picked up somewhere along the way.

   We love our bread
   We love our butter
   But most of all,
   We love each other.

- And finally, here's a simple prayer filled with plenty of gratitude:

Thank God for dirty dishes; they have a tale to tell.
While other folks go hungry, we're eating pretty well.
With home, and health, and happiness,
We shouldn't want to fuss;
For by the stack of evidence, God's very good to us.

~ Anonymous

Show up to your next meal centered on grace. It's important for us not to view heaven as somewhere "out there" any longer. It is meant to be our daily experience—an intimate, powerful illumination that fills our every cell and courses through our veins, not some sterile bliss that happens somewhere over our heads. To recognize a sense of heaven on earth, we must fill our bodies with Light and Grace, and one of the best places to start is at mealtime.

SOMETHING TO CHEW ON

"(Grace is) the outward expression of the inward
harmony of the Soul."
~ William Hazlitt

When was the last time you thought about the "greater graces" of living in such an abundant world and being able to eat such an amazing variety of food. Thank God!—literally. **We only truly realize that we have anything, if we give thanks for it.**

SOUL-FULL EXERCISE #12

Take a look at some of the above prayers and see if any of them resonate with you. Next, begin to say it at your meals with gratitude—especially if it's not a prayer from your own Spiritual tradition. Or take some time this week to compose your own heart-felt mealtime blessing. Who knows, maybe it will even become part of your dining traditions for decades to come!

Know Thy Food

"When you ask for guidance and assistance, simply assume that it is immediately pouring forward... Do whatever it is that you need to do in order to relax your mind... but live in the total assumption that the moment you ask for guidance it is pouring in."
    ~ Gary Zukov, author of *The Seat of the Soul*

I FEEL COMPELLED TO REMIND YOU now that although each of the guidelines and beliefs put forth in this section is useful and in my experience healthful, *I am not advocating any single strict approach to eating.* The needs of one person's body are different from that of another's. Based upon your metabolism, genetics, lifestyle, the climate you live in, etc., you have your own unique set of nutritional needs. The only person who can tell you what best sustains your body and what connects you to your Soul is you—and you can know! You only have to pay attention and listen to your body's clues. I suggest considering the information that follows and experimenting a little, then you can decide how to integrate the information into your own diet.

The only real truth is what each individual finds for themselves based on their careful and conscious exploration, intuition, and questioning. My only goal is to give you as much accurate, well-researched information as I can and let you decide how and what you will eat. I do know what works for me. And I'll also share that along the way.

CHAPTER THIRTEEN

Dead and Live Foods

"Food is a living, powerful force that interacts with us on a physical, mental, emotional, vital and Spiritual level."

FOR ONE YEAR after graduating college, I was a junior-high-school general science teacher. I loved the interactive learning that teaching science afforded. We blew up, dissected, mixed and measured everything we could get our hands on. While we were studying the human digestive system, the topic of enzymes came up. I described enzymes to the class as being the life-force found in our cells and in living foods. Some children had a hard time grasping this concept, which is understandable since enzymes can't be seen with our naked eye. We can only see the life and energy that is the result of an enzyme's presence.

So to clarify the concept of enzymes and make it more concrete, we did a little experiment. I gave each of the students two almonds, both of which looked very much alike. However, there was one substantial difference—one was raw and the other was roasted. In other words, the raw one was alive and the roasted one was dead (having had the enzymes, its life force, cooked out of it).

"It can be said that the greatest single cause of degeneration in man is the use of fire in the preparation of foods."

~ Arnold De Vries, author of
The Fountain of Youth

Then I gave each student two plastic cups filled with potting soil. I told them to label one with a "D" for Dead and the other with an "L" for Living, and then plant their almonds in the appropriate cups. We placed them on the windowsill in the direct sun and then each day, at the beginning of class, the students would water and observe their almonds. Lo and behold, after approximately three weeks, the raw almonds sprouted and began to grow, while nothing at all appeared to be happening in the cups that held the dead, roasted almonds.

I told the students to take both cups containing the almonds back to their seats and to turn the soil in the cup labeled "D" that contained the roasted almond. When they did, my students oooh-ed and ahhh-ed when they saw that for the last three weeks the dead, roasted almonds had been decaying, and had already begun to disintegrate into the soil. Then they noted the vivid contrast between the contents of those cups and the bright new green life sprouting from their cups which were marked "L" for living. I further drove the point home by telling them that since it was springtime, once the seedlings got a little larger they could each take one home, plant it, and water it. With care and luck, each live almond could eventually give birth to a beautiful almond tree that could hold thousands of almonds and perhaps even parent other almond trees. That's because the imperative of the invisible life-force in every living thing is to share with life and add to it—to create ever more growth, expansion and vitality. Life naturally begets more life.

However, notice that even the dead, roasted almond contained energy that was compelled to add to life. By its death, it added its nutrients to the soil, and that soil then could be used to support more life. So the cycle of life will always continue… life prevails, that is clear. But now ask yourself, which side of this coin would you choose to be on? The side that is supported by living foods and their present, available life-force, which allows you to thrive, and grow more vibrantly each day—*right now!* Or do you choose to eat dead foods and right now feel less alive due to daily fatigue and mood swings and all manner of "dead feelings"?

There is an answer. You can add more spark to your life by eating more living foods today.

BENEFITING FROM LIVE FOOD

Our bodies are made up of living cells, so it is logical that these cells are best nourished by living foods, with all of their natural nutrients and energy intact. It is also important that the food be untainted by artificial processes. The body benefits most from simple foods, which are easier to digest and contain the most nutrients. Human life cannot be sustained at optimal levels by dead foods that have been denatured and depleted of their natural energy and vitality.

In my opinion, your entire diet needn't consist of entirely raw fruits and vegetables, but it is a healthy base to keep in mind. One guideline for a healthy approach to a raw food diet is about 80% raw foods, and 20% cooked. Overcooked and processed dead foods, as well as artificial chemicals and preservatives, are obviously not as healthy as simple, unprocessed raw fruits and vegetables, and they contain nowhere near as much nutrients and natural energy. But once again, it is up to you to make your own decisions about what you want to eat, based on what makes you feel the best. In our culture, many people find that avoiding all processed foods is largely unrealistic. It just may be helpful for you to keep in mind the raw, live-food guidelines, and to be conscious about what it is that you are putting into your body.

Cooking by baking, boiling, and steaming reduces the nutritional value of most foods. For this reason, foods are most beneficial when eaten raw, if possible. When cooking food, it is best to do it at the lowest workable temperature. Steaming is more beneficial than either boiling or frying, and should be considered if cooking is required. Eight to ten times more nutrients are available from uncooked vegetables than from the same vegetables cooked, and the overall nutrient destruction from cooking is estimated to be about 85%. Plus, eating too much cooked, enzyme-depleted food drains the body's natural store of enzymes that aid our body's digestion.

When being fed live-foods, the body needs less to satiate its appetite and fulfill its energy needs. A person living on this kind of diet will find themselves able to eat smaller amounts, at the same time feeling greater energy and vivacity. Therefore a frequent side effect is that excess weight naturally leaves the body when more raw foods are consumed.

SOME HELPFUL GUIDELINES

Here are some things to be aware of when shopping for and preparing your food:

- **Vegetables are best when fresh and vibrant with color.** For example, leafy green lettuce contains more nutrients than iceberg lettuce, and it tastes better too.

- **There are various ways to assess how ripe or fresh a particular type of fruit or vegetable is.** For example, to test the ripeness of both pineapples and cantaloupes, you sniff them to see if they smell sweet. However, you gently squeeze the cantaloupe to look for some "give" as an additional test, just as you do an avocado. Squeezing is not as effective a barometer for freshness with pineapple. For pineapple, just gently pull a leaf from the crown of the pineapple; if it comes out easily, it's ripe.

    I've found that there is a "trick" for assessing quality for every fruit and vegetable. But far and away the best way I've discovered for discerning which produce to choose is to cultivate a trusting relationship with your store's produce manager or local farm-stand owner and staff. Then ask them what's fresh, what's in season, and what selections they recommend.

- **Fruits are most "alive" and full of nutrients when they are allowed to ripen on the tree or vine.** And you want to eat ripened fruit because the body can't break down the starches and sugars that are in unripe fruit. Tomatoes and bananas are two examples of produce that is often picked before it is ripe. On large corporate farms, produce is commonly picked by machine, and it is much easier to pick hard, unripe tomatoes, for example, without bruising them than it is to pick tender, juicy ripe ones. Note that tomatoes can be stored for long periods of time when refrigerated well. And if they are not organically grown, they are often treated, and even gassed and colored to give them an appealing color and texture.

- **Eating a lot of leafy greens in addition to citrus fruits is very beneficial to the body.** The citrus helps to draw the calcium out of the greens.

- **If you eat bread at all, try eating sprouted, yeast-free whole grain breads.** They are available now even in most supermarkets, in the health food freezer section. *Essene Bread* is a very good brand. All other bread should be cooked or toasted until dry. Dry breads sweep out the system, as opposed to mushy or doughy breads, which only clog it up. Whole grain and sprouted grain breads are best. See Chapter 32, "The Ying/Yang Energies of Food," to read more about grains and Macrobiotics.

- **Soak nuts and seeds in water before eating them. Nuts and seeds naturally contain enzyme inhibitors.** By soaking them, you not only release these toxic enzyme inhibitors, but also increase the life and vitality contained within the nuts and seeds! The purpose of these enzyme inhibitors is to protect the nut and/or seed until it has what it needs for growing (i.e. sunlight, water, soil, etc.). Since the soak water will contain the enzyme inhibitors, and is very acidic to the body, be sure to rinse your nuts and seeds well after soaking.

"And God said: Behold, I have given you every herb bearing seed which is upon the face of the earth, and every tree, in which is the fruit of a tree yielding seed, to be your food."

~ Genesis 1:29

HOW TO SOAK NUTS AND SEEDS

Soak the nuts and seeds in mason jars, and then drain and rinse them after 12 hours. If you don't eat them immediately, store them in the refrigerator without a lid so that air can get to them. They will stay fresh for a few days this way, but it is vitally important to rinse them at least once (preferably twice) a day with fresh water, draining the water each time. Why? Well, as with any live food, mold tends to set in within days if you're not careful.

You can also soak a couple of pounds of nuts at a time (raw almonds, walnuts, pecans, sunflower seeds, pumpkin seeds, etc.) if you dehydrate them afterwards. To do this, soak them overnight in glass jars or large bowls (or for a minimum of 12 hours), then rinse them well in the morning. Set your dehydrator at 118 F or below—dehydrating foods at such low temperatures keeps the enzymes in the food alive. Eighteen to 24 hours later, they'll be ready. Check the nuts near the end to be sure that they are dry and crunchy. When they're ready, you can store the dried nuts and seeds in jars with lids (you could also use plastic bags or containers) in the refrigerator or cupboard, and they are ready to use in any recipe!

A RAW TRUTH ABOUT DEAD FOODS

Technologies used to process food not only reduce its nutritive value, but also its flavor. Hence, the need for the flavor industry. This is the business of making food taste good. Is it any surprise that dead foods are flavored chemically? These products can offer nearly a blank palate to which the chemicals necessary to give them a specific taste are added. Yummy.

In his book, *Fast Food Nation*, Eric Schlosser warns the consumer to be wary when seeing the phrases "natural flavor" or "artificial flavor" included in the list of ingredients on the back of a package. Know that these short and sweet, yet peculiarly mysterious phrases often stand for a long litany of human-made chemical additives. The term "natural flavors" can be especially confusing, as most natural and artificial flavors contain the exact same chemicals. The only difference between them is that natural flavors are obtained through the use of a natural distillation process rather than by chemical extraction. This does not make them any more healthy or "natural." The term "spices" on some ingredient lists can also be misleading—sometimes they masquerade for chemical compounds and additives.

MAKING A STATEMENT

By choosing healthier foods, we can make a statement to those who are now capitalizing on the unconscious consumer. We hit food companies in their pocketbooks, the place they look to measure their success, every time we choose simpler, raw fare. We can all make more enlightened food choices, allowing producers to see our preferences.

It might appear from the above that choosing food is similar to negotiating a minefield on a pogostick. Relax! Knowing what is available in the marketplace is just an important prerequisite to making good choices—choices that you only have to answer to yourself for making, no one else. With availability and quality of whole foods improving all the time, everyone has the opportunity to take advantage of the many benefits they have to offer. Have fun. Experiment. And enjoy!

SOMETHING TO CHEW ON

Just as we have subtle energy inside of us, so does every other living thing. This energy is called "chi" in Chinese medicine, "prana," "tapasya" or "hara" in the Vedic and Hindu traditions, "ki" in Japan, and a variety of names in other traditions. Our Soul's fire, the Light within us, is a pilot light if you will. It is from this place that the body's subtle energy flows. This fire is what ultimately keeps us connected with our Soul, and other living organisms. When we eat live foods, we can actually assimilate and combine that food's subtle energy with our own.

I've personally found that the raw food diet coaxes your inner fire to ignite and actually fans this flame which exists within us. "The fire" and living Light of an uncooked food has not been extinguished. The food is very much still animated with sunlight and filled with living water. Think of how enlivening it is to consume that energy while still in its un-tampered-with state. Direct from the Sun, from the Light of God, to you!

We can lighten up all other areas of our lives—on emotional, mental and Spiritual levels—but if we forget about fueling the Light in our body, we've left out a very tangible part of the picture of who we are. Our fire needs kindling on the physical plane as well as on the more subtle, ethereal planes of existence. Eating raw, whole foods is a way of providing that kindling.

In his book, The Sunfood Diet Success System, raw food enthusiast David Wolfe writes, "Cooked food is addictive (there really is no softer way to phrase it)." He goes on to say that an addiction is a desire for a substance that has no connection to the true needs of the body, noting that certain cooked food behaviors have all the marks of a physio-chemical addiction. Although many people eat their favorite foods for flavor or fun, he notes that in his experience most people are usually addicted to and have trouble releasing five or six cooked foods, including bread, baked potatoes, coffee, potato chips, corn chips, tofu, candy (cooked chocolate), cigarettes (although not a true food), and/or fish.

Think about the food you eat most often and why you are eating it—could you be addicted to certain tastes and textures? Then think about how much of the food you eat that is alive. Could you benefit from more raw food in your daily menu? Can you see how adding more raw food to your diet might affect your typical preferences and alleviate some cravings? This week add at least one raw food item to every meal and have your in-between-meal snacks be some kind of raw food treat. Some of the books listed at the end of Chapter 27, "The Raw Food Diet," can help you get started.

CHAPTER FOURTEEN

The Importance of Enzymes

"When enzymes are in ample supply, their work keeps your body running at an optimal level."

~ Patricia Fitzgerald, author of *The Detox Solution*

LET'S TAKE A MORE IN-DEPTH LOOK at the enzymes we spoke about as being so vital to life in the previous chapter. As we now know, the nutrients in food are not the only aspect of it that vitalizes our bodies. In addition, we get sustenance from the subtle energy in the food. This fine, vital energy is carried by enzymes.

Enzymes, which are found in every cell of the body and in all living things, can be viewed as little energy-releasing life packets or fire-stokers that animate and free the life-force in an organism. As all body processes depend upon and are sustained by enzymes, it can be said that all life does as well.

The word "enzyme" comes from the Greek word "enzymas," which means "to cause change" or "to ferment." In a more physical sense, when enzymes act upon matter, they stimulate chemical-changes causing a tangible release of heat and energy. Enzymes are the substances that ripen fruit, and make milk sour. During digestion, the natural enzymes in food and your body's enzymes work together to process what you eat.

Because enzymes are the force of life and are needed for every biological and chemical action of the body, we literally can't do anything—read, drink, laugh or breathe—without them.

Raw and whole foods contain all of their natural enzymes. Enzymes, like all other living things, begin to die at temperatures beyond 118 degrees F. That is why raw foods are viewed as more beneficial to the body than cooked foods.

BENEFITS TO THE BODY

Enzyme-rich meals add life to our bodies. They make us feel lighter and more energetic. They make it easier for us to maintain our ideal weight. You'll look and feel more vibrant if you eat a diet rich in enzymes. And there's one added benefit that I find distinctively different from any of the diets that are built on restricting the quantity you eat instead of focusing on the quality of your food; due to the large amount of fiber you consume when eating raw foods, your eliminative processes improve. For instance, digestion is smoother, faster, and more efficient.

When your enzyme supply is low, you can feel sick, lethargic, achy and dull. Conversely, as you build up the enzyme level in your body, you may notice that you become free of some aches and pains that you were beginning to accept as "part of life." You will begin to crave activity, as the added life force courses through your being.

When you eat foods that still contain their natural enzymes, the digestion process gives energy to your body rather than sapping it. This way of eating also reinforces the body's immune system and healing processes.

"Enzymes are substances that make life possible. They are needed for every chemical reaction that takes place in the human body. No mineral, vitamin or hormone can do any work without enzymes. Our bodies, all our organs, tissues and cells are run by metabolic enzymes."

~ Edward Howell, author of *Enzyme Nutrition*

THE THREE TYPES OF ENZYMES

There are three classes of enzymes—metabolic, digestive and food.

- **Metabolic enzymes** are an essential part of every biological activity and are found in every cell, organ and tissue of the body.

- **Digestive enzymes** are found in and produced by the alimentary organs (the gastrointestinal tract). They are *amylase*—the enzyme responsible for digesting carbohydrates, *lipase*—which digests fat, and *protease*—the enzyme that digests proteins.

- **Food enzymes** are found in all raw, whole food, where they are available in proper proportions to help digest the food (or to help the food to ripen, or decompose it if not eaten).

INCREASING YOUR ENZYME SUPPLY

The three main ways to maintain and increase enzyme energy in the body are: (1) eating a raw food diet—which supplies us with the unadulterated, natural enzymes inherent in each food, (2) taking enzyme supplements—which complements the body's natural ability to produce enzymes, and (3) juice fasting—which not only allows you to benefit from drinking the most easily assimilated fruit and vegetable enzymes, but also stimulates the body's natural ability to produce enzymes by ridding it of excess waste.

If you are ill, or just not feeling up to par, taking enzymes is a must. Even if your diet is ideal, unless you live in an entirely pollution-free, stress-free environment, and eat an almost all-raw organic vegetarian diet, you can still benefit from taking a good plant-based digestive enzyme supplement with any cooked food.

Be sure that the quality of the enzyme you take is good. Enzymes are frequently prepared on beds of yeast, and it is very important that purification and testing are done during manufacture to insure that no organisms, spores or other by-products remain in the final product. I personally have found a great difference between enzyme brands. The pure brand I take now gives me so much energy I can only take it in the morning or I will not be able to sleep at night! (For those readers who are interested, they are available on my website at *www.experienceaxiom.com* or at *www.Soul-Fulleating.com.*)

Specifically, digestive enzyme supplements may help to:

- **Reverse the digestive upsets that can occur with normal aging**. Supplemental enzymes help to restore good digestion by replenishing these dwindling supplies.

- **Treat heartburn, irritable bowel syndrome, flatulence and other digestive complaints**. Nearly all types of digestive problems can benefit from enzyme therapy because enzymes are an essential part of the digesting process.

- **Control the ruddiness of rosacea**. Taking a small amount of digestive enzyme supplements with meals may improve this chronic skin complaint.

- **Provide nutritional support for cancer patients**. Enzymes have been used in Europe in cancer treatment for many years. Although U.S. studies are still underway, some practitioners prescribe high-dose enzyme therapy as adjunctive (supportive) treatment for cancers of the pancreas, colon, lung and other organs. Enzymes are also given to soothe side effects from harsh chemotherapy and radiation regimens.

- **Ease symptoms of candida overgrowth syndrome**. This controversial illness, featuring runaway growth of Candida yeast in the intestines, can cause diarrhea, gas, bloating, joint aches, and many other discomforts. Plant-based digestive enzymes can help to restore good digestion, in combination with beneficial bacteria supplements (probiotics) including acidophilus. One good brand of probiotics is Jarrow-Dophilus EPS. (It does not need to be refrigerated, so it travels well.)

PURCHASING TIPS

When buying a digestive enzyme product, look for one that mixes several enzymes (enzymes all end in the letters "ase"). The highest quality products contain amylase (for starches), lipase (for fats), protease (for protein), and lactase (for dairy). Bromelain (from pineapples) and papain (from papayas) are two plant-based digestive enzymes frequently found in enzyme mixtures as well. If you know you have a particular problem with a certain food (say dairy), look for that specific enzyme (lactase helps digest dairy products).

GUIDELINES FOR USE

For digestion-related complaints, like gas or bloating, take an enzyme product at the start of a meal. For non-digestive complaints, such as skin inflammation, doctors typically recommend taking digestive enzyme supplements on an empty stomach to enhance absorption. If you don't like swallowing pills, buy a powder, or sprinkle the contents of a capsule over your food. Probiotics are often taken in combination with supplemental enzymes to help bring the body back into balance.

"A good way of boosting your enzyme potential is to eat foods raw, because in this state they contain significant amounts of enzymes."

~ Patrick Holford, founder of the Institute for Optimum Nutrition

Wait a couple of hours after taking digestive enzymes before taking an antacid, since acid neutralizers (such as TUMS or Mylanta) may interfere with the activity of certain enzyme supplements. Also, if you're on anticoagulants or other blood-thinning medications, consult with a health-care professional about taking enzymes. Some enzymes, such as bromelain, can thin the blood further and possibly cause complications.

Whatever digestion is accomplished by the food enzymes contained in raw food, enzyme supplements, or fresh juices does not have to be done by the digestive enzymes of the body. This results in an overall energy boost and the conservation of your enzyme potential which allows your body to produce more metabolic enzymes for other uses by your organs and tissues. This savings alleviates a lot of stress on your system.

Dr. Edward Howell, who has written books on enzymes, notes that humans are given a limited supply of enzyme energy at birth, and that it is up to us to replenish our supply of enzymes to ensure that their vital jobs get done. If we don't replenish our supply, we run the risk of ill health. The capability to manufacture enzymes is different for each individual, but dwindles with age for everyone. So you can see how important it is to conserve and, wherever possible, boost our body's enzyme supply.

SOMETHING TO CHEW ON

It's key is to keep in mind that food enzymes are destroyed at temperatures above 118 degrees F. Freezing and refrigeration also hinder enzymatic activity. Freezing food destroys at least 30% of its enzymes and up to 66% if frozen for an extended period of time. This means that cooked and processed foods contain few, if any, enzymes. When we eat that type of diet, we could well be eating for a shorter and less-than-healthy-life. This points back to the importance of eating lots of raw fruits and vegetables because they are "live foods"; that is, foods in which the enzymes are active. This was discussed thoroughly in the last chapter.

For now, remember that the more enzymes you get, the healthier you will be. And the more raw foods you eat, the more enzymes you get. If you eat primarily cooked foods, consider taking enzyme supplements.

SOUL-FULL EXERCISE #14

For one day, while eating what you'd normally eat, see how much of the food you choose that has been heated above 118 degrees F or was frozen. This should give you a good idea of the percentage of the food you eat that contains active enzymes.

RESOURCES

Enzyme Nutrition by Edward Howell

*Enzyme and Enzyme Therapy: How to Jump-Start Your Way to Lifelong
　　Good Health* by Anthony J. Cichoke

*The Enzyme Cure: How Enzymes Can Help You Relieve 36 Health Problems
　　by Lita Lee*

Food Enzymes for Health and Longevity by Edward Howell

CHAPTER FIFTEEN

The Question of Genetically Engineered Foods

"It presents the largest ethical problem that science has ever had to face."
~ Dr. George Weed, Nobel Laureate

THINK YOU'RE NOT EATING genetically engineered food? Think again. If you live in the US, Canada and Argentina—the countries that account for 96% of the world's genetically engineered food—chances are quite likely that you are the unwitting consumer of GEs.

Genes are the building blocks of life; they give specific characteristics to living things. They make a potato a potato and a human-being a human-being. Genetic engineering is the science of cutting, splicing and transferring genes between unrelated living things to produce combinations that would never occur naturally. I find it astounding to realize that scientists can actually change the genetics of living things.

I feel that at our best, we are co-creators with the Divine, always serving the greater cause with utmost humility. Today, however, humility and reverence seem absent in some of the uses and advancements in genetic engineering technology. Chicken genes have been used in growing potatoes, tobacco genes are

"What the public fears is not the experimental science, but the fundamentally irrational decision to let it out of the laboratory into the real world before we fully understand it."

~ Barry Commoner, renown cellular biologist

used in vegetables such as cucumbers and lettuce, and viruses are regularly used in a variety of foods. Why are these genes being used so casually? The governments and food industries of Europe and Japan frequently reject our genetically engineered exports unless they are separated and clearly labeled. And yet, these foods have been approved by the FDA and by our own industry-financed government, even though sufficient scientific testing for unwanted side effects have yet to be completed.

There has actually been an ongoing trade dispute in the World Trade Organization involving GMOs (Genetically Modified Organisims) for the last few years. Free Trade agreements between the US and Europe state that companies from those countries can import and export anything they want, with no restrictions made by the governments. But many European countries have put bans on unlabeled GMO products. The US says that such a restriction is a violation of the trade agreement. The European countries say that imported products should have to live up to the same standards and integrity as domestic ones.

Interestingly, genetic engineering technology was actually first developed by European companies. However, by the mid-90s, European activist groups and consumers were speaking out about it. In contrast, 20% of US farmland had already been planted with genetically modified seeds by 1997, with hardly any knowledge about it by consumers, and no major reporting by the news media. Today, in the US, genetically engineered foods are sold in supermarkets nationwide, *unlabeled and unmarked*. An exception can be genetically modified fresh produce. (More on this later in the chapter.)

A MULTI-PRONGED CONTROVERSY

Scientists and farmers across the country are sounding off against genetically engineered foods. These scientists are stressing the fact that this new technology has been put to use too early, without adequate knowledge and testing. Gary Kaplan, MD, PhD, Associate Professor, New York University School of Medicine, points out that "the technology itself is imprecise, uncontrolled and random—it's like performing heart surgery with a shovel." Dr. George Wald, Nobel Laureate in 1967 and a former Higgins Professor of Biology at Harvard University, has commented: "It presents the largest ethical problem that science has ever had to face… Restructuring nature was not part of the bargain."

History is full of scientific inventions that were marketed prematurely, leading to disastrous, unforeseen side effects on both the environment and the human race. For instance, only half a century ago, the pesticide DDT was widely acclaimed by both the government and scientists as a benefactor to humanity. Nuclear power was once praised as the cleanest energy source on earth and advancement pushed it ahead of other possibly more viable and "earth friendly" sources of power.

Biotech companies and their PR firms have constantly exalted genetically engineered foods as the solution to world hunger. Yet many opponents say it's a myth that we need genetically engineered food and state that there is more than enough food on the planet.

Actually the problem is not that we don't have enough food, it is that we have a hard time getting the food to the people who need it. (For more information on world hunger, see Chapter 9, "Recognize Your Blessings.") According to Peter Rosset, Director of the Food First's Institute for Food and Development Policy, "Studies continue to demonstrate the success of small farmers using simple farming techniques like crop rotation and integrated pest-management. These solutions may not be high tech, but they are highly productive. They don't make big companies rich, but they make family farmers self-sufficient, ensure soil protection and conservation, and enhance agrobiodiversity—which results in high-quality natural food, and reduces poverty by increasing food access, reducing malnutrition, and improving the livelihoods of the poor."

Despite this, the biotech industry has been pushing its lab-created processes and products on third-world countries, now that most developed nations have rejected them. In 1998, 24 African delegates made a statement to the Food and Agriculture Organization of the UN saying, "We do not believe that such companies or gene technologies will help our farmers produce the food that is needed in the twenty-first century. On the contrary, we think it will destroy the diversity, the local knowledge, and the sustainable agricultural systems that our farmers have developed for millennia and that it will thus undermine our capacity to feed ourselves." The widespread use of patented seeds in developing countries bars farmers from using traditional growing practices, instead forcing them to buy new seeds from bio-tech corporations each year.

Indeed, a major aspect the ethical dilemma surrounding GMOs centers on *the patenting of living things*! In 1970, the Plant Variety Protection Act allowed individuals and companies to patent the seeds of plant varieties they had developed in the lab. Today, just five companies sell all genetically modified seeds worldwide. Under patent laws, a farmer cannot reuse or save seeds without the patented company's permission. Many genetically modified seeds are designed to be fertile for only one growing season, forcing farmers to buy a new batch of seeds each year. Monsanto, a company whose seeds account for more than 90% of all acreage planted with GMOs worldwide, has sued hundreds of farmers for patent infringements.

ETHICS OF THE MATRIX CHANGES

Noting that humankind has a propensity to push the limits of its boundaries, we might consider whether we are going too far, too fast, in this area. Is it ethical for us to produce genetically engineered foods to the extent that we have, simply in the name of increased profit and consumer convenience? Humans are taking the responsibility upon themselves to *redesign nature*, manipulating the genes of species that have required millions of years of evolution to achieve their present adaptations. In the words of Dr. Joseph Moorman, "Food is part of a matrix in which everything has a purpose. Everything has a role. What will happen to that matrix if we put fish genes in tomatoes? We don't know."

In this day and age when our power to change and control our environment supersedes anything previously experienced, it is important that our consciousness keeps pace with our power. It is not just for a select few to change the biology of our entire world overnight, without the knowledge, or consent, of the other five billion people on the planet.

The fact is that both sides of the GMO debate have their arguments, and as of yet nothing has been proven. But it is also important to realize that the people who control the food and agriculture industries in America are all coming very much from the same world, with similar perceptions and points of view. Executives of bio-tech and food corporations and the government officials charged with regulating them often work closely, therefore sharing the same opinions regarding the GMO debate. For example, Michael Taylor, who supervised matters relating to GMOs for the Food and Drug Administration, had previously been a partner in the law firm that represented Monsanto in their dealings with the US government. (The source for this information is a book called *Hope's Edge* by Frances Moore Lappe, one of the co-founders of Food First.) It is up to you, the consumer, to make informed decisions on GMOs, without relying on government regulations or FDA standards.

According to Mothers For Natural Law, a group that closely monitors GMOs, if you really want to avoid the influence of genetic engineering, buy fresh organic produce. If you want to buy processed foods and avoid genetically engineered ingredients, you will have to read product labels. If the label mentions any of the ingredients listed below without explicitly qualifying it as organic, then the product is likely to contain genetically engineered ingredients.

The most common genetically engineered foods in the world presently are:

- **Soy** and its derivatives, including **soy flour** and **soy oil** (sometimes sold as oil for cooking without specification of its source). Soy is very common in processed foods, bakery goods, meat products and pet food. It is also common in infant food.

  Soy is also used as animal feed. If feed contains a harmful substance, it may appear in considerably higher concentrations in the meat than in the feed.

"We've developed technology faster than we have developed the safeguards to protect our common assets— air, water, soil and more—from technologies unintended consequences."

~ Anna Lappe and Bryant Terry, authors of *Grub*

- **Animal Products**. Because animal feed often contains genetically engineered organisms, most animal products or by-products may be affected.

- **Dairy Products**. If the cows are not being fed organic grains, chances are very good that they will be eating genetically engineered animal-feed.

- **Corn** is also a common GE food. You can expect to find GE corn in, for example, corn flakes and other common corn foods. Corn is also used widely as animal feed.

- **Cotton** oil and fabric. Products that may contain GE cotton or its derivatives are clothes, linens, chips, peanut butter, crackers and cookies.

- **Canola** (rapeseed) used most commonly as oil for cooking and in margarines and "lean" butter substitutes. (Which is why I recommend canola oil made strictly from organic rapeseed in Chapter 20, "Here's the Skinny on Fats and Oils.")

- **Papaya**, if not organic, is very likely to be genetically engineered.

In addition, the following GE vegetables, crops and plants have been approved by the FDA for commercial use:

- Tomato
- Potato
- Rice
- Cantaloupe
- Sugar beet
- Radicchio
- Flax (linseed)
- Squash

Applications to the FDA for marketing GEs are rapidly increasing and the number of genetically engineered foods that are now being submitted to governmental agencies is on the rise. However, recently Monsanto's application for genetically engineered wheat was denied—a major coup for GE opponents.

SOMETHING TO CHEW ON

At your local supermarket, every piece of fruit and all of the vegetables should be tagged with little stickers—that's the PLU code. Knowing how to read the digits on these PLU codes is helpful. For example, all produce with codes beginning with the number 9 is organic—that means they have never been touched or tainted by genetic engineering. All codes that begin with the number 8, however, are genetically modified.

SOUL-FULL EXERCISE #15

Do a search on the Internet. Look up "PLU codes." Find out everything you need to know to shop your produce section wisely. And while you're at it, why not look up "genetic engineering" as well. With the insidious way that GMOs are being introduced into our food supply, it's important that you be well informed.

RESOURCES

The best book I've found on genetic engineering is:

Against the Grain: Biotechnology and the Corporate Take Over of Your Food
    by Marc Lappe and Britt Bailey

To be certain that you are not purchasing from companies that support GMOs, you can look at the list of companies that belong to the *Alliance for Better Foods in the USA*. This Alliance is known to be "a heavy propaganda-machine" for GE foods. GMO opponents say its information is unscientific, flawed and seriously misleading. The Alliance maintains that GE foods are as safe as non-GE foods, which cannot be proven since we don't have the scientific research available yet.
    www.betterfoods.org

To see a full list of genetically engineered vegetables, crops and plants that have been approved for commercial use in the US according to the Food and Drug Administration, see the *"Completed Consultations on Bioengineered Foods"* list on the FDA website:
    www.cfsan.fda.gov/~lrd/biocon.html

Greenpeace has the most extensive list for genetically engineered foods worldwide on their website. They also have lists that inform about "GE free alternatives"—non-genetically engineered foods. In addition, you can also get active by signing petitions, taking online action, and joining their network at:
    www.truefoodnow.org

Mothers for Natural Law has very extensive lists of genetically engineered foods as well as a listing of companies that support the use of genetic engineering. They also have a very expansive and user-friendly list of genetically free brand names. Check them out.
    www.safe-food.org

You can voice your opinion about genetic engineering on the Citizens for Health website:

www.citizens.org

Green People is the world's largest directory of eco-friendly and holistic health products that I've seen. There you can find sources for non-genetically engineered items.

www.greenpeople.org

Physicians and Scientists for Responsible Application of Science and Technology has a very interesting website that addresses genetic engineering. Check it out at:

www.psrast.org

CHAPTER SIXTEEN

The Truth About Protein

"Given today's typical diet, people should be concerned about eating too much protein rather than not enough."

AS A MOSTLY RAW FOOD VEGAN, my opinions about protein consumption may be a bit biased. I don't eat the traditional meat-based sources of protein and I find that my health is superb. Personally I don't understand all of the excitement about insuring that we are getting enough protein. I think it's easy, and I hope you will too—no matter what source you decide to get your protein from after reading this chapter and the next one. Again, the main thing I am advocating is that you eat consciously—that you not take any nutritional information as law until you've thoroughly explored its validity for you.

As I researched this chapter, I found that information regarding protein consumption can be conflicting. However, I will impart it as objectively as I can. If you find yourself wanting to know more about healthier meat sources of protein as you read Chapter 16, move on to Chapter 17. However, my suggestion is that you read this chapter with an open mind.

THE PROTEIN REQUIREMENT DEBATE

"It is now known that any normal selection of plant foods provides more than enough protein."

~ Neal Barnard, M.D., President of the Physicians Committee for Responsible Medicine

One of the greatest controversies about diet and eating involves proteins—how much is enough? Well, the average American lives on a meat and potatoes diet, consuming over 100 grams of protein a day. This is at least double what many nutrition experts now say is necessary. In their book *The Nutrition Desk Reference*, Robert Garrison and Elizabeth Somer state, "Americans eat far more meat than their bodies require. This excessive protein consumption taxes the kidneys and can contribute to degenerative diseases and obesity." Some experts say that our daily need of protein can be as little as 20 grams. Yet the World Health Organization recommends an intake of .75 grams of protein for each kg of body weight, or more depending on the age, energy needs, and stress of a person's lifestyle. The US government mandated Recommended Dietary Allowance (RDA) is similar at .8 grams per kilogram or .36 by your weight in pounds. According to this model, for a person weighing 130 pounds, the recommended protein intake would be around 46-50 grams each day. The average American easily meets and more often greatly exceeds this requirement each day.

Here's a chart that lists the amount of protein in some popular foods. It will help you discern how much you need to eat to get the amount of protein you require each day.

APPROXIMATE PROTEIN IN SELECTED FOODS

Foods	Protein Content
Beef	7 grams per ounce
Poultry	7 grams per ounce
Fish	7 grams per ounce
Large egg	7 grams per 1 egg
Milk	8 grams per cup
Cheese (i.e., Cheddar)	7 grams per ounce
Bread	4 grams per 1 slice
Cereal	4 grams per 1/2 cup
Vegetables	2 grams per 1/2 cup
Soybeans (dry)	10 grams per ounce
Peanuts	7 grams per ounce
Lentils (dry)	6.5 grams per ounce
Red beans	6 grams per ounce
Baked potato	9 grams per ounce
Cashews	5 grams per ounce

Note that there are some conditions in which you may need more protein, but not much more—for instance, during pregnancy and lactation, intense athletic or strength training, and if you are a growing child, adolescent or an elderly adult. In these cases, multiply .8 gram by your body weight in pounds—but don't overdo it. Because, remember, as stated earlier, your body cannot use excess protein and over consumption can tax your kidneys and liver—the organs which help you rid your body of wastes. A single serving of meat based protein need only be 3 ounces, about the size of a deck of cards. This is because there is protein in many other foods that you eat.

SURPRISING THINGS ABOUT PROTEIN

Many of us know that protein *is* essential to our bodies, but what many people don't realize is that too much protein can also be hazardous to our health. And what may be even more surprising to some is that you can get fat eating a high-protein diet if you stay with it too long for weight loss. That's because excess protein intake increases the body's use of amino acids as an energy source, thus decreasing the body's need to break down fat for energy. So the body's fat content can increase.

Something else which may come as a surprise to you is that meat, dairy and eggs are not essential as protein sources. That may be difficult for many Americans to believe. It's estimated that the typical American gets a whopping 72% of protein from animal products and only a meager 29% from plant foods. Interestingly, the idea that meat is an all-important addition to the human diet is based upon a now discredited experiment that was conducted on rats in 1914. Two researchers named Mendel and Osborn found that rats grew faster on animal protein than plant protein. However, since then researchers have realized that the nutritional needs for humans are very different from those of rats. Illustrative of this is the fact that the breast milk of rats contains 49% protein, while that of humans only contains only 1.4%.

To think this through further, consider the silver-back gorilla, which is one of humankind's closest relatives in the animal kingdom, much closer than rats. Their digestive systems closely resemble ours. In the wild, these gorillas thrive primarily on a herbivore diet consisting of bamboo leaves and fruit, and their diets average between .2 to 2.2% protein—about the same amount of protein found in human breast-milk. Are silver-back gorillas weak because of this "lack" of protein in their diet? No, far from it; in general the gorilla is the strongest animal on earth for its size, having 10 times the strength of human beings. In fact, most herbivores in the animal kingdom—such as cattle, oxen, horses and elephants—have been known for their strength and endurance. What carnivore has had the strength and endurance to be used as a beast of burden?

Given today's typical diet, people should be more concerned about physical problems related to consuming *too much animal protein* rather than not enough.

Additionally, in population studies and animal studies comparing meat-eaters to vegetarians, there is evidence that it is not just a matter of protein quantity which is important but the food source of the protein as well. Excess animal protein has been found to promote the growth of cancer cells, and it is known to cause liver and kidney disorders, digestive problems, gout and arthritis, osteoporosis and other mineral imbalances. Populations that live on high-protein diets have higher cancer rates and lower life expectancies than those existing on a low-protein vegetarian diet.

RETHINKING YOUR PROTEIN SOURCES

Contrary to widespread belief, a vegetarian diet can more than meet our daily protein requirements. The tide has turned and now national health organizations recommend that protein intake should be somewhere between 2 1/2 to 8% of our daily caloric intake. Even a strict vegan diet of fruits and vegetables can easily meet this. The percentage of calories provided by protein in spinach is 49% of its total calories, broccoli 45%, lettuce 34%, potatoes 11%, green beans 26%, strawberry, watermelon and peach 8%, pear and banana 5%. Therefore we can satisfy our protein needs without food combining or added protein supplements.

Our bodies derive eight of their essential amino acids from the foods that we eat, and every one of these amino acids can be found in fruits and vegetables. Carrots, brussel sprouts, cabbage, eggplant, corn, cucumbers, potatoes, peas, tomatoes and bananas all contain these needed amino acids. In his book *Are You Confused?* Paavo Airola states, "It is virtually impossible not to get enough protein, provided you have enough to eat of natural, unrefined foods."

The best and cleanest sources of protein are seeds—such as poppy, sunflower, sesame, hemp and flax—as well as green vegetables and superfoods. **Superfoods** are aptly named since they are plant foods with extraordinary properties. They contain a wide array of nutrients (some found nowhere else on earth), high levels of minerals, and usually all of the essential amino acids.

"Protein is necessary for the structure of almost every molecule of the body."

~Michael Murray ND, author of *The Encyclopedia of Healing Foods*

Some of my favorite superfoods are:

- **Spirulina:** A spiral algae, it contains the highest concentration of protein on earth. Spirulina has been consumed for thousands of years by indigenous people in Africa.

- **Blue-green Algae:** Considered by some to be the perfect food for humans, blue-green algae is an excellent source of chlorophyll, trace minerals and amino acids. It is high in Beta-carotene and other carotenoids, making it an excellent source of vitamin A. It benefits immune system function, heart and circulation, digestion, and helps to increase memory.

- **Chlorella:** A high-protein algae.

- **Wild Coconuts:** For those lucky enough to have access to tropical abundance, wild coconuts are one of the most astounding foods on earth. I often drink a smoothie of the flesh and water combined. They are electrolyte and mineral-rich. Truly a delicious superfood!

- **Hemp Seed:** Hemp seed contains a unique and wide-array of minerals. It is perhaps the most bio-available source of protein (edestin) as well as rejuvenating sulfur-bearing amino acids.

- **Bee Pollen:** Considered by many to be nature's most complete food, bee pollen is best from the wild and not from cultivated sources.

- **Maca:** Although it's still mostly undiscovered by the masses and seen as somewhat on the fringe, in the high Andes where it grows, maca is well known. It is a radish-family root, not only rich in protein, but high in mineral content as well.

- **Goji Berries:** Originating from the Tibetan plateau, goji berries
  are considered to be one of the world's most nutrient-rich fruits.
  Legendary in Tibetan and Chinese medicine, the goji berry has
  been honored for its strength-building properties and and properties associated with longevity. Not only are they rich in
  anti-aging agents but in anti-oxidants, vitamins and minerals.

So you can see that there is a wide and interesting variety of plant-based
protein sources. If you do eat meat however, it is important to look at all the
factors surrounding such a lifestyle—including what types of meat you are
eating, where it comes from, how you prepare it, and what you eat to supplement it.

As I have mentioned before, and will explain in detail in following chapters,
the quality of much of the meat found in today's supermarkets is appalling.
Animals are kept in conditions that drastically lower the quality of the meat and
provide a breeding ground for many diseases. Chemical pollution to the earth's
rivers, lakes, and oceans makes eating even wild-caught fish a risk, while fisheries produce farm-raised fish that is pronounced toxic by some standards.

In addition to eating less-optimal-quality meat, many people do not
support a high-protein diet with mineral-and-vitamin rich fruits, vegetables,
and grains. Protein is important, but it is by no means the only nutrient our
body needs. Animal sources of protein do not offer the same amount and array
of minerals and vitamins that vegetable protein sources do. Because of this, a
person eating a high-protein diet can easily ignore the other aspects of nutrition
needed by their body.

Of course, it is easy for someone on a vegetarian diet to neglect certain
aspects of nutrition as well. Cutting out meat alone will do nothing to improve
health if it is not supported with a good amount of unprocessed, whole foods.
"junk food vegetarians" who replace meat with large amounts of processed
carbohydrates, sugar, and vegetable oils can equally compromise their health.

WHICH PROTEIN? YOU CHOOSE

The very reason we are so concerned with getting enough protein is that proteins contain amino acids which are used for the growth and repair of cells. There are 25 amino acids. Eight of those are "essential," meaning that your body cannot manufacture them, but they are needed by your body. Some proteins are considered complete proteins, meaning that they contain all 8 essential amino acids. Complete-protein foods include meat, fish, eggs, dairy products and a few vegetable proteins such as quinoa and avocado, as well as nuts and seeds.

Here is a quick reference list that shows some common protein sources of all 8 essential amino acids:

PROTEIN SOURCES CONTAINING
ALL 8 ESSENTIAL AMINO ACIDS

Animal	Vegetable
Meat	Quinoa
Dairy	Avocado
Eggs	Millet
Fish	Hemp
Milk	Soy

The complete proteins also include *superfoods* like spirulina, blue-green algae and chlorella.

You can be creative with certain vegetable combinations and get all eight amino acids from them as well. For instance, you could eat whole grains (brown rice, chapati, whole grain bread) and legumes (lentils, peas or beans), or whole grains and nuts (such as whole grain bread with any kind of nutbutter).

HEALTHIER MEAT CHOICES

If you do want to include meat protein in your diet, consider specific sources. Meat from animals that are raised entirely on pasture can taste noticeably different from that found packaged in plastic from an industrialized source. Meat from such animals is growing in popularity, not only as a far superior dining experience, but also a healthier choice.

You'll find such meat products at some health food stores and gourmet markets and increasingly in traditional supermarkets (especially if you ask the management to stock them!) as well as on the Internet. You'll also discover more on this in the next chapter.

IN CONCLUSION

It is wise to ensure that the proteins you ingest—like all other nutrients you consume—are in a natural, living form that can easily be assimilated in order to build healthy new living cells, and to sustain your body on that cellular level. It is to our greater benefit to focus on the quality rather than the quantity of nutrients in our foods—especially with regard to protein. In my opinion, raw fruits and vegetables are a much healthier protein source than animal products.

Note that many people find they have less of an appetite and feel more satisfied, energized, and more able to cope with stress when they eat an adequate amount of protein. So, just as with any other type of food, check in with your body and ask your own Intuition what your nutrition needs are. Chances are, if you find yourself craving meat or other high-protein foods, your body is in need of a protein boost.

No matter how it may appear in this day and age where the "super-sized" meal has become the norm, a healthy serving size is not the size of an entire platter. You may want to keep these images in mind as you eat protein.

- 1 serving size of beef, chicken and/or fish = 1 deck of cards or the size of the palm of a woman's hand

- 1 serving of meatball = a ping-pong ball

- 1 serving of cooked ground meat (i.e., a burger—a substitute could be soy) = a hockey puck

- 1 serving size of nut butter = a ping-pong ball

Take a minute to calculate your protein requirements as recommended by the US government standards. The amount you need is usually considerably less than the amount most Americans typically take in. The RDA is as follows:

Multiply .36 by your weight in pounds or .8 by your weight in kilograms. The result will equal the amount of protein you need each day as measured in grams. (See chart earlier in the chapter for the number of grams in typical foods.) You can round off your answer to an approximate amount.

For example, a woman who weighs 125 pounds would require about 45 grams of protein a day. (125 X .36 = 45 grams)

A man who weighs 62 kilograms would require about 50 grams of protein a day. (.8 X 62 = 49.6 grams)

CHAPTER SEVENTEEN

Home Free
on the Range

"The greatness of a nation and its moral progress can be measured by the way its animals are treated."
~ Mahatma Gandhi

I WAS DRIVING UP ROUTE 5 in California on my way to Mt. Shasta with a friend. I looked out at a picture perfect day, featuring a blue sky dotted with puffy white clouds, and then on the horizon I spotted something I couldn't quite make out. At the very same time, I caught whiff of a stench so putrid I had to bury my nose in my sleeve. Pointing to the blackened landscape, I cried out, "What the heck is that!?" We squinted until the thousands of specks of black came into focus and we realized that they were cows, lined up in stalls for as far as the eye could see, standing shoulder to shoulder in tight quarters, in what turned out to be their own feces. Not a spot of green grass was noticeable on the site. My friend replied, "That's a cow conglomerate—a commercialized feedlot." My jaw dropped as I stared in disbelief. The place reminded me of a concentration death camp. I said, "That's not just inhumane, it's repulsive."

That's just a small snapshot of what's happening today, in not only the cattle industry, but with poultry and hogs as well.

Like most corporate conglomerates, the meat industry is driven by profitability and efficiency, so acting with humane sensibility and conscience is not high on the list of priorities. In short—there's little love in evidence.

A CLOSER LOOK

What's natural for cows is to eat grass. They have a four-chambered stomach, which can easily convert grasses into protein. However, when they are fed the rich, starchy corn-based feedlot diet, all manner of health problems ensue—which are most often addressed with daily doses of antibiotics. This diet is also augmented with a variety of additives designed to grow an animal as quickly as possible, such as liquefied fat and protein. In addition, the animals are routinely injected with growth hormones. But that's not the worst of it—the cows barely move, let alone graze—because the only important factor to the industrialized farmer is how fast the cattle can reach a profitable weight.

As if that's not bad enough, there is an even worse-case scenario—industrialized poultry and pig farming. At least the cattle are out in the open air and sunshine. Chickens are housed in metal cages, crammed in so tightly they often peck at and kill each other. The solution—remove their beaks! Hog's tails are removed for the same reason; they're under such stress that they chew up their cage-mates. These caged animals also endure broken bones, skin problems, open sores and tumors—to name but a few of their ailments. And the industrialized slaughterhouse scenes are even worse.

You get the picture.

In a Soul-Full diet—which is based on eating what is grown with love, selected with love, prepared with love, and served with love—these methods of farming are simply not acceptable.

"It is hard to deny that animals deserve some measure of compassion, and the technology for slaughtering farm animals has grown increasingly inhumane over the past two decades."

~ Erik Marcus, author of *Vegan—The New Ethics of Eating*

A BETTER WAY

Fortunately for those who still wish to eat meat, there are some ranchers who practice a right-minded, compassionate way of raising livestock. Just as there are organic choices for produce, there are healthier and more loving choices in the meat and dairy department as well. In his book, *Fast Food Nation*, Eric Schlosser writes about his visit to the ranch of Dale Lasater in Matheson, Colorado. The cattle on the Lasater Ranch never spend any time at a feedlot, instead they graze on the open plains. Dale raises his cattle in a way that does not harm the consumer, nor the land.

This rancher has committed himself and his business to producing meat that is friendlier, healthier and safer. His cattle are raised without the use of hormones or anabolic steroids. Even the grass that they eat is natural, never having been treated with chemical fertilizers or pesticides. Compare that to the hormone and steroid-laced, synthetically based diets fed to conventionally bred livestock.

Striving to preserve a natural balance in the area, the ranch never kills coyotes or any other local predators. The philosophy of the ranch, Schlosser writes, is "Nature is as smart as hell."

Allowing animals to eat the diet that is the most intrinsically natural to them is not only most humane but also the healthiest for the consumer. When the animals peck, graze or root for their food, they are following their basic instincts, and this coupled with exposure to fresh air and sunshine promotes a stress-free existence. As a result, the necessity for damage control, such as the use of antibiotics, is lessened greatly.

When you consume these free-range and grass-fed animal products, as opposed to factory-farm-raised meats and dairy, you'll notice a conspicuous difference from its mass produced counterpart—the taste! I believe it's because the cells of the meat are not interlaced with additives and toxins. According to meat eaters I've talked with, the free-range meats are noticeably more robust.

There is no nationally enforced standard for labeling free-range and grass-fed products, so it's important to know your source. Here are some ideas for finding and selecting suppliers:

- **Buy direct**—See if you can find a farm close by, using a national directory of producers of grass-fed meats from Jo Robinson, author of *Why Grassfed Is Best!*
  www.eatwild.com

- **The Eat Well Guide**—Check out this national search engine developed by GRACE—The Global Resource Action Center for the Environment.
  www.eatwellguide.org

- **Find a butcher you trust**—They are the ones who have long-standing relationships with the food growers. They are skilled in their profession and can tell you what's fresh and exactly where the meat came from.

- **Shop in a health food supermarket**—There are meat departments in most of the larger organic markets, such as Whole Foods or Wild Oats. Don't be afraid to ask the person behind the counter about the meats they stock.

IT HELPS TO READ LABELS

Here are the USDA definitions used to describe some of the meats you may be purchasing from a larger organic market or supermarket chain:

- **Certified**—This term implies that the USDA's Food Safety and Inspection Service and the Agriculture Marketing Service have officially evaluated a meat product for class, grade and quality characteristics.

- **Organic**—As this applies to meat, the National Organic Standards require:
  - No antibiotics
  - Animal are fed only an organic diet.
  - Animals are not fed animal by-products.
  - No bio-engineering
  - No growth hormones
  - No treatment with ionizing radiation

All of these requirements must be documented by the farmer and veri-fied on site by a government certified inspector—only then does it get the USDA Certified Organic seal.

- **Kosher**—This label may only be used on meat and poultry products prepared under Rabbinical supervision. (See Chapter 28, "Kosher Eating.")

- **Fresh**—Refers to poultry whose internal temperature has not been below 26 degrees Fahrenheit.

- **Free-range or free-roaming**—Producers must demonstrate to the USDA that the poultry has been allowed access to the outside. Note: Having access does not necessarily mean that they have been outside!

- **Hormone-free**—This means raised without the use of hormones. The producer must submit documentation, but there are no tests done to verify this.

- **No antibiotics**—This label may be used if sufficient docu-mentation is supplied by the producer to the USDA, but the facilities are not inspected.

"The quality of the meat is directly influenced by the quality of the life of the animal itself."

~ Heston Blumenthal, author of *Family Food*

- **Natural**—This applies to a product that has been only minimally processed and contains no artificial ingredient or added color. It applies only to the handling of the meat after slaughter, regardless of how it was raised.

SOMETHING TO CHEW ON

Jane Goodall is the world's foremost authority on chimpanzees. In 1984, she received the J. Paul Getty Wildlife Conservation Prize for "helping millions of people understand the importance of wildlife conservation to life on this planet." Her other awards and international recognitions fill pages. Goodall's research and writings have made, and are still making, revolutionary inroads into scientific thinking regarding the evolutions of humans. Now she's written a new book titled *Harvest for Hope*; in it, she advocates the humane treatment of animals as a way of healing our planet. Goodall's text also provides further thinking on mindful eating. I highly recommend Goodall's latest book and it's available on Amazon.com.

> *"Most people are basically decent; most people do not like to think of animals suffering at our hands; most people want to do their bit to make this a better world for all—only they don't know quite what they can do. So let us join forces, let us not turn away from this torture of millions of animals. Each one of us can do our bit. We can change the way we eat. We can refuse to buy animal food produced by inhumane farming methods, thus lobbying for a change with our purse."*
> ~ Jane Goodall

SOUL-FULL EXERCISE #17

If you are a meat eater, find a source of free-range products and do a taste test using all five of your senses. While you eat the meat, realize that you are not only feeding your body, but also making a statement and taking a stand for a more conscious and sustainable world.

RESOURCES

Vegan—The New Ethics of Eating by Erik Marcus
Mad Cowboy by former cattle rancher Howard Lyman
Pasture Perfect by Jo Robinson
Fast Food Nation by Eric Schlosser

If you are a meat-eater, here are some websites where you can purchase quality free-range, organic meat.

Wholesome Harvest is a coalition of over 40 concerned small family farms. Since 2001, Wholesome Harvest has been offering premium organic certified poultry and meats to grocers, chefs and households. Their commitment to quality extends above USDA organic standards to additionally include pasture-based production methods—and no feed lots or confinement/factory farms. They carry beef, chicken, lamb, pork and turkey that you can purchase online to be shipped to your door.

   www.wholesomeharvest.com

Shelton's is a family-owned company that makes their products from all-natural free-range poultry. Their products are available nationwide in health food stores, natural foods supermarkets, and regular supermarkets with natural foods sections.

   www.sheltons.com

Go Dairy Free sells meat and fish from various sources that qualify as free range, organic, and/or free of antibiotics and hormones.

www.godairyfree.com

American Grass Fed Beef not only sells natural, dry-aged, grass fed beef and steaks, but grass fed, raw dog food as well.

www.americangrassfedbeef.com

And finally our friends at **Newman's Own**, which was founded by Paul Newman produces organic cat and dog food that can be purchased at many health food stores, such as Wild Oats and Whole Foods. To find a store near you that carries their organic pet foods, visit their website at:

www.newmansownorganics.com

If you feel the inclination to find out more or to get involved in supporting animal rights, here are some websites you may want to check out:

Meet Your Meat—Be certain you have a strong stomach to view this website. It is billed as the site the meat industry doesn't want you to see. It contains graphic footage of "life" for the animals in factory farms.

www.meat.org

PETA—People for the Ethical Treatment of Animals

www.peta.com

Vegetarian 101—Offers information on vegan and vegetarian diets and a free vegetarian starter kit.

www.goveg.com

CHAPTER EIGHTEEN

Got Organic Milk?

"Whoever is kind to the creatures of God is kind to himself."

THINK OF "THE GOOD OLE DAYS" on the farm and chances are that among the images you'd conjure up would be some of Farmer Joe in his overalls, his wooden footstool pulled up alongside Bessie, where he would be seated, happily milking away. You might also envision a warm, frothy white stream of milk hitting the side of a tin pail, eventually filling it, and cream floating to the top.

Milk is one of the world's favorite foods. But today down on the dairy farm it's not quite so warm and fuzzy. Instead, dairy is big business. In the United States alone, dairy is an 18 billion dollar industry.

Just as in years past, many people rely on milk as a source of high-quality protein. However, there's a relatively new twist to the business, now that *natural dairy* has arrived—front and center—into the mainstream. In fact, it's likely that you'll find not only several brands of certified organic milk but organic butter, yogurt, cheese products and ice cream at your local health food store and also in your neighborhood supermarket if you're lucky. Even though the cost of conventional milk products is significantly less, the demand for organics has soared over the last 10 years. Why?

Aisha Ikramuddin is with Mothers and Others for a Livable Planet, publishers of the Mother's Milk List, which keeps track of certified organic and hormone-free dairy products. She notes: "People are concerned about having hormones and antibiotics in their milk. Even though the FDA says that [conventional] milk is safe, consumers aren't so sure."

"What will it take to draw more scientific attention to pasture-based ranching? Pressure from an enlightened public."

~ Jo Robinson,
author of
Pasture Perfect

WHY ALL THE CONCERN?

Consumers are chiefly apprehensive about a genetically engineered drug called rBGH, or bovine growth hormone, which is administered to an estimated 30% of conventional dairy cows. This growth hormone has been shown to increase milk production up to 15%. And although the drug has been outlawed in Europe and Canada, it has been used in the US since 1993 when it was first approved. There is much controversy over its use and speculation that drinking milk from cows injected with rBGH can cause hormone-related cancers.

Another prominent reason for disapproval of the hormone's use is the many adverse effects it has on the cows. Increased mastitis (inflammation of the mammary gland or udder) and stress are just some of the symptoms these animals suffer as they stand side-by-side hooked up to enormous steel milking-machines, barely surviving, in often very inhumane living conditions. Reports are that one out of every four dairy cows in the state of California is a "downer." That means they fall down from exhaustion unable to support their own weight.

Even if there were no health concerns surrounding the use of rBGH, or questions about its effects on animals, it's evident that we do not need our cows to produce more milk. The US government is currently subsidizing the dairy industry by buying 2 billion dollars of milk surpluses each year!

MILK IN MODERATION

Is milk really good for the body? Perhaps, but not necessarily to the degree that we've been lead to believe through massive advertising campaigns.

Dairy Management Inc., the dairy industry's promoter, has one purpose, and that is "to increase the demand for US-produced dairy products." In 2003, they had a marketing budget of more than $165 million. This, from a Soul-Full and non-manipulative perspective, is suspiciously excessive. Their target milk consumers?—children, ages 6 to 12, and their mothers. To influence buying decisions, they market in schools to teachers, students, educators, and food-service professionals. They make the presence of dairy known not only in the lunchroom but also in the classroom.

In fact, the very reason so many people believe they can't get adequate protein or calcium without dairy is because this industry has been teaching their own version of nutrition for decades—and quite successfully.

Just in recent years, nutritional education programs such as "Pyramid Café" and "Pyramid Explorations" reached over 12 million students, teaching them that dairy products are key to their health. Meanwhile, in his book, *The China Study*, research scientist T. Collin Campbell has stated: "The dairy industry spends $4 to $5 million a year to fund research towards the goal of finding something healthy to talk about."

Actually, the fact is that many people are allergic to, or intolerant of, milk.

THE SCOOP ON MILK INTOLERANCES

While cow's milk has been a traditional food in areas with long winters, such as northern Europe, it has not been traditionally consumed at all in other areas of the world. Digesting milk requires an enzyme called *lactase*, which babies naturally have but which decreases in the child after the age of two. Milk can be tolerated by adults who are descended from areas where it was traditionally consumed, but many people of South East Asian or African descent have a low tolerance for milk products.

Milk allergy is the most common food sensitivity in the United States, followed by wheat. When someone consumes a food allergen, such as milk, it produces a powerful immune response in the stomach. As white blood cells rush to the stomach, they leave other areas of the body deficient, and infections of the tonsils, sinuses, and ears often set in. Also, many people find that dairy overstimulates mucus production in their body as well. In his book, *The Healing Power of Minerals and Trace Elements*, Paul Bergner, a naturopath and therapeutic nutritionist, writes about an encounter he had with an ear, nose and throat specialist: "[The specialist] received many referrals from general practitioners to surgically place tubes in the children's ears. He told me that he could prevent 25% of the surgeries by screening for cow's milk allergies."

Traditional peoples who consume milk make fermented milk products, such as yogurt and buttermilk, which predigests the milk proteins and makes them easier for the body to break down. In contrast, the process of pasteurization destroys the enzymes inherent in milk, making it even harder to digest than raw milk in its natural state. Individuals who are sensitive to butter can often eat ghee (clarified butter—see Chapter 20, "Here's the Skinny on Fats and Oils.")

THE UDDER TRUTH

Whole milk products and cheeses are loaded with fat and cholesterol, and they can be tainted with pesticides, antibiotics and contaminants—all of which can lead to health consequences. And although milk fat can be one of the most nutritious sources of fat available to humans, as it is rich in vitamin A and its essential fatty acid balance is ideal (about 1:1 omega-6 to omega-3 fatty acids), that's true only if it is from cows that graze on pasture. Take away one-third of the grass and replace it with grain, and the omega-3 fatty acid content of the milk goes down while the omega-6 fatty acid content goes up, upsetting an essential balance. If you replace two-thirds of the pasture with a grain-based diet, the milk will have a very top-heavy ratio of omega-6 to omega-3 fatty acids—a ratio that has been linked to a wide-range of health maladies including depression, diabetes, obesity, allergies and various cancers. Much of the milk on the supermarket shelves has an even more lopsided ratio because the cows producing it get no pasture whatsoever.

As far as milk contributing to the growth of strong bones and good teeth—ironically there is now good evidence that consuming milk actually increases the risk of osteoporosis. In his book, *Healing Foods*, Michael Murray ND says, "One of the first clues that milk consumption may not be beneficial for bone health is data showing that countries with the highest dairy intake have the highest rate of hip fracture per capita." Findings from the Nurses Health Study, a study involving 77,761 women, even showed the more milk a woman consumed, the more likely she was to have a hip fracture! (Weight bearing exercise, plus eating calcium-rich foods like spinach, kale and almonds, are actually more important factors in preventing osteoporosis.)

So you decide. And if you want to eat dairy and tolerate it well, then partake mindfully and with moderation. But whenever you can, go organic.

ORGANIC DAIRY FARMS

Fortunately, developments on the organic side of the dairy industry are encouraging. For instance, Amy Barr, spokesperson for *Horizon Organic Dairy*, the nation's leading producer of organic milk and dairy products, has remarked, "We feel that agriculture should be done in a way that does the least amount of damage to the environment as possible." She adds, "It's a mission for us. If we lose our vision of what organic is, we lose the heart of our business." Horizon's cows receive no antibiotics or hormones and survive, quite happily, on a chemical-free diet of open air, sunshine and organic feed.

Another farm that operates on a much smaller scale is the *Straus Family Creamery*, which centers on a family-owned dairy farm located just north of San Francisco. The operation makes everything in small batches, sells its milk in glass bottles, and instead of using antibiotics—as is so widely practiced in the conventional dairy world—it relies on homeopathic remedies.

These businesses, and many others like them, are illustrating that working compassionately with their animals is affording them not only

"We're being sold that our industrial approach to farming—with the latest genetically modified twist— is the avatar of progress, but sorry, folks, this might just be the grandest illusion of all."

~ Anna Lappe and Bryant Terry, authors of *Grub*

great success, but also a deeper sense of connectivity to the entire planet. They help us to see that showing respect, gratitude and love for the animals that serve us so well is not unquestionable, and that the insensitive, conglomerate approach does not have to be accepted as the only way.

Here's a list of resources to help you find out more about organic dairy and where you can find it in your area:

- **Brown Cow**—(925) 757-9209; *www.browncowfarm.com*
- **Organic Valley**—(608) 625-3025; *www.organicvalley.coop*
- **Cascadian Farms**—(800) 624-4123; *www.cascadianfarm.com*
- **Horizon Organic Dairy**—(303) 530-2711; *www.horizonorganic.com*
- **Stonyfield Farm**—(603) 437-5050; *www.stonyfield.com*
- **Straus Family Creamery**—(213) 481-0745; *www.strausmilk.com.*
- **Nature by Nature**— *www.deliciousorganics.com*

For a full list of certified-organic and rBGH-free dairy producers in the United States, contact **Mothers and Others for a Livable Planet** at (212) 242-001 or visit *www.mothers.org.*

Note: Unfortunately, the labels on milk cartons won't tell you whether the cows were fed grass or grains. Even on organic labels, there's no guarantee that the cows grazed on pasture. To my knowledge, at the present time there are only two large dairies that make a point of raising their cows on pasture: **Organic Valley** and **Nature by Nature**.

WHAT ABOUT GOAT MILK?

In the US, we most often think of goat milk as an alternative to cow's milk, but in many parts of the world the opposite is true. Worldwide, more people drink goat milk than cow's milk. Perhaps that's because goats eat less and occupy less grazing space than cows, so in some families throughout the Third World the backyard goat supplies all the milk for the family's needs. In fact, while traveling in the countryside of India, I found it was fairly common in farm villages to find a three-generation family and their goat all happily occupying a small hut home together!

Goat milk has a reputation of being a highly digestible dairy product—even more digestible than cow's milk—and less allergenic as well.

Here are the facts:

- **Vitamins and minerals—***Goat milk* contains 47% more vitamin A, 13% more calcium, 25% more vitamin B-6, 134% more potassium, 27% more selenium and three times more niacin. It is also four times higher in copper.

- *Cow's milk* contains five times as much vitamin B-12 as goat milk and 10 times as much folic acid. That's why you may see "supplemented with folic acid" on popular brand goat milk cartons.

- **Protein—**The composition and structure of the protein of goat milk is different from cow's milk. It forms a softer curd when acted upon by stomach acid, which makes it more rapidly and easily digestible. Goat milk also lacks casein, a protein found in cow's milk that may precipitate allergic reactions.

- **Fat—**Goat milk contains about 10 grams of fat per 8 oz. serving, as opposed to 8 to 9 grams of fat in whole cow's milk. But it is believed that since the fat globules in goat milk do not cluster together, they are easier to digest.

The goat milk industry in the United States is a relatively small one at the present time. However demand is increasing. Be sure of the quality of the goat milk you purchase, just as with cow's milk. Although I've found it difficult to find organic goat milk, some sources are certified free of antibiotics and bovine growth hormones (BGH).

Here are some resources for goat milk.

- *Redwood Hill Farm*—Located in Sonoma County, California, this is a small family farm that has been producing goat milk products for over 35 years. Although their products are not "certified organic," they use a natural approach to animal husbandry and state, "our dairy goats are raised 'free range' and humanely."
  www.redwoodhill.com

- *Meyenberg*—Headquartered in Santa Barbara, California, Meyenberg began operations in 1934. Their products are not "certified organic"... however, the milk produced for Meyenberg is free of antibiotics, pesticides, preservatives and bovine growth hormones.
  www.meyenberg.com

SOMETHING TO CHEW ON

Traditionally, the cow is considered to be sacred in India (bringing to mind the expression, "Holy Cow!" The ancient Vedic Spiritual texts praise milk as a miracle food, proposing that it contains all the nutrients needed for good health. The Vedic scriptures add that milk develops the fine cerebral tissues needed for understanding Krishna (God) consciousness. In the Vedic age, many yogis lived only on milk, which was so abundant that householders gave it away freely. Because milk nourishes human beings both physically and Spiritually, Vedic culture considers it the most important of all foods, essential to civilized society. So to millions of Hindus, the cow is seen as a gift of the gods to the human race. This sentiment has far deeper nuances when you realize that the cow is not just seen as a provider of life-sustaining milk, but also as the symbol of the Divine Mother. In India, the treatment of cows, the Earth and ourselves has always been connected. It's interesting to note that the Greek word *gaia* and the Sanskrit word *gau* refer both to the earth and to cows.

Is large-scale milk production really the best way to respect Mother Cow and Mother Earth?

SOUL-FULL EXERCISE #18

Rent the movie, The Corporation, to find out more about rBGH and the dairy industry. It's a real eye-opener!

If you haven't already, begin to transition to organic dairy. As you do, try doing a comparative taste test between them and the conventional dairy products you had been eating and drinking in the past.

CHAPTER NINETEEN

Eating Fish

There's a Catch

"In a handful of ocean water...a handful of God...you could not count all the ecstatic life that is dancing there. There is no loneliness to the clear-eyed mystic in this luminous, brimming playful world."
~ Hafiz, Sufi poet

LIVING ON THE OCEAN, I've experienced many moments of deep communion with this watery world that from a surface perspective often seems so devoid of life. I swim in it, become one with it, every single day, come rain or shine, when I am in Florida. At dawn, I am quite often the only one I see for miles and miles in "my" ocean.

I've been infused with the majesty of the sea, and never more than when such placid moments have been interrupted by a giant manta ray or a dolphin leaping before me from the depths and into the sun's expanding light. At these times, it seems as if a messenger has been sent from God to defy me to continue the human delusion of it being "my" ocean any longer. It's a symptom of the human condition that this "I, me, my mentality" can appear connective on the surface. But actually it's a signal of a separation from the whole, and the deep humility and connectedness that arises when all of the "I", "me" and "my" words are choked into silence, and we are transported beyond time and space into the Awwwwwwe of God.

Living as I do, it's hard for me to imagine a world without this incomparable glory. Yet the life of our seas is in jeopardy…

A CHANGING WORLD

All over the world, people are eating more seafood than ever. This is not only because the Earth's population is increasing, but also that health-conscious folks are choosing seafood as their protein source more often. Partly that's the result of a growing awareness of the benefits of omega-3 fatty acids.

If you are one of these fish eaters, you may want to know that the single most important question to ask when ordering seafood is "where did it come from?" You may think that's a crazy question—it comes from the deep blue sea, doesn't it? Maybe, maybe not. While the majority of seafood is still caught in the wild, nearly one-third comes from fish farms. This sourcing can have some adverse consequences, both ecologically and health-wise, for the consumer. Also, remember that the widespread effects of industrial pollution lingers in our waterways. Another consideration about fish consumption is the ecological impact that overfishing and trawling is having in some areas. So it's critical that you ask about the source of the fish you're considering.

FEED-LOTS OF THE SEA

Farm-raised fish are grown in net pens near the shorelines, and currently they rely on the surrounding waters to dilute waste. We're not talking about small, innocuous amounts of waste either. According to Tony Brookhart of the Seafood Alliance, "A single farm can produce as much waste as a city with 62,000 people. All of which is untreated and discharged directly into surrounding water." Additionally, the way the fish are fed reduces their food value. Farm-raised salmon, when tested, had up to ten times higher levels of PCBs and dioxins than their wild counterparts. Living in such close quarters also promotes diseases which are then treated with antibiotics, fungicides and paraciticides. The farm-raised fish are exposed to an entire array of other chemicals such as disinfectants, and even anesthetics to reduce stress. Escaping fish can transmit diseases and parasites to wild salmon too.

AVOIDING THE HEALTH RISKS

It's not only farm-raised fish that has health-researchers raising their eyebrows. Due to the widespread contamination of our oceans, fish are absorbing inordinate amounts of toxic chemicals, such as PCBs and mercury, from the water around them. Since big fish eat little fish, and thus absorb all of the chemicals the smaller fish ate, chemical levels become more concentrated as you move up the food chain.

All of this begs the question, is it possible to find fish that is relatively clean and healthy to eat without damaging the environment? Fortunately, you can. The fish that carry the highest health risks are also those that are typically over-fished and among the most endangered. These tend to be the larger, older fish at the top of the food chain like shark, swordfish and marlin. So taking them off your food list for health reasons also helps impact the environment in a positive way. Some of the best fish to keep on your list are catfish, Pacific cod, Pacific halibut, Alaskan salmon, and trout.

Another helpful approach is reading food labels. That's right—in 2004, the United States Congress passed a labeling law for seafood requiring disclosure of the food's source. Now packages must state a fish's country of origin and whether it is farm-raised or wild. So your retail market and restaurants and their suppliers should know when you ask them.

In addition, an easy-to-remember rule of thumb for choosing seafood is: Thumbs up for wild Alaskan salmon, Pacific Albacore tuna, Pacific Halibut and farm-raised mussels, clams and oysters. Thumbs down for bluefin tuna, shark, swordfish and farm-raised salmon.

Turn the page for a more detailed chart:

FISH LIST

Enjoy	Just OK	Avoid
Anchovies	Caviar (farmed)	Alaska King Crab
Bluefish	Flounder: "Summer Flounder" Fluke	Caviar (wild sturgeon)
Catfish (farmed)	Lingcod	Cod (Atlantic)
Clams (farmed)	Lobster (Atlantic)	Flounder: Yellowtail
Crab: Blue, Dungeness, Stone	Mahi Mahi or Dorado	Grouper
Crawfish	Octopus (Atlantic)	Haddock (Atlantic)
Dogfish	Prawns (US farmed or wild)	Hake
Halibut (Pacific)	Rainbow Trout (farmed)	Halibut (Atlantic)
Herring (Pacific)	Salmon (wild from WA, OR, BC Canada)	Hoki (Atlantic, New Zealand)
Mackerel: Atlantic, Spanish	Salmon (farmed from Chile or WA)	Monkfish / Goosefish
Mussels (Black, Green-lipped)	Scallops (Sea, Bay)	Orange Roughy
Octopus (Pacific)	Shrimp (domestic, trawl-caught)	Pacific Rockfish (Rock Cod)
Oysters (farmed)	Snow Crab	Pollack
Pacific Black Cod (sablefish)	Sole	Prawns (imported, tiger)
Prawns (trap-caught, Pacific)	Squid (Atlantic)	Red Snapper
Rock Lobster (Australian)	Swordfish (Pacific)	Salmon (farmed from Scotland)
Salmon (Wild Alaskan)	Tuna: Yellowfin or skipjack	Scrod
Sardines		Seabass: Chilean
Squid (Pacific)		Shark: all species
Striped Bass (farmed)		Skate
Sturgeon (farmed)		Swordfish (Atlantic)
Tilapia (farmed)		Tuna: Bluefin
Tuna: Pacific Albacore		Turbot
Uni (sea urchin)		

INFORMATION SOURCES

US National Marine Fisheries Service
UN Food and Agricultural Organization
Institute for Fisheries Resources
Citizens Guide to Seafood—Sierra Club
EPA Fish Contamination Program
Audubon's Guide to Seafood
Monterey Bay Aquarium's Seafood Watch

For a wallet copy of a similar list, visit www.mbayaq.org

More resources for obtaining pocket-sized sustainable seafood guides and detailed information about your favorite seafood choices are provided in the resources section at the end of this chapter.

When incorporating fish into your diet, eat a variety of it rather than concentrating on just one type. Also, don't necessarily go for "the whopper"—the smaller and the younger the fish, the less toxins they likely will have accumulated.

"Contaminants work their way up the food chain as tainted organisms are eaten by smaller fish who then become a food source for a list of increasing larger fish."

~ Edward R. Blonz, PhD, author of *The Really Simple, No Nonsense Nutrition Guide*

ASSESSING FRESHNESS

So many times, people ask the waiter in a restaurant or the person behind the fish counter about the fresh fish that are available. However, the question to ask is "When was it caught?" not "Is it fresh?" Technically, "fresh" refers to fish that has never been frozen or subjected to any heat treatment—not fish that was just caught yesterday.

Under proper temperature control (between 30-32 degrees), lean fish can last up to 10-12 days and oily fish about 6-8 days. So don't discount frozen fish altogether. Many modern fishing boats have state-of-the-art equipment that freezes fish right on board. So if you find out that a fish you'd like to purchase has been previously frozen, you may want to ask, "Where?" If this was aboard the ship, that's good news. If possible, find out how long ago.

When buying fish in a market, a guide to freshness will be the fish's appearance. For example, whole fish should have eyes that are convex, not sunken, and the flesh should be firm and springy when pressed. In addition, the color of the filets should be translucent and light. Clams, mussels and oysters should be alive with shells that are tightly closed.

FISH PREPARATION TIPS

If serving raw fish—such as sushi—always be certain it is fresh, from a clean source, and then prepare it consciously. After handling raw fish, wash your hands and all surfaces that came into contact with it well. Seafood poisoning is the *number one* cause of food poisoning in the United States.

When cooking seafood, always cook it well. Contaminants are mostly stored in fatty tissue, so grilling and broiling when cooking fish is recommended to allow fats and juices to drain away. Deep-frying can seal in toxins which may be stored in the fat. In general, cooking fish (as opposed to eating it raw) can reduce contaminant levels by about 30%.

Note: In doing the research for this chapter, I discovered some very good news—it turns out that those who make their living from the sea have a strong interest in conservation! So green-business partnerships related to fish are being cultivated more and more worldwide.

SOMETHING TO CHEW ON

The United States Food and Drug Administration (FDA) and the Environmental Protection Agency (EPA) have both issued warnings about mercury in some fish. They say some fish have so much mercury that eating them could be dangerous to the developing brain of a fetus as well as hazardous to our autonomic nervous systems. Therefore the FDA recommends that pregnant women, women who might become pregnant, and young children shouldn't eat fish with high levels of mercury—such as shark, swordfish, king mackerel or tilefish—at all and shouldn't have more than two meals a week of any kind of fish. According to EPA scientist, Elsie Sunderland, you'd have to drink 2,641 gallons of water to get the amount of mercury in just one 3.5 ounce piece of shark or swordfish.

SOUL-FULL EATING EXERCISE #19

When at the fish counter, choose your fish with Soul. Use all five of your senses and even your sixth sense to discern whether or not any piece of fish is healthy for you and your family. Cultivate a relationship with the person behind the counter; they should know about every catch that's delivered there. If not, find a fish counter with clerks who do know. When it comes to eating fish, having information about where it's from, where it's been, and how it was handled is important. Plus, consumer concern is the best promoter of sustainable fishing practices.

RESOURCES

Seafood Choices Alliance
Their message is "Everything we serve, everything we eat, has an impact on the environment." Stop by their site to learn more.

www.seafoodchoices.com

Blue Ocean Institute

The Blue Ocean Institute, based in Cold Spring Harbor, New York, is focused on building "a more inspired cultural atmosphere for ocean conservation through science, art, and literature." They research and evaluate fisheries to help people confidently select, enjoy and discuss sustainable, healthy seafood. You can get smart about your seafood by downloading your own *Mini-Guide to Ocean Friendly Seafood* from their site.

www.blueocean.org

Environmental Defense's Seafood Selector

This site has a "search by fish" engine, as well as a recipe of the week button, and it allows you to find out about other issues relevant to the fishing industry by reading articles such as "Health or Hazard" and "Troubled Waters."

www.oceansalive.org/eat.cfm

Audubon's Seafood Lover's Guide

The message of Audubon's Living Oceans Seafood Lover's Guide is that consumers' decisions can encourage sustainable seafood. When visiting the site, you can download seafood cards and be linked to the Audubon Society's home page.

www.seafood.audubon.org

Monterey Bay Aquarium's Seafood WATCH

Check out their "All-Fish List" and hook on to the latest scoop on over 35 fish species. This site is the home of the downloadable wallet-sized "Seafood Card," a handy reference guide that ranks fish choices.

www.mbayaq.org

Here's the Skinny on Fats and Oils

"By our most conservative estimate, replacement of partially hydrogenated fat in the US diet with natural unhydrogenated vegetable oils would prevent approximately 30,000 premature coronary deaths per year, and epidemiologic evidence suggests this number is closer to 100,000 premature deaths annually."
~ The Harvard School of Public Health

IN 1994, MY FATHER HAD A HEART ATTACK. He was rushed to the hospital, and after testing, his doctor told him he would have to have balloon angioplasty—a fairly common procedure—to open up his clogged arteries. There was only one catch. Six months earlier, my father's sister had gone into the hospital for the same "easy" operation after doctors found that her arteries were clogged. However, the balloon dislodged a clot which traveled to my aunt's brain, causing her to have a massive stroke. In one single day, she went from being a World-Class Master's Swimming Champion to not being able to walk. Needless to say, my father was not thrilled at the prospect of suffering the same consequences—so he flatly refused the operation.

Before I went to see him in the hospital, I stopped at a bookstore to see if I could find any information at all about a "natural approach" to healing heart disease. I had never heard of Dr. Dean Ornish before that day, but his name became a household word of ours over the next few months.

"Suffice it to say that trans fatty acids are b-a-a-a-d. They raise your total blood cholesterol level and your LDL, or bad cholesterol; lower your HDL, or good cholesterol; and are suspected of contributing to obesity and diabetes."

~ Robert L. Wolke, Professor Emeritus of Chemistry, University of Pittsburg

If you don't know of Dr. Ornish, he is the research and medical doctor who authored the best-selling book, *Eat More, Weigh Less*. In the book's Introduction, he writes, "Our research, called the 'Lifestyle Heart Trial,' was the first randomized, controlled clinical study scientifically demonstrating that the progress of even severe coronary heart disease can often be reversed by making lifestyle changes alone (including [a no-fat] diet, stress management training, smoking cessation, moderate exercise, and emotional support) without cholesterol lowering drugs or surgery." Voila!—a whole body approach to healing. I also find it interesting to note, that in the Acknowledgements, Ornish states that much of what is written in his book is an outgrowth of his 20 years of study with the renowned Spiritual teacher, Swami Satchitdananda.

The gist of the program Ornish teaches to others is how to make and maintain comprehensive lifestyle changes while living in the real world. In other words, his program is about *transformation*—not just losing weight.

I thumbed through the book in the bookstore and decided to bring it to my father along with a pot of vegetable soup. I'd made the soup for him because I wanted my father to have something to eat other than the cheese omelet breakfast and roast beef smothered in gravy and mashed potato with butter dinner that was on his hospital menu for the day. Even before reading the book, I knew that those meals were less like nourishment and more like feeding a ticking time-bomb to an artery-clogged heart patient.

While he was still in the hospital, my father read the Introduction to Ornish's book and was sold. His doctor, however, was not. The physician tried every fear-promoting tactic he could come up to get my father to "come to his senses" and have the operation. This included telling him, "If you don't have this operation in less than a year, you'll be dead!"

That didn't shake my father; he resolved to try the diet and became the ideal Dean Ornish dieter—"a poster boy" adherent to the no-fat way of eating—and my mother joined him. Less than a year later, my father wasn't dead—far from it! He'd lost 25 pounds and lowered his cholesterol from 240 to 160.

By the way, at the time I'm writing this book, 11 years later, my father is still healthy and very much alive. Why? He listened to his Soul.

And the heart doctor who was adamantly opposed to my father trying the no-fat diet? Ironically enough, he's the one who died.

THE BIG FAT MISCONCEPTION: LOSE THE FAT, LOSE THE FLAVOR?

"Ah, come on," you may be thinking. "No fat! I'll give up anything, but not the fat."

I completely understand. When I first became a vegetarian, I went through what I fondly call my "Fettuccini Alfredo phase." Everything I ate, although sans meat, included lots of dairy and butter. I also loved potato chips and ice cream. Needless to say, my cholesterol level hovered somewhere around 240. Today, I can barely remember the last time I opened a tub of margarine or unwrapped a stick of butter. But I didn't try to make those dietary changes; I just evolved into them naturally.

Remember, I am not in the business of making you give up anything. The Soul-Full approach is an approach of abundance, not one of deprivation. So you'll see as you read on that there are plenty of ways to keep the flavor while you forgo the perils of fat. It just takes a bit of awareness and a slight shift in perception about what fat is. Soon you'll see that you can eat very delicious foods that naturally have either no fat, little fat, or "good fat." And it will be your choice—based on what you feel is most whole for you—and you won't feel deprived of anything. You'll be able to eat the foods you love most, maybe with some slight modifications, and at the same time you'll experience an abundance of good health and feelings of well-being.

A CRUCIAL ISSUE

There's probably no other aspect of eating that has people feeling more interested, confused or obsessed than the issue of fat. When I was doing research for this chapter, I found 12,867 pages of websites related to fats and oils!

As recently as just a few hundred years ago, humans ate very little fat. Prior to that, much of the fat and oil in the human diet came from nuts, seeds and grains. However, today, millions of people are eating their food smothered in fat.

Why? Because as inferred earlier, fat can make food taste good.

But the primary reason that many people feel it's necessary to overindulge their taste buds with so much fat is because they have become accustomed to eating dead food that needs a lot of added flavor. The reason fats and additives appear to be so necessary is that a good deal of the flavor is taken out of foods, via cooking and processing. Then, of course, a modified version of the flavor has to be put back into them.

Many people are not living off the land, but living off the "fat of the land" and paying a dear price for it—with serious health consequences. We toss salads in fat, serve our bread and vegetables with fat, and indulge in rich, fat-laden desserts. The fast food industry, which has now made its mark worldwide, makes billions of dollars a year satisfying the world's hunger for grill-fried and deep-fried foods that are saturated in fat. Looking at that, one may ask, "Are we still food eaters, or fat and oil eaters who have a little bit of food on the side?"

SKIMMING THE FAT

Of course, fat, like everything else, is okay in moderation. And the right kind of fat is actually beneficial and necessary for our health. However, because fat makes food taste good, it is being commercially fed to us, more and more, and in all the wrong forms.

Let me give you some facts about fat and then you can decide how to put them to best use.

WHAT IS FAT?

Body fat serves several important functions. In addition to protecting our bodies in certain vulnerable areas, such as around vital organs, fat is the body's main source of stored energy. If we go without eating, our bodies will mobilize the fat to provide energy. So it's easy to see that fat in our bodies is a necessary thing. It is excess fat that causes us problems.

Fat reserves do not just come from the fat that is eaten. Excess carbohydrates that are not used immediately by the body are stored as fat as well, so it is not necessary for us to consume fat in order to have an adequate store of it. A little fat consumed goes a long way, so it is best used sparingly. Therefore when it comes to eating healthily, it is wise to become a fat connoisseur.

THE "GOOD" ESSENTIAL FATS

Essential Fatty Acids are fats which must be consumed in the diet because the body has no mechanism to manufacture them. The two families of essential fatty acids (each of which must be consumed independently) are *omega-3* and *omega-6* fatty acids. Omega-3 fatty acids have anti-inflammatory, anti-clotting effects in the body. Omega-6 fatty acids have the opposite effect, promoting inflammatory and pro-clotting effects. Both are necessary to the body under different circumstances, and a proper ratio of Omega-6 to Omega-3 is absolutely crucial to proper health. A ratio that is too high in Omega-6 fatty acids can have pro-inflammatory, pro-clotting, pro-heart disease, and pro-cancer effects.

An ideal ratio of Omega-6 to Omega-3 is between 2:1 to 3:1. Most cultures eating long-standing traditional diets have this ratio naturally. For example, the New Zealand Maoris, living a traditional lifestyle on the coast and eating a diet predominantly of seafood, have a ratio of about 2.8:1. The Japanese, who also eat a diet high in fish and low in processed carbohydrates,

"Truly fat-free foods, like people, tend to lack personality. Fat is comparable to the volume knob, because without it our taste buds are incapable of distinguishing flavors but in and of itself it is almost flavorless."

~ Stewart Lee Allen, author of *In the Devil's Garden*

have a ratio of about 4.6:1. By contrast, the average American eating a diet high in carbohydrates, vegetable oils and commercially raised meats has a ratio of 17.6:1! In fact, the main reasons why our society is so dependent on many painkillers and anti-inflammatory drugs such as aspirin and IB Profin is precisely because our bodies are lacking in Omega-3 fatty acids, a natural anti-inflammatory agent.

Omega-3 fatty acids are found in the fat of animals that eat green things, and can also be obtained through flax, borage and hemp seed oil. Omega-6 fatty acids are found in the fat of vegetables, such as nuts, seeds and avocados. So why does the average American have a ratio so high in Omega-6 and so low in Omega-3? The excess of Omega-6 comes from refined vegetable oils. Processed foods are full of them. We are lacking in Omega-3 because our meat is no longer grass-fed. Even animals raised for free-range, organic meat are often fed dried grains, and therefore the meat does not contain Omega-3 fatty acids. Wild-caught fish, and to a lesser extent wild game, are the only animal sources of Omega-3 available to us. So fish oils, such as cod liver oil, are a good supplemental source of Omega-3 fatty acids.

To restore your ratio of Omega-6 to Omega-3 to a healthy level, start by cutting out vegetable oils from your diet—including corn oil, safflower and sunflower. Organic olive oil and organic canola oil (which would not be genetically engineered) are OK, as they contain only low levels of Omega-6 fatty acids, and have little effect on the ratio. Olive oil also contains no saturated fat and so it's great for cardiovascular health. Canola oil is even lower in saturated fat than olive oil, and its smoking point makes it good for cooking. It is made from rapeseed. These two oils are the best choices for salad dressings, stir fries, and other recipes calling for oil. All other types of processed vegetable oil should be avoided, especially those in commercially prepared foods and baked goods, which are often hydrogenated (more on that later). It is ideal to get your Omega-6 fatty acids from raw nuts, seeds, and fatty vegetables such as avocados and olives.

To increase your levels of Omega-3 fatty acids, I would suggest taking a supplement of fish oil (such as cod liver oil) if you are not vegan or adding more flax seed oil to your diet if you are vegan or prefer this choice. Eating fresh fish is obviously a more natural way to go about ingesting fish oils, as well as being a healthy source of protein; however, as discussed earlier, environmental pollutants have made eating large amounts of fish risky. Metals such as mercury are not fat soluble and therefore not found in the oil of fish as they are in the meat of fish.

As I said, for vegetarians, vegans and other interested readers, it is possible to get Omega-3 from flax seed oil, although this is a bit more inefficient and can take more effort. The conversion of flax oil into Omega-3 can be easily inhibited by vitamin deficiencies, by excess Omega-6 fatty acids and hydrogenated oils, and by diabetes. It is necessary to ingest 2 to 3 tablespoons of flax seed oil each day, and to make sure you are eating a mineral-rich diet or taking a mineral supplement, and to cut back on vegetable oils and processed foods containing hydrogenated oils. Taking an algae-based DHA supplement will also help in the conversion.

"Cold-pressed, uncooked oils will increase thermogenesis, a process that revs up fat-burning cells. They also send a message of satiety to the brain to create a feeling of fullness so there is less desire to eat fat."
~ Gary Null, Author of *Kiss Your Fat Goodbye*

Here is a chart showing the percentage of omega-3 fatty acids in the fats of fish and meats (as 100g in weight).

Fishes and Meats	Total Fat (g)	% Omega-3 fatty acids
Salmon (wild)	6.34	4.65
Salmon (cooked)	8.13	4.60
Sardine (canned)	11.45	4.35
Trout	3.46	3.44
Halibut	2.29	2.84
Deer	2.42	2.89
Elk	1.45	2.76
Catfish	2.82	2.52
Lamb	21.59	1.81
Bison (wild)	1.84	1.63
Beef (retail cuts)	19.2	1.19
Salmon (canned)	6.05	0.95
Chicken	15.06	0.93
Salmon (farmed)	10.85	0.93
Shrimp	1.73	0.87
Bass	2.33	0.64
Pork (retail cuts)	14.95	0.6
Beef (ground)	26.55	0.6
Clams	0.97	0.41
Snapper	1.34	0.3
Tuna (canned)	0.82	0.2
Shrimp (fast food)	15.1	0.17
Cod	0.67	0.15

Here is a chart showing the amount of omega-3 fatty acids in one tablespoon of various sources:

Flaxseed Oil	7 grams
Flaxseeds	3 grams
Cod Liver Oil	2.43 grams
Canola Oil	1.5 grams
Canola Oil Mayonnaise	1 gram
Walnut Oil	1.3 grams
Walnuts	0.7 grams

THE PROBLEM-CAUSING FATS AND OILS

Hydrogenated

> *"Transfat is bad fat. The less transfat people eat, the healthier they will be."*
> ~ Tommy G. Thompson, Secretary of the
> US Department of Health and Human Services

On January 12, 2005, the US Department of Agriculture and the US Department of Health and Human Services issued dietary guidelines urging the public to "keep trans fatty acid (found in hydrogenated fat) consumption as low as possible." And a recent article in *The New York Times* indicated that on August 10, 2005, the New York City Department of Health and Mental Hygiene asked city restaurateurs and food suppliers to voluntarily eliminate partially hydrogenated vegetable oils from the kitchen. Although it appears that things have gotten out of control when it comes to the consumption of hydrogenated fats, that was not the initial intention.

The method of hydrogenation was originally developed to produce low-cost soap. Then during World War II, when the butter supply was at a low, scientists discovered the same process could be used to make a spreadable shortening. Today it is used to make not only margarine but most of the oils used to make commercial baked goods.

In hydrogenation, the oil or fat is exposed to high temperatures and extreme pressure. Hydrogen is then bubbled through the fat to make it hard. The end product is then treated with various chemicals to make it appealing to the consumer. One result of the hydrogenation process is the formation of trans fatty acids (TFAs), a type of fatty acid.

To say the least, hydrogenated fats and TFAs are unhealthy and harmful to your body. (You can check ingredient labels on foods to avoid hydrogenated fats.) Yet they are extremely popular in the commercial cooking industry because these fats can last for years, even under poor storage conditions and harsh temperatures. (You can imagine how long they stay in your body and clog up your system when you ingest them!)

Hydrogenated fats also contain a number of chemical residues left over from processing. For instance, here are some of the things that can be found in a typical tub of margarine (a type of hydrogenated fat):

1. Benzoate of soda
2. Dyes and other coloring
3. Artificial flavoring
4. Saturated fats
5. Pulverized nickel
6. Fragmented aluminum
7. Other chemical additives

Up until now, there has been little or no control over most of the additives used in margarine. Chemicals are used in the extraction of oils and fats from seeds, in neutralizing, bleaching, deodorizing, and at the stage where the final consistency of the margarine is improved. Antioxidants are used to improve shelf life, and antimicrobial agents also may be added.

Animal Fats

Animal fat is obtained, as one might assume, from the fatty tissues of animals. It includes tallow (beef fat), lard (port fat) and chicken fat. And just like humans, animals store accumulated pesticides and other toxins from their diets in their fat tissue. As a result, such fats, when they come from non-organic, non-grass-fed animals, contain high concentrations of environmental poisons and waste products. Animal fats are also usually super-heated during processing to prevent rancidity. (The most harmful form of fat for your body is that which is heated. When fats and oils are heated, they can become more difficult to digest, and toxic to the body.)

A large component of these animal fats is saturated fat. The saturated fat in our diet also comes from fatty meats or animal products including dairy, such as butter, cheese, milk, and eggs. In addition, many commercial baked goods contain saturated fat in the form of hydrogenated (heated) palm and coconut oil. Saturated fats are usually solid at room temperature. They raise cholesterol and should be avoided in hydrogenated form and eaten in moderation otherwise while making organic and grass-fed choices. In addition, non-organic butter, a popular form of fat from animals, is usually colored and salted and likely contains hormones and additives that come from the cow's exposure to these substances.

Vegetable Oils

As mentioned earlier, excessive consumption of vegetable oils can lead to an inflammatory, pro-disease environment in the body. Non-organic vegetable oils often contain pesticide residues from the plants used to make them, in addition to chemicals to keep them from going rancid or becoming cloudy.

The best quality oil to look for is the organic, cold-processed variety. For olive oil, look for extra-virgin as well. Extra-virgin olive oil is the highest quality available and contains many of the nutrients removed during the refining of virgin-quality oils. Olive oil labeled simply "pure olive oil" is of the lowest quality.

Many modern refined oils are treated with chemicals and boiled until virtually all nutritive value has been eliminated. Only avocado oil and olive oil, when labeled "cold-pressed," are extracted without the use of heat. Macadamia oil is good to use in cooking because it is heat-stable and canola oil (organic) is good to use in salad dressings because it is light in color, flavor and saturated fat.

STEPS IN THE REFINEMENT OF VEGETABLE OILS

Stage	Description	Nutrients
Starting material	Seeds, nuts, beans	Oils, protein, minerals, fiber
Step 1	Clean and hull.	No effect
Step 2	Add solvent.	Lose protein, fiber, vitamins, minerals.
Step 3	Distill and degum.	Lose chlorophyll, calcium, magnesium, copper, iron
Step 4	Refine.	Lose phospholipids, more minerals.
Step 5	Bleach.	Lose more chlorophyll, beta-carotene, flavor compounds.
Step 6	Deodorize.	Lose vitamin E.
Step 7	Add preservatives.	
Step 8	Hydrogenate.	Lose essential fatty acids.

End product: Margarine and shortening

Some of the best sources of good vegetable fats are young coconut meat, durian, avocado, soaked nuts (especially macadamia, which are highest in fat) and seeds—which are higher in protein than nuts. The seeds highest in fat are also some of the most delicious such as pumpkin, sesame, sunflower, hemp, and flax.

EFFECTS OF EXCESS FAT ON THE BODY

Excess fat can actually cause red blood cells to stick together. When red blood cells clump together, they are unable to fit through the tiny capillaries supplying many of the body's vital organs, including those that supply the brain with sufficient oxygen. Red blood cells are forced to reroute through larger blood vessels, therefore leaving parts of the body neglected. The larger vessels themselves can become blocked, leading to severe medical complications.

Processed fats can also hinder white blood cells in fighting infections in the body. People who eat high-fat diets have a greater risk of skin cancer when exposed to the sun. Excess fats settle in the skin tissue and bake there.

AN ALTERNATIVE TO BUTTER OR MARGARINE— GHEE (CLARIFIED BUTTER)

Ghee has been an esteemed cooking medium since the ancient Vedic times in India, when it was counted among the riches of the household. Ghee is the *essence* of butter—pure butterfat—and so many believe it to be the very best of all cooking mediums. Since it has no milk solids to turn rancid, it will keep for months, even without refrigeration. It is viewed as ideal for cooking because the nonfat ingredients (water, proteins and carbohydrates) are separated from the fat of the butter when it is melted to make ghee. As a result, ghee can be heated at much higher temperatures without burning. Bringing out the sweet, nutlike flavor of the melted butter requires long, slow cooking to fully evaporate the water and to allow the milk solids to separate and float to the surface, leaving the clear amber-colored ghee.

According to a study published in the *American Journal of Clinical Nutrition*, there was a dramatic difference between the heart-disease rates of populations in northern and southern India. The northerners were meat-eaters and had high cholesterol levels. Their main source of dietary fat was ghee (clarified butter). The southerners were vegetarians and had much lower cholesterol levels. Present-day "wisdom" would predict the vegetarians to have the lower rate of heart disease, but in fact the opposite was true. The vegetarians had 15 times the rate of heart disease when compared to their northern counterparts! What was the reason for this surprising difference? Aside from meat versus vegetables, the major dietary difference was that the southerners had replaced their traditional ghee with margarine and refined polyunsaturated vegetable oils. Twenty years later, the British medical journal *The Lancet* noted an increase in heart-attack deaths amongst the northern Indians. By this time, the northerners had also largely replaced the ghee in their diets with margarine and refined vegetable oils.

Ghee contains cholesterol, but not oxidized cholesterol or the hydrogenated trans-fatty acids that cause free-radical damage in the body.

HOW TO MAKE GHEE (CLARIFIED BUTTER)

Place 1 pound of unsalted butter in a saucepan and heat it until it boils. Lower the heat and allow foam to accumulate on top.

When the foam begins to thicken, skim it off, being careful not to stir up the butter. Be watchful so the butter, and the solids, which adhere to the bottom of the pan, do not burn. When the foamy milk solids are all skimmed off and a clear liquid remains in the pan, turn off the heat.

Let the ghee rest for a few minutes and then carefully pour it into a metal or earthenware vessel. Since clarified butter will last for weeks without refrigeration, you can keep it near your stove for ease in cooking.

KEY GUIDELINES FOR FAT

The following guidelines can help you develop healthy habits regarding your fat intake.

- **Limit your fat consumption to no more than 30% of the calories you take in.** Based on a standard 2,000 calorie a day diet, that's 400 to 600 calories. Also, reduce the amount of saturated fats in your diet. Animal products are generally high in fat and plant products are generally low. However nuts and seeds are high in monosaturated fats and should be eaten in moderation.

- **Use alternatives to margarine** such as ghee and eliminate foods containing trans-fatty acids (TFAs) and partially hydrogenated oils. Trans-fatty acids are formed during the hydrogenation process. Both TFAs and hydrogenated oils interfere with the body's healthy utilization of essential fatty acids.

- **If you are a meat-eater, increase your intake of fish and reduce the amount of meat and dairy products you consume.** Particularly beneficial are cold-water fish because of their high levels of omega-3 fats.

- **Use supplemental oil.** Take 1 tablespoon of flaxseed oil or eat 2 to 3 tablespoons of ground flax seed daily. Or take a high-quality fish oil supplement that provides you with 600-1,200 mg. of omega-3 fatty acids.

- **Use healthier oils for cooking.** Ghee, olive oil, canola, coconut oil or macadamia nut oil are good choices. And remember to buy cold-pressed and organic oils.

How much fat do you consume in a day? Some people are consuming virtually none, because they are being extremely selective about what they eat. Some are consuming more than 20 grams of transfat a day! The trick is not to be afraid of fat or avoids fats altogether—which could actually be harmful to your health—but to eat the right kinds of fat, from natural and unprocessed sources.

In his book, *Fats That Heal, Fats That Kill*, author Udo Erasmus states that highly unsaturated oils are as vital to our health as is sunlight. He proposes that sunlight and highly unsaturated oils not only compliment each other, but can substitute for each other to some extent, although both are necessary. "Every region of the globe gets a little light, and every area grows organisms that contain at least some EFAs," he says. "The more light there is, the less EFAs seem to be needed. The less light there is, the more fatty acids appear to be necessary in the diet (and the more unsaturated they must be). If an Inuit ate only fruits and vegetables during an arctic winter, he would starve. If a Samoan ate the Inuit's protein and marine oils under a hot tropical sun, he would suffer. Each, in his place and in his native diet, thrives."

Now that you are a fat connoisseur, you can decide just what's right for you. Enjoy!

Think about whether you have a favorite food you like to prepare that is just chock-full of saturated fat. If so, maybe you don't have to give it up completely. Instead, see if you can make it using some form of "friendly fat"—either cold-pressed oils, ghee or ground nuts and seeds.

CHAPTER TWENTY-ONE

Sugar,
The Not-So-Sweet Truth

"That stuff [sugar] is poison. I won't have it in my house, let alone my body."
~ Hollywood Legend Gloria Swanson

IF YOU'RE EATING the typical American diet, then it is quite likely that you're ingesting *a whopping 42 teaspoons of sugar a day*! My farmer friends tell me that if you were to eat this amount of sugar in its natural form, you would be eating approximately 90 feet of sugar cane! How on earth do people manage to consume so much of the white stuff?

Well, first of all, it's not all white. The major percentage of our sugar intake comes from eating prepared foods. For example, did you know that one chocolate bar has 7 teaspoons of sugar; a stick of gum has 1/2 tsp.; a half-cup of ice cream, 5 to 6 tsp.; a slice of apple pie, 12 tsp., and a half-inch piece of chocolate cake, 15 tsp.? Even though that's a lot of sugar, you do expect to find sweetener in those items. However, it may surprise you to discover sugar in foods you'd never suspect—such as frozen dinners, cereals, breads, many canned fruits and vegetables, even French fries and ketchup!

"It's as addictive as nicotine or heroin and as poisonous, responsible for modern plagues ranging from depression to coronary thrombosis."

~ William Duffy, author of *Sugar Blues*

The sugar in prepared foods is often masked by a variety of different names, so be sure to look out for the following ingredients: cane sugar, evaporated cane juice, corn syrup, high-fructose corn syrup, dextrose, fructose, lactose, levulose, maltose, rice syrup, succinate, sucrose, and turbinado sugar. Because ingredients are listed in order of their significance (if the first ingredient is white flour, that product contains more white flour than anything else), some companies try to mask the amounts of sugar in their products by using two different types of sugar and listing them separately. For example, a list of ingredients may read: flour, almonds, high-fructose corn syrup, milk, turbinado sugar. This makes it seem that flour is the most-used ingredient, when in reality it is sugar.

Nutritionally speaking, the sugar added to foods adds little or nothing. And when you eat sugar, you are stoking your inner fire with empty calories. Sugar is an empty fuel. It flares up and burns off quickly.

A high sugar intake does not only promote tooth decay (that seems to be its least detrimental effect), it also elevates the serum lipoprotein. This substance has been implicated as being just as bad, if not worse, than fat as a leading cause of heart disease. Gallbladder disease, various skin disorders—including acne—diabetes, indigestion and hypertension have all been associated with excessive sugar consumption.

In general, eating too much sugar lowers our resistance to disease. White blood cells, which fight infection in the body, become sluggish and cannot destroy as much pathogenic bacteria and other invaders when blood-sugar levels go up.

SUGAR QUIZ

Try this simple quiz to determine if you are eating too much sugar. Answer "Yes" or "No" to each question below:

1. I feel dull, heavy or sluggish in the morning.
2. I lose concentration from time to time.
3. I typically need more than 7 hours sleep a night.
4. I urinate frequently.
5. I need a pick-me-up to start the day (coffee, tea, a cigarette).
6. I drink coffee and tea throughout the day.
7. I drink alcohol every day.
8. My palms sweat whether I am active or not.
9. I smoke.
10. I drink sugary drinks such as sodas throughout the day.
11. I feel sleepy during the day.
12. I avoid exercise, due to tiredness and lack of motivation.
13. I crave sugar, bread and carbohydrates.
14. I get very thirsty, but it is not quenched by drinking water.
15. I get dizzy or irritable if I don't eat often.

Have you answered "Yes" to three or more of these questions? Then you may have a blood-sugar management problem. It's a good idea for you to begin to cut back on your sugar intake and see if that helps you feel better. If you've answered "Yes" to five or more items, than you more than likely *do* have blood sugar problems. Follow the suggestions offered in this chapter, and if symptoms persist, see your health care practitioner.

So what did you discover? Do you need to cut back on sugar? Only you know what sugar intake is right for you. Your preferences, lifestyle, attitudes, and overall state of health will determine your response to sweeteners in general. If you live a balanced, healthy, happy life with little stress, chances are you'll react to the intake of any type of sugar with relative equilibrium. However, if you are under duress, overworked, in emotional turmoil and/or your overindulgences have been pushing your adrenal glands to the limit, there's a good chance that you'll feel the loss of your normal resilience when you give in to even periodic cravings for sweets.

Because sugar is an addictive substance, and our intake of it is often driven by cravings, it may take some time to gain a healthy perspective on how sugar consumption affects your daily life. Once you are sure that your diet is supplying you with your proper nutritional needs (remember, it is so much harder to quit addictive substances if we are not receiving the proper support from our diets), try gradually cutting out all sugar, including natural sweeteners and fruit juices, from your diet. This will probably be hard at first, and as you become more mindful of it, you may realize how much of your diet contains sugar. You may experience withdrawal symptoms such as fatigue, lack of concentration, and intense cravings, but try to counter these with satisfying nutritious meals and fresh fruits or berries. After living a largely sugar-free lifestyle for a couple of weeks, you will be amazed by how intensely sweet a simple chocolate chip cookie, or even a dried banana will taste. A few bites of cake will be more than enough sweetness, when your tolerance for sugar has been lowered to a healthy level.

WHAT GOES UP MUST COME DOWN

Hypoglycemia (Low Blood Sugar)

You take a bite of a gooey, scrumptious sweet thing and your taste buds immediately stand at attention. As you chew, your senses begin to come alive, and you feel brighter, more energetic. And that's just what's going on with your body that you're aware of. Meanwhile, on the inside, with each bite, your blood sugar is rapidly rising, which triggers the release of insulin in your body. This sharp increase will later cause your blood-sugar level to come crashing down, leaving you feeling tired and craving something to alleviate the dramatic drop in energy and to get yourself going again. This is the blood sugar roller-coaster that so many people experience on a daily basis and think is normal. It has become an addictive pattern for many.

A related condition, hypoglycemia—an abnormally low concentration of sugar in the blood—is a major problem in this country, and yet only a few doctors recognize it. In his book, *Spiritual Nutrition*, Gabriel Cousens, MD, refers to hypoglycemia as "the great mimicker" stating: "It can manifest in a variety of symptoms such as chronic fatigue, exhaustion, weakness, depression, headaches, unexplained mood changes and anxiety attacks, concentration difficulties, transitory meal confusion, and even allergies."

If you've found yourself with any of the above symptoms, hypoglycemia may well be the culprit.

Cousens believes that hypoglycemia is the result of so many people's desire to keep up with and live the "All-American Dream"—moving faster, wanting more, believing bigger is better, and living a highly competitive and aggressive lifestyle. All of this is out of harmony with our inner Self and Mother Nature. In order to keep up with the frenetic pace, many turn to quick energy foods, including sugary treats as I described above.

When I was a model, I was one of the lucky ones who was drawn to finding out about food and nutrition in order to stay slim. That is not typically the case. Despite their svelte figures, I found that many models ate lots of sweets.

 Modeling is a superficial life, and staying on the surface of things is quite typical. Because sugary foods provide a "fast-burn" high and the ability to keep up with the fast pace, it's often a preferred food for models. However, it's a method that takes its toll physically, emotionally and mentally. There was frequently a lot of erratic behavior on sets. As we all know, pretty on the outside doesn't always mean it's so pretty on the inside.

"Sugar has been shown to shorten life in various animal experiments."

~ Sally Fallon, author of *Nourishing Traditions*

SOME SOLUTIONS

Hypoglycemia is very easy to treat. A holistic treatment includes six small meals per day, with lots of raw fruits and vegetables and a small amount of protein. Patients usually heal very quickly. It's important to know that if you begin your day with sugar-laden cereals or other carbohydrates such as muffins and pastries, you are essentially jumping on the high-low blood sugar roller-coaster first thing in the morning.

Instead, you could eat a breakfast consisting of whole foods, such as fruits, whole grains and/or a small amount of protein. That way, you would most likely find yourself with less cravings and in an overall more well-balanced state of being. What protein should you consider? Well, although it's not typical in America to have protein other than eggs and meat for breakfast, eating fish for breakfast is the norm in Japan. And in many other countries, people start the day with grains, beans and other legumes.

It's also helpful to know that all foods have what is termed a "glycemic value"—the higher the value, the more quickly the food's sugars will affect your blood-sugar levels. Most beneficial are the foods that contain moderate to slow-release sugars, providing a consistent release of sugars throughout the day.

Here's a chart that can help you discern which types of food to eat in order to avoid the sugar surges that deplete the body's energy reserves.

Quick-Release Sugars	Moderate-Release Sugars	Slow-Release Sugars
Honey	Chips	All root vegetables
Sweets and chocolate	Dried fruit	Fresh fruits
White flour products	Pasta	Legumes
White sugar	Popcorn	Whole grains

Notice in the above chart that fresh fruit has a slow-release sugar time. That is because, even though the fruit is sweet, its fiber content slows down the digestion process and thus the sugar-release as well. Fruit still digests fairly rapidly though, particularly when eaten on an empty stomach. So people who suffer from fluctuations of energy, swings in mood, and other hypoglycemic symptoms should eat fruit in moderation while they're attempting to balance their blood-sugar levels.

ARTIFICIAL SWEETENERS—THE BIG NO-NO

Contrary to what many people seem to think, artificial sweeteners are not the answer to satisfying a sugar craving. Because these are high-intensity sweeteners—ranging anywhere from 30 to 600 times the sweetness of table sugar—many people like to use them to lose weight. But they most definitely will not help you to tame your desire for sugar; more likely, artificial sweeteners will exacerbate it.

There is also an increasing number of problems currently being reported by artificial sweetener users. These include seizures, mood swings, headaches, blurred vision and, surprisingly, *weight gain*!

SOME HEALTHIER ALTERNATIVES TO WHITE SUGAR

So what types of sugars are best to choose when you do consume them? Various options are discussed below.

Honey

Honey is one of the least refined sweeteners we have available. It is about 25 to 50% sweeter than sugar. It is actually nectar from flowers that has been transformed by the addition of bee enzymes. Therefore, it is not only a healthy, alternative sweetener, but also a great enzyme source. Good-quality honey is natural and unrefined, heated only enough to extract it from the honey comb and to strain it to remove the wax. If you want to eat honey with the enzymes intact, be sure to use raw unpasteurized honey. But as with all other foods, it's important to know your source to insure its purity.

Date Sugar

This sweetener is made from dates that are dehydrated down to a 3 to 5% moisture level and then ground into a powder. It contains all of the flavor and minerals supplied by dried dates. Date sugar tastes great on cereals, and it can be used in baking.

Maple Syrup

Don't confuse real maple syrup with "pancake syrup," which is actually flavored, colored corn-syrup and sugar. Pure maple syrup is concentrated from the sap of maple trees, which flows in the late winter and early spring. Maple syrup is two-thirds as sweet as white sugar, and it is metabolized in a similar way to white sugar in the body. It is highly and distinctly flavorful and comes in grades ranging from AA—which is pale gold, delicate and very sweet—to D which is dark with a strong caramel flavor. Maple syrup offers a high concentration of minerals, and it is a good source of both manganese and zinc.

Molasses

Molasses is manufactured as a by-product of sugar refinement, created when the sugar cane or sugar beet is boiled. It is a thick, strong-tasting syrup. Blackstrap molasses is produced in the third boiling. Light molasses comes from the first boiling, and a darker molasses from the second. Molasses is not as sweet as white sugar, however it contains many minerals, including calcium, magnesium, potassium and iron. Since molasses is a by-product of sugar processing, it can also contain contaminants so be sure of its source and purity.

Agave Nectar

This is a fairly new sweetener commercially that is naturally extracted from the pineapple-shaped core of the Agave, a cactus-like plant native to Mexico. It has a 90% fruit-sugar content. Although it is 35% sweeter than sugar, Agave nectar is absorbed slowly into the body, decreasing the highs and lows associated with intake of some other types of sugars.

Stevia

This intensely sweet natural substitute for sugar is obtained from an herb grown in South America known as *yerba dulce* or "sweet leaf." Its flavor is similar to dark molasses, and it is 100-200 times sweeter than sugar, so very little is needed in a recipe.

Brown Rice Syrup

This is one of the most balanced, unrefined sweeteners. The process for making it uses whole or partially polished brown rice, and the syrup is completely devoid of chemicals. Brown rice syrup is slowly and steadily absorbed by the body, making it extremely easy on blood-sugar levels.

Barley Malt

I've saved what is considered to be one of the best whole-food-based sweeteners for last. When barley is sprouted, the grain's starch is transformed into a sweetener consisting primarily of complex, slow-digesting sugars. Barley malt has a strong flavor and can be used well in baking.

SUGAR AND THE WILD CHILD

Many children who are labeled as hyperactive or said to have Attention Deficit Disorder crave sugar. Could it be that they are actually craving something else... perhaps some sweet attention to their Soul? Such a true craving is dramatically demonstrated in the following story.

A client once shared with me that overall he felt he was doing well with his Spiritual practice of being present with and accepting of most everything in his life. Still there was one area that he was continuing to find particularly challenging. This client constantly craved sweets. He'd tried paying attention to what he ate, cutting back on sugar, and even going cold turkey from it while eating a diet consisting of primarily protein. Still none of it had worked.

I asked the client if this was a fairly new development for him or if he was always this way. He said that as long as he could remember sugar had been an obsession with him. He was quite fit and trim so if he hadn't revealed his dilemma to me, it would not have been evident.

I said, "Let's try a little meditation." We both sat down and began to breathe deeply. When I could see that he was relaxed and in touch with his body, I asked him to close his eyes and listen to me as I spoke to him. I began to ask the client about his first memory of feeling a need or affinity to sugar. An image came to him immediately. He remembered one Christmas Eve, when his older brother had stolen one of his gifts out from under the tree. "My brother saw my name on the tag and he knew it was the fire engine I'd wanted most of all. In fact, I hadn't even asked for any other gifts. He took it just to spite me, to ruin my Christmas. He just opened the box and began playing with the fire engine. When my father found out, he scolded him a bit. But then my father just sort of half-wrapped it back up and stuck it back under the tree, like everything should be alright. That made me feel even more devastated. What's worse is that the only thing my father did to console me as I sat there crying was to pick a candy cane off the tree and shove it into my mouth. As he did this, my father said, 'Here, that'll shut you up.' As you can see, I didn't grow up in a very sweet environment."

With the last comment, my client's teary eyes flew open in shock. I looked back at him smiling and asked, "So what do you do now with that little epiphany?" He replied, "I'm not sure." As we discussed it further, my client realized that the only thing he could do was to begin now to give himself the love he'd felt deprived of all of his life—that was his real craving.

My client said he knew just where to start. He told me, "I hate my mother-in-law. Up until now, I've never been able to say one nice thing to her, and she lives with us! My life now is a repeat of the same family hell I grew up in."

He went home and opened a whole new chapter in his life. And during our next session, he very animatedly related what had happened. My client had gone home and walked into the kitchen only to find his mother-in-law icing a cake! Instead of ignoring her as he stuck his finger in the bowl to grab a taste of the icing, as he would have done in the past, he said, "Hey Ma, you look great." Then he got himself a drink of water and engaged her in genuinely joyous conversation. In our session, he remarked, "You know what? I never even looked at the cake; before that's all I would have seen."

My client told me two years later that he never had a sugar craving again!

Sugar can be physically addicting, but all addictions happen to bodies. When you begin to realize that you are so much more than your physical experience, it's easy to see that on a Soul level sugar-cravings often have deeper meaning—i.e., craving to BE sweet, kind, caring, considerate of others, or having a need to give or receive more love.

NOTE ON ALCOHOL

All forms of alcohol behave like simple sugars. Alcohol is absorbed directly into the bloodstream through the stomach, and from there, it goes straight to the brain, giving the drinker a feeling of elation or "high"—a state of mind that becomes addicting to so many.

Notice how many drinkers "loosen up" and become "sweeter" when they have their first couple of drinks. Yet most alcoholic addictions progress from being a "fun experience," as a result of feeling less inhibited and more expressive, to being an experience of finding it even more difficult to communicate and go out into "the world." The sad end-state is an amplification of unforgiven past pain—and of the underlying feelings that sparked the "need" to drink to begin with.

HEALTHY WAYS TO DEAL WITH SUGAR CRAVINGS

The best ways I've found to alleviate severe sugar cravings and most withdrawal symptoms as you wean yourself off of a high-sugar diet are to eat a well-balanced diet, with plenty of fresh seeded fruits (apples, pears, and grapes, for example), vegetables and whole grains. The seeded fruits and grains especially will greatly help to satisfy most sugar cravings. (*Seedless* fruits are genetically altered as is their sugar content, which is most often much higher in non-seeded fruits than in seeded fruits.) You can also eat dried fruits (dates, figs, apricots, etc.) *in moderation*. These are both sweet and healthy if eaten with mindfulness. Also, when eating dried fruits be sure to drink water afterwards, since all of the moisture has been taken out of these fruits. Other healthy sugars are found in vegetables like carrots and beets, so eating them or drinking their juice is quite satisfying to a sweet tooth—but again in moderation.

Interestingly, by far the most healthy and effective way I've found to cut right through sugar cravings is to add large portions of dark green-leafy vegetables and a variety of raw plant foods to the diet. Also drinking fresh green-leafy vegetable juices (rather than fruit juices) such as kale, cucumber, celery and lemon juice is particularly excellent. As is drinking plenty of water to flush excess sugars out of your system.

Wheat grass juice is a quick, "sweet" alternative boost of energy, for those addicted to candy or soft-drink energy highs. Have a shot when you feel intense cravings. (There's more information about wheatgrass in Chapter 34, "Getting on the Fast Track.")

And finally, add spice to you life! Foods such as cayenne and jalapeño peppers and ginger are more deeply stimulating and satisfying to the body than sugars, and they help to alleviate cravings for superficial stimulation.

SOMETHING TO CHEW ON

One of Mahatma Gandhi's favorite stories was about a mother who was worried that her son was eating too much sugar. So she took the child to the village priest and asked for advice. But the priest only said, "Come back in two weeks." Upon their return in two weeks, the priest told the youngster: "Please reduce your sugar consumption." When the mother asked why the priest did not say that the first time, he said: "Two weeks ago, I was eating a lot of sugar myself. I had to reduce my own sugar consumption before dispensing such advice." Moral: Listen to your instincts! What are they telling you about your sugar consumption?

Something that's interesting to note with objectivity is that the sugar trade has had far-reaching negative effects for our entire world. Imperialism and colonialism were largely driven by the hunger for coffee, tobacco and sugar, plus the money that came with these goods. The Caribbean slave trade was built almost exclusively on sugar plantations. In fact, if you look at the history of sugar and the way it has been produced and traded throughout history, it very closely resembles the trade of illegal substances such as heroin and cocaine (which are coincidently white powders as well). Part of eating mindfully is to consider the global impact of the foods you choose to buy and eat. Considering the historical impact of foods means you pay attention to the connotations and "charge" that can surround certain foods. In the case of sugar, a history of blinding greed and cravings comes along with the sweetness.

SOUL-FULL EXERCISE #21

I may not be the village priest dispensing advice. However, I suggest that for two weeks you reduce your sugar consumption so you can begin to better feel your body's instincts about sugar. Once you feel you are more in touch with your natural cravings and have somewhat kicked all of your sugar "addictions," introduce some of the natural sweeteners recommended in this chapter. My favorite is Agave Nectar!

Or, if you're really brave…Avoid all sugar for two weeks. Then first thing in the morning, on an empty stomach, try eating a spoonful of white sugar—the taste will be quite overpoweringly sweet! This can help put your relationship with sugar in perspective and thereafter help you to kick the sugar habit entirely.

RESOURCES

Sugar Blues by William Dufty

Get the Sugar Out: 501 Simple Ways to Cut the Sugar Out of Any Diet
by Ann Louise Gittleman, MS, CNS

The New Sugar Busters: Cut Sugar to Trim Fat by H. Leighton Steward,
Morrison Bethea MD, Sam S. Andrews MD and Luis A. Balart MD

CHAPTER TWENTY-TWO

Salt—Easy Does It

"We add more salt to food than any other condiment."
~ Edward R. Blonz, PhD, nutritionist

SALT—SOME PEOPLE LOVE IT so much they put it on just about everything they eat.

But think of this the next time you reach for the salt shaker or a bag of chips—too much of a good thing can wreak havoc within our body's many systems. Meanwhile, on the other hand, sodium, or salt, is vital for maintaining the health of every cell in our bodies.

Yes, sodium is not just a tasty seasoning. It's a vital component of the fluid that bathes each and every cell of your body. Along with potassium, it is needed for the proper functioning of your nerves and the contraction of your muscles (such as your heart!). It's also necessary to maintain the delicate balance of fluids, electrolytes and pH in your body. With no sodium, you couldn't exist… however, too much of it is detrimental.

So how do you avoid the perils of eating too much salt? Here are some tips:

"Salt is cheap and plentiful; it all too easily becomes a habit, if not an addiction. As you use it, your numbing palate demands more and more."

~ David C. Anderson and Thomas D. Anderson, authors of *The No-Salt Cookbook*

- **Eat fresh, whole foods**—The less processing there is, the better. Don't eat canned foods, particularly soups or vegetables, as these are high in sodium.

- **Substitute unrefined sea salt** or Himalayan rock salt for common table salt. (See information on them later in this chapter.)

- **Cook with less salt** and eliminate it entirely from recipes whenever possible.

- **Check labels**—Seek out products that are low in sodium or have no salt added. Look for the words that signal a high-sodium content such as "barbecued," "broth," "pickled," "cheddar," "Parmesan," "smoked," "marinated" and "tomato-based."

- **Use savory seasonings and fresh herbs** whenever possible. But go easy with (or avoid altogether) those condiments that have a high-sodium content such as mustard, soy sauce, barbecue sauce, cocktail sauce, teriyaki sauce and many bottled salad dressings.

- **Learn to recognize ingredients that contain sodium**, such as soy sauce, salt brine, or any ingredient with sodium in its name, such as monosodium glutamate, or baking soda (sodium bicarbonate).

Craving salt is one of the easiest tendencies to overcome. As Andrew Weil, MD, author of *Natural Health, Natural Medicine*, expresses it—no matter how much you like or crave salt, this love is the result of a learned behavior and you can easily unlearn it.

SEASONING WITH HERBS

You don't have to give up salt, or anything you love. But if you find you are experiencing problems from an overexuberant affinity for it, just develop an even greater love—a love for herbs and spices.

I used to have a magnificent herb garden and I can truly say that there isn't much on earth that's closer to experiencing heaven than to sit among that wild greenery and notice the seductive scents emanating off each leaf. I learned a lot from my garden about the subtleties of nature and how even a little of a *very good thing*, such as fresh seasoning, can go a long way.

Use herbs and spices imaginatively. If you're like many people, you haven't even begun to explore the possibilities of these gifts from the garden. From pungent mustard to sweet marjoram, they run the full gamut of flavors. Even the smallest pinch can pack a provocative punch. So don't be surprised if your taste-buds thank you when you introduce these wonderful, fresh sensations into your cooking instead of using salt. Preparing meals with fresh herbs and spices opens up a whole new world of culinary pleasures. (*If you use fresh herbs, as opposed to dried, use two to four times the dried amount specified in recipes.*)

Herbs and spices are rich in nutrients, and can be very beneficial to your health. For example, tarragon is rich in potassium, while fresh mint helps calm an upset stomach. According to a USDA report, an ounce of many dried herbs contains a far higher mineral content than even three ounces of fruits, vegetables or other plant foods—sometimes even 10 times the amount!

Now that I live by the ocean, I grow my herbs in containers. And once they are picked, I dry and store them. You'll learn how to prepare fresh herbs for later use yourself in the next sections.

PREPARING YOUR OWN DRY HERBS

It's easy to preserve herbs by drying them. Simply expose them to warm, dry air.

Herbs are best harvested for drying just before the flowers first open when they are in the bud-stage—this is usually in the late summer. If you grow your own herbs, gather them in the early morning after the dew has evaporated and before the plants are wilting in the afternoon sun.

Use a sharp knife or scissors to cut healthy branches from your herb plants and remove all dry, bruised or imperfect leaves (and insects!). Rinse them in cool water and shake gently or pat dry to remove excess moisture. Wet herbs will mold and rot.

Remove the lower leaves along the bottom inch or so of the branch, then gather the stems into small bundles. Hang the herbs upside-down to dry. This way, the oils will go into the leaves and not the stems which will most likely later be discarded. You can air dry them outdoors, however better color and flavor retention usually results from drying indoors and away from the sunlight—which depletes the oils. So you can either leave the herbs out in a dark, dry place, such as an attic, or place a bunch upside down in a large paper bag into which you've punched or cut several holes for ventilation. Put them where air currents will circulate through the bag. Any leaves and seeds that fall off will collect in the bottom of the bag. If you're drying many different kinds of herbs at the same time, be sure to label each bag with the name of the herb that's inside.

With either process, check the herbs in about two weeks and they should be ready to use or store. Depending on the humidity in your area at the time, this process can take a little longer or a little less time. Also, some herbs dry faster than others.

STORING DRIED HERBS

Store your dried herbs in air-tight containers. Ziplock plastic bags will do or I like small canning jars. Place them in a cool dry place away from the sunlight. Dried herbs are best if used within a year and will retain more flavor if you store the leaves whole and crush them (using a mortar and pestle is best) only when you are ready to use them.

Use about 1 teaspoon of crumpled dried leaves in place of a tablespoon of fresh leaves. Also, note that you can use the same amount of your personally dried herbs as the amount called for in a typical recipe.

FREEZING HERBS

You can freeze fresh herbs as well. Gather, wash and then pat or shake them dry as described above. While it is possible to place herbs right out of the garden into the freezer, the quality in terms of taste and color will not be quite like fresh herbs; slightly bitter flavors and drab grayish-green colors are common.

Frozen herbs can be improved by blanching before freezing. Just dip them in boiling water briefly; swish them around a bit. and then when their color brightens, remove them from the water. Cool the herbs—either by holding them under running water and then blotting them dry with paper towels, or by placing them on towels after taking them from the boiling water to let them air cool.

You can either place the dried, cooled herbs in small freezer bags in the amount that you feel you will use for a single recipe or serving, or place them in a single layer on wax paper. Roll or fold the paper so that there is a layer of paper separating each layer of herb. Then place the herb packs, paper and all, in freezer bags or wrap them in freezer-rated plastic wrap.

To use, break off as much herb as you need for any recipe.

"If you find you are experiencing problems from an overexuberant affinity for salt, just develop an even greater love—a love for herbs and spices."

~ Maureen Whitehouse

SEAWEEDS

I also use a lot of dried and powdered sea vegetables—such as dulse and kelp—which I find at my local health food store. They can easily satisfy salt cravings and are rich in not only natural sodium but all kinds of beneficial minerals—including calcium, magnesium, potassium, iodine and iron. In fact, sea vegetables offer the broadest range of minerals of any food since they contain virtually all of the minerals found in the ocean—the same minerals that are found in human blood!

Anthropologists have found that throughout time human beings have traveled great distances to include such fare in their diet. The renowned researcher and nutritionist Weston Price traveled the world in the 1930s studying the dietary habits of different cultures, and he came across an

Indian high in the Andes Mountains—hundreds of miles from the sea—who had kelp and fish eggs in his pack, having traded for them. During time of famine, the Irish used kelp and other seaweeds as supplemental foods. In the dead of winter, Eskimos break through the thick ice to gather seaweeds.

Eating sea vegetables has been shown to help those with heart and cardio-vascular system ailments since they contain therapeutic levels of folic acid and magnesium. Sea vegetables can support thyroid function since they are rich in iodine. Their high magnesium and lignan content can help prevent cancers and aid women experiencing menopausal symptoms. But perhaps the most interesting fact about sea vegetables for many is that their high B vitamin, riboflavin and pantothenic acid content can be very helpful to those who suffer from stress and anxiety, both of which deplete these nutrients.

Because seaweeds grow in coastal waters, be sure to get seaweed from clean sources.

Here is a list of some sea vegetables you may like to try:

TYPES OF SEAWEEDS

RED SEAWEEDS

Dulse: Reddish-brown in color with a soft, chewy texture, dulse is available in large, dry pieces or ground flakes—used to sprinkle on food.

Nori: Dried dark purple sheets that turn to phosphorescent green when toasted, nori is famous for its use in making sushi rolls.

BROWN SEAWEEDS

Arame: Lacy and wiry in texture, arame is sweeter than many of the others.

Kelp: Dark green to light brown in color, kelp is often found in flake form.

Kombu: Found in strips and in sheets, kombu is very dark and typically used in soups and stews.

Hijiki: Strong flavored, green to light brown, hijiki looks like small strands of wiry, black pasta.

Wakame: Similar to kombu, wakame is commonly used to make miso soup.

HERB AND SPECIALTY SALTS

If you are going to use salt, I suggest you try Himalayan Crystal Salt or Sea Salt. They differ from table salt, which is mainly sodium chloride, in that they are nature's original crystal salts and contain trace elements and minerals.

Himalayan Crystal Salt

Himalayan crystal salt is purportedly one of the most beneficial and cleanest salts available on the planet today, as it contains no impurities from environmental pollutants. This salt is becoming famous for its abundance of minerals and life-sustaining properties. It is taken from sources where the energy of the sun has dried up the original, primal sea millions of years ago or from veins in salt mountains where sufficient pressure was available to form the crystalline structure. Himalayan crystal salt contains a very high mineral content with all of the elements found in the human body, and these are easily absorbed and metabolized by the human cells. Most types are stone-ground, hand-washed and prepared. This has been called the "king salt" because it was historically reserved for royalty. It can be found in most health food stores and gourmet specialty stores.

Sea Salt

Sea salt is a broad term and generally refers to unrefined salt derived directly from a living ocean or sea. It is harvested through channeling ocean water into large clay trays where the sun and wind evaporate the moisture naturally. Manufacturers of sea salt typically don't refine sea salt as much as other kinds of salt, so it still contains traces of other minerals. Celtic Sea Salt is most popular but other types include French, Italian, Hawaiian and New Zealand.

Herb Salts

There are also all kinds of wonderful herb salts, which are made up of sea salt, dried herbs and even dehydrated vegetables. My favorite brand is *Herbamare.* You can make your own herb salt by mixing sea salt or Himalayan rock salt and your favorite dried herbs—experiment, you may find many different combinations you like.

PASS THE POTASSIUM!

A good way to gain balance as you cut back on your salt intake is to increase your potassium intake. If you are like most Americans, you have a potassium-to-sodium intake ratio of less than 1:2. In other words, you eat twice as much salt as potassium. Many nutritional experts believe the optimum daily potassium-to-sodium ratio is more than 5:1 (five times more potassium than sodium), which is 10 times higher than the average intake of potassium.

In general, if you want to insure that your potassium-to-sodium ratio is optimal, just eat lots of fresh fruits and vegetables. Most fruits and vegetables have a potassium-to-sodium ratio of at least 50:1.

Common (and delicious!) examples of potassium-rich foods		
Ratio of Potassium to One Part of Sodium		
	Postassium	Sodium
Apples	440	1
Bananas	260	1
Oranges	110	1
Potatoes	90	1

Or, if you own a dehydrator, you can dry celery, which is naturally high in sodium, and therefore adds a salty flavor. Grind the dried celery up in a food processor and sprinkle the result on your food for a very satisfying salt substitute.

As you can see, it won't be that difficult after all to kick the salt habit—that is once you incorporate the use of these many alternatives into your life! Be creative and have fun. For instance, one other salt-substitute you may have never thought of is to serve lemon wedges with meals. The tart lemon juice makes a great salt substitute (and it's loaded with vitamin C!). And here's one last tip: There's nothing better than having several shakers full of dried spices on the table. Try onion and garlic powders, or cayenne, my personal favorites when I visit up north in the winter!

SOMETHING TO CHEW ON

Once again, I'd like to stress paying attention to your own body's signals. There is a "just right" amount of salt for you.

If you feel that you may have a sodium imbalance in your body, there is a way to determine whether or not that is true—get a simple nutrient analysis test done. If you have a sodium level below 137, you may need to increase your sodium intake slightly. If your sodium level falls between 137 and 144, you will most likely do best with moderate levels of sodium in your diet—which is about 2,000 milligrams a day. If you have a sodium blood-level above 144, it's best for you to eliminate unnecessary salt from your diet.

Now remember to be kind to yourself as you make this change in your diet, or in any area of your life. Loving yourself is the key and having an intention to change is 90% of the battle. I used to be a salt addict, and because of that, I sprinkled nearly everything I ate with it. Plus I ate at least a handful of potato chips almost every day! Now that I live near the ocean and I swim in the salt water each morning, I find that my salt craving has naturally lessened. And even if you don't live by the ocean, you can get your "taste of the sea" by using sea salt as opposed to iodized table salt.

At this point, I can't remember the last time I held a salt shaker.

SOUL-FULL EXERCISE #22

Try using fresh herbs and spices in some of your favorite dishes—instead of salt. See this as an experiment in creativity, instead of a dry mandate to give up something. In fact, you don't have to give up salt at all; just begin using more herbs and see if you feel satisfied using less salt after introducing the variety of new tastes into your life.

It's best to use herbs and spices that are fresh and at their peak flavor. You can tell a fresh herb or spice by its fresh, strong, distinctive aroma. A wide variety of fresh herbs and spices are available in most health food stores and supermarket produce sections. Buy organic herbs and spices whenever possible.

CHAPTER TWENTY-THREE

Kicking Caffeine

Grounds for Change

"Caffeine can't provide energy, only chemical stimulation and an induced emergency state that can lead to irritability, mood swings, and panic attacks."
~ Stephen Cherniske, author of *Caffeine Blues*

CONSIDER COFFEE CONSUMPTION as an illustration of the inseparable link between the individual and the collective whole. The love of coffee is crossing all boundaries as well as bridging the gap between generations.

For instance, go into any java joint, such as Starbucks, and it seems that at any time of the day or night, you could easily see a group of college students cramming for exams—their bikes chained to the meters out in front—and then at the tables right next to them, professionals—whose Volvos and Jaguars are parked next to the bicycles. Inside they all sit side-by-side, drinking their lattes, espressos and mochaccinos.

And recently, due to the politically correct theme adopted by Starbucks and so many of their competitors, terms such as "certified organic," "shade grown," and "fair trade" are becoming increasingly mainstream. So is expecting the hefty price tags that come with "guaranteeing farmers a living wage." Could it be that through this latest caffeine consumption craze, the public is waking up to more than they'd expected—perhaps global awareness?

That is the best case scenario.

A SOUL-FULL LOOK AT YOUR CUP OF JAVA

"After a prolonged 'caffeinism,' your body enters a state of adrenal exhaustion. Your caffeine consumption has simply pushed your adrenal glands so much that they've burned out."

~ Gayle Reichler, MS, RD, CDN

Actually, the average consumer is entirely oblivious to the fact that coffee is the root of widespread social ills, such as deforestation, pollution and loss of biodiversity—or that it also has the potential to reverse these problems. The real reason that there seems to be so much "consciousness speak" at most coffee establishments is that coffee growing is greatly affecting our environment.

This shouldn't be a surprise. What is not Soul-supportive of the microcosm (the little world) is not Soul-supportive of the macrocosm (the larger world), and visa versa. Your body is one of the microcosms, so when you've had one too many cups of coffee or tea and then go out to greet the world—the macrocosm—the caffeine you've consumed affects your ability to make sound decisions—let alone Soul-Full ones. But due to the widespread lack of mindfulness, most people don't equate that second or third cup of coffee with getting irrational and irate when they are cut off in traffic, or when they blow up at their children, or just feel overall tired and lousy at certain times throughout the day. And according to a recent study done at Johns Hopkins University, which examined over 170 years of research on caffeine, true caffeine addiction can occur from drinking only one cup of coffee a day.

Caffeine stresses your body and numbs your emotions with a surface solution—*a quick fix.* The more effective you are at running from yourself, the harder it becomes to be in touch with your Soul (or to recognize your True Self). Relationships suffer, and ultimately the world suffers, when we collectively have no baseline of peace upon which to build our personal connections and society.

So many people tangibly feel the sub-par quality that their lives have taken on, and that one extra cup of coffee does not help matters. It just helps to numb us to the reality of a less-than-fulfilling life.

Beyond the need to silence their inner warning system, another reason that many people find themselves attached to the "small" addictions of caffeine is that their bodies are not receiving the proper nutrition they need to feel energetic and awake in a natural way. For this reason, trying to quit caffeine—or anything—without first having the support of a nutritious diet that provides you with all necessary vitamins, minerals and proteins can seem like torture. You would be surprised to discover how easy it is to feel vibrant, alert and satisfied when having nutritious meals instead of running through the day propped up on caffeine.

CAFFEINE AND YOUR HEALTH

Many health professionals are now advising their patients to cut down on caffeine consumption or eliminate it from their diets entirely. And for good reason! Just one cup of coffee, tea or other caffeine-containing beverage can lead to an increase in blood pressure and provoke feelings of stress. Plus, with that cup of morning coffee, you set a pressured tone for your entire day. Alternatively, many who've cut back their caffeine consumption find that they feel better physically and emotionally. Their energy levels increase, and they have less headaches. Without the caffeine, people feel more balanced and optimistic.

So there's a lot more to consider than just flavor when buying your cup of 'joe'. Consider your health and the health of the planet as well.

EMERGING OPTIONS

Is your coffee organic, shade grown, free trade, and supportive of giving the growers a living wage?

Most of the big coffee companies appear to be moving in a sustainable direction. However, consider the fact that while a number of small companies sell 100% fair trade coffee, larger companies, such as Starbucks and Green Mountain, buy just 1 to 12%. Plus it has been difficult for consumers to know which locations of these chains offer these options and when.

With such larger companies, we see marketing dollars go to small projects that look good; however, this is largely because activists have forced the environmental issues and many core issues still remain unaddressed. As a consumer, see to it that the momentum towards sustainability continues by voicing your opinion—and through your spending. Applaud and support those companies that make an effort toward sustainability.

Shade Grown

Traditionally, coffee plants are grown in the shade under the canopy of taller trees in tropical rainforests, and they share the same space with orchids, orange and lime trees, and bananas. They support a plethora of wildlife—from salamanders to parrots and a vast array of other exotic birds, to bats, monkeys, anteaters and wild boars. The Audubon Society reports that a shade coffee-farm may have more than 100 species of plants, and one study counted 793 species of insects and spiders on a single farm.

But as demand for coffee has increased, coffee farmers have been replacing native shade-grown coffee over time with a high-yield, low-quality hybrid. And with the help of industrial chemicals, the new plants can be grown in open fields. These monocultures have almost no biodiversity value at all! In fact, to grow coffee in full-sun, farmers must kill all other forms of organisms in their fields—not just insects, but also competing plants.

According to the Rainforest Alliance, the switch to monocultures has led to increased runoff and erosion, as well as the reduction of wildlife habitat and deforestation. Environmentalists see habitat loss as one of the planet's biggest threats, and coffee production has engulfed and destroyed its share. It has been the second leading cause of rainforest destruction in recent years. In heavily deforested Haiti, almost 80% of their tree-cover loss comes from coffee production.

Note: Another reason to purchase only shade-grown coffee is pleasing the connoisseurs. It not only has a higher quality, but also tends to taste better.

Organic

Shade-grown coffee is much more likely to be organic coffee. Since full-sun plantations are not protected by the rich rain-forest canopy, they lack the natural fertilizer and pest control provided by the surrounding environment. As a result, they require heavy loads of chemical pesticides and fertilizers. While research suggests that these chemicals pose little risk to consumers (since they may be burned off in the final product during the roasting process), they can have a huge effect on the environment and on workers in host countries.

"Caffeine is the #1 cause of headache."

~ Gary Null, author of *Kiss Your Fat Goodbye*

Free Trade and Living Wage

Coffee is the principal commercial crop of over a dozen countries, half of which earn 25 to 50% of their foreign cash from its export. Unfortunately for the world's java growers, less than 10% of the commodity's $60 billion annual value makes its way into the hands of the farmers. About half of the world's coffee has been controlled by four corporations: Nestle (Nescafé is the world's number one java brand), Kraft (brands include Maxwell House and Kenco), Procter and Gamble (Folgers and Millstone) and Sara Lee (Chock Full o'Nuts and Hill Bros.). Despite the hardships faced by coffee growers in recent years, these companies have earned robust profits, with profit margins as high as 25% according to the publication, *The Washington Monthly*. This is much higher than those for most other food products.

Tea

Like coffee, the temporary relief from fatigue that tea provides is a big reason for its popularity. On average, tea offers one-half to one-third less caffeine than coffee.

All teas have roughly the same caffeine content. However, how much caffeine a particular cup of tea contains depends on the brewing technique and time as well as the leaf size and variety.

To reduce the amount of caffeine in the tea you drink, brew the tea with slightly cooler water and for a shorter period of time. Green, white and lightly oxidized oolong teas are good choices, as they tend to benefit from lower-water temperatures and shorter steeping times.

To avoid caffeine altogether when drinking tea, try the decaffeinated or herbal tea products. You can find a vast array in any supermarket. Kombucha (pronounced kom-Boo-cha), which is fairly new on the market, is one of my favorite herbal teas. It is a handmade Chinese tea that is delicately cultured for 30 days. During this time, essential nutrients form like active enzymes, viable probiotics, amino acids and antioxidants. Instead of sapping your body of energy the way caffeine does, this elixir works with the body to restore balance and vitality. You can find it at health food stores, such as Whole Foods.

Although I have read many reports of the benefits and healing properties of green and white tea, my personal preference is to avoid caffeinated teas altogether.

KNOW YOUR CAFFEINE DRINKS

Coffee and tea are not the only beverages that contain caffeine. Here is a list showing the caffeine content of any popular drinks:

Caffeine Content of Beverages

Sodas, Energy Drinks	*Mg. per 8 ounce drink*
7-Up	0
A&W Creme Soda	29
A&W Diet Creme Soda	22
A&W Root Beer	0
Aspen	36
Barq's Root Beer	23
Big Red	38
Canada Dry Cola	30
Canada Dry Diet Cola	1.2
Cherry Coke	34
Coca-Cola Classic	34
Coke C2	34
Diet Barq's Root Beer	0
Diet Cherry Coke	34
Diet Coke	45.6
Diet Coke with Lemon	45.6
Diet Coke with Lime	45.6
Diet Dr. Pepper	41
Diet Pepsi	36
Diet Pepsi Twist	36
Diet RC	43
Diet Rite Cola	0
Diet Sunkist Orange	41
Diet Vanilla Coke	45.6
Diet Wild Cherry Pepsi	36
Dr. Pepper	41
Fresca	0
Jolt	71.2
Kick Citrus	54
Lemon Coke	34
Lipton Brisk, All Varieties	9
Mellow Yellow	52.8
Minute Maid Orange	0
Mountain Dew	55
Mountain Dew—Diet	55
Mountain Dew Code Red	55
Mr. Pibb	40
Mug Root Beer	0
Nestea Sweet Iced Tea	26.5
Nestea Unsweetened Iced Tea	26
Pepsi One	55.5

Sodas, Energy Drinks	*Mg. per 8 ounce drink*
Pepsi Twist	37.5
Pepsi—Wild Cherry	38
Pepsi-Cola	37.5
RC Cola	43
Red Bull (only 8.2 ozs!)	80
Red Flash	40
Ruby Red	39
Shasta Cherry Cola	44.4
Shasta Cola	44.4
Shasta Diet Cola	44.4
Sierra Mist	0
Slice	0
Slim-Fast Cappuccino Delight	40
Slim-Fast Chocolate Flavors	20
Snapple Flavored Teas	31.5
Snapple Sweet Tea	12
Sprite	0
Storm	38
Sugar-Free Mr. Pibb	40
Sundrop Orange	0
Sunkist Orange	40
Surge	51
Tab	46.8
Vanilla Coke	34

Coffee, Teas	*Mg. per 8 ounce drink*
Coffee, Brewed	80 to 135
Coffee, Brewed Decaf	2 to 4
Coffee, Drip	115 to 175
Coffee, Espresso (only 2 ozs)	100
Coffee, Instant	65 to 100
Coffee, Instant Decaf	2 to 3
Hot Cocoa	14
Tea, Brewed, imported (avg.)	60
Tea, Brewed, U.S. brands (avg.)	40
Tea, Green	15
Tea, Iced	47
Tea, Instant	30

Note: When discerning whether or not you will give up that caffeinated soda, consider this as well. A glass of Coke is the equivalent of a piece of chocolate cake, in terms of sugar.

Chocolate

> *"Research tells us that fourteen out of any ten individuals like chocolate."*
> ~ Sandra Boynton

Like coffee, chocolate is popular in developed countries, but grown largely in the developing world. It is also derived from what are known as beans, and grown traditionally under the canopy of taller trees in the shady tropical rainforests, sharing its home with a wide range of wildlife.

Another parallel with coffee is that chocolate farmers have also discovered they can successfully grow a high-yield, albeit low quality hybrid cocoa, in open fields with the help of industrial chemicals. In order to make a living in this highly competitive market, many farmers have been replacing native shade-grown cocoa with a product that is not only inferior, but that has a detrimental impact on the environment. Again, just as with coffee, this switch has led to increased runoff and erosion, deforestation and reduction of wildlife habitat.

And there's another, even more devastating woe. While the many privileged children in the world munch on their chocolate bars, they are oblivious to the fact that hundreds of thousands of children are being exploited on African cocoa farms. These African youngsters are foregoing an education to do what is often dangerous work, only to take home from $30 to $108 per year. This is despite the fact that the major food company's profits are astronomically higher in comparison.

THE GOOD NEWS

Many coalitions and cooperatives have been started in hopes of abolishing unsustainable practices related to the growth of coffee and chocolate. They are helping to establish new standards for worker treatment and conservation of wildlife, water and soil. Find out more about them.

And if you feel an inner urge to be of help or service in the world, think of this chapter the next time you are about to grab that second or third cup of coffee. Ask yourself if doing so is in your best interest. Also, consider this: *"When thinking of helping to solve the world's problems, that on a large-scale may appear unsolvable, perhaps the best place to start is with ourselves."*

Finally, remember, you can mindfully eat chocolate by purchasing only fair trade and organic certified chocolates. They are increasingly available from a number of companies, such as Rainforest Chocolates, Newman's Own, Yachana Gourmet, Dagoba, Equal Exchange, and Ithaca Fine Chocolates.

RESOURCES

—*ORGANIZATIONS*

The Institute for Coffee Studies
www.mc.vanderbilt.edu/coffee; phone: (615) 322-3527

National Coffee Association
www.ncausa.org; phone: (212) 766-4007

Oxfam America
Oxfam is a confederation of 12 organizations working together with over 3,000 partners in more than 100 countries to find lasting solutions to poverty, suffering and injustice.
www.oxfamamerica.org; phone: (800) 77-OXFAM

Rainforest Alliance
www.rainforest-alliance.org; phone: (888) MY-EARTH

National Audubon Society
1901 Pennsylvania Ave. NW
Suite 1100
Washington, DC 20006
www.audubon.org; phone: (202) 861-2242

—*SUSTAINABLE COFFEE*

Audubon Coffee
Audubon-branded coffee is 100% organic, shade grown and habitat friendly.
www.auduboncoffeeclub.com; phone: (800) 829-1300

Café Canopy
Offers shade-grown, organic coffees certified by the Smithsonian Migratory
Bird Center's standards.
www.shade-coffee.com; phone: (858) 449-4033

Café Campesino
Specializes in organic, fair-trade coffee directly imported from single locations,
as opposed to blends.
www.cafecampesino.com; phone: (888) 532-4728

Caffe Sanora
Organic coffee that is roasted using a patented method to preserve more
natural antioxidants.
www.caffesanora.com; phone: (512) 732-8300

Dean's Beans
All Dean's coffees are 100% fair-trade, and the company supports small-scale
assistance projects in producing regions.
www.deansbeans.com; phone: (800) 325-3008

Equal Exchange
The US's oldest and largest fair-trade seller, Equal Exchange offers a range of certified goods from coffee and tea to chocolate and t-shirts.
www.equalexchange.com; phone: (781) 830-0303

Grounds for Change
This Pacific Northwest-based company hand-roasts organic, fair-trade and shade-grown coffee to order, and offsets its greenhouse gases from operations.
www.groundsforchange.com; phone: (800) 796-6820

Jim's Organic Coffee
Jim's was one of the first to roast organic coffee, and the firm continues to offer 100% organic, shade-grown coffee that is bought at fair prices. They donate to Child Aid, WaterAid and other charitable efforts.
www.jimsorganiccoffee.com; phone: (866) 546-7674

Peace Coffee
All coffees are shade grown, organic and fair-trade.
www.peacecoffee.com; phone: (888) 324-7872

Thanksgiving Coffee Company
Sells shade-grown, organic and fair-trade coffees, as well as other "cause coffee," such as a line aimed at ending the embargo against Cuba and one from a Ugandan co-op of Jewish, Muslim and Christian farmers.
www.thanksgivingcoffee.com; phone: (800) 648-6491

Wild Forest Coffee
Diego Llach's El Salvador coffee is grown under Rainforest Alliance principles.
www.wildforestcoffee.com; phone: (503) 263-4284

—*CHOCOLATES*

Organic Chocolate—The Definitive Guide (in the UK) from
Organicfood.co.uk.
www.organicfood.co.uk/inspiration/chocolate.html

Dagoba Organic Chocolate Company
www.dagobachocolate.com/

Newman's Own Organic Chocolate
www.newmansownorganics.com

Nature's First Law
For the serious chocolate lover—raw cacao (chocolate) beans and powder.
www.rawfood.com

SOMETHING TO CHEW ON

Caffeine withdrawal headaches can be incapacitating. Often they are accompanied by fatigue as your body starts to recuperate from its former caffeine-driven pace. It may interest you to know why you get a headache when you cut back on coffee consumption. Caffeine acts as a powerful vasoconstrictor in the brain. That is, it constricts blood vessels in the brain and decreases circulation! When caffeine is not present, the sudden increased circulation causes headaches. While this keeps millions of people addicted to the caffeine habit, the good news is that you can avoid this pitfall by slowly weaning yourself off caffeine over a two-to-three week period.

In an article in EMagazine, researcher Thomas dePaulis of Vanderbilt University's Institute for Coffee Studies (which receives funding from the coffee industry) remarked: "Caffeine is classified as a stimulant, but its effects come from a different mechanism than cocaine or amphetamines, and it is not addictive the way those stimulants are. Caffeine is addictive on a cellular level, in that your blood vessels get addicted, which explains the headaches and other withdraw symptoms when you quit." He added, "Coffee is a health food, and my personal view is that anyone can drink as much as they can stand." Go figure that one out!

SOUL-FULL EXERCISE #23

Do you need a caffeine fix to wake up in the morning? Does your energy take a nosedive in mid-afternoon? Do you crave chocolate? Do you find yourself having trouble concentrating? Do you have caffeine breaks strategically placed throughout your day in order to "keep going"? Pay attention to what it is you are doing when you are tired. Instead of automatically reaching for the caffeine, do something Soul-connecting, such as taking a break to practice presence, journal about your feelings, stretch, walk, deep breathe or drink water. These things help you reconnect to life and feel naturally invigorated.

CHAPTER TWENTY-FOUR

Do Drink The Water

"It indeed requires much effort to find 'natural' water in the true sense of the word."
~ Dr. Masaru Emoto, author of The Hidden Messages in Water

AS PART OF MY WORK, I lead *Miracle Journey Tours* to sacred places all over the world. Over the past few years, we've visited some astounding sites in which the powerful energies present were amplified by the presence of water. In Lourdes, France, the healing waters have been flowing ever since a young girl, Bernadette, saw an apparition of the Divine Mother. This mystical figure told her to dig in an area of the dirt from which a spring of healing water began to flow. Since then, it has become one of the most visited places on earth, with more than 4 million people from all corners of the planet making pilgrimages there each year to drink and immerse themselves in the water with the intention of healing their bodies and connecting with the Divine.

In Avebury, England, there is the Chalice Well, which is fed by two springs of "living water"—one "red" with iron and the other "white" with calcium. Is it coincidence that this sacred locale is also the place where the Holy Grail is said to have been taken after it left the Holy Land? While in England, I heard there is scarcely a well of consequence that has not been solemnly dedicated to some saint.

In Brazil, waterfalls abound with delightful little energy orbs of Light evident to the trained naked eye and visible on film. There, a group of us was also touched by an amazing healer, John of God, and within "The Casa," we drank blessed holy water to open us up to grace and facilitate healing. In India, I've watched village women and young girls fill their jugs with water in the dawning light at the community-well amidst chatter and smiles. Then with agile ease, they balanced the jugs on their heads as they walked home to prepare their family's morning meal. It is evident that this hole in the ground is the village life-spring.

To me, it's no wonder that springs and wells of water have been greatly valued in all lands and in all ages; in some, they've been regarded with a feeling of veneration little, if at all, short of worship.

Interestingly, water conducts energy. When our bodies are well hydrated, we feel better physically. Moreover, on subtler levels, we are also more in sync with "the flow" of life. As a mother, I found out early on that one of the best ways to soothe an inconsolable child was to place them in water. And quite often, when one of my daughters was feeling out of sorts and tired—mentally, vitally or emotionally—just offering her a big glass of water did the trick and set her straight.

Water is *The Great Purifier*.

WATER'S INTELLIGENCE

Clean, fresh water is as vital to the health and survival of our bodies as it is to the survival of the planet. Our bodies, just like the earth, are made up of 65-70% water.

As I write this book, our planet is going through many changes, and water seems to be playing a powerful part in the process. Throughout the year 2005, low-lying coastal areas in various parts of the world have been affected, and in some cases devastated, by tsunamis, storms and hurricanes. Other areas have experienced unprecedented flooding due to excessive

"Our bodies need more water than any other thing we ingest."

~ Edward R. Blonz, Ph.D, nutritionist

rains. Some say it's due to changing earth cycles and global warming, and it's quite possible that those things are having an effect. However, could it be that these changes are also due to a factor that is less scientific and measurable and more subtle? Could it be that the Soul of our planet is calling us to a greater awareness of the need of a greater energy flow in our lives?

Whether we like it or not, the tides are "turning" and we are collectively being called to wake up to *love*. Through these events, a silver lining has become evident; a love has begun to flow towards areas of misfortune. These tides turned a world's focus in many areas from consumption and selfishness to compassion. They moved love into areas that had little established connection to the great flow of the rest of humanity. Then, literally overnight, a surge of goodwill poured forth to these places.

Yes, water is The Great Purifier.

WATER'S MESSENGER—DR. MASARU EMOTO

Many people are now familiar with the work of an eminent scientist, Dr. Masaru Emoto. I first heard of him in 1999 when a Japanese friend showed me his book, *Messages from Water*. I was so impressed with the book's images that I immediately tried to find a copy for myself and discovered that only a limited number had been published and that it was out of print. Since then, Dr. Emoto's work has been widely recognized, and a series of his books are now available in most any bookstore.

For those of you who have not yet had the opportunity to view the miraculous images of water that Dr. Emoto and his colleagues have captured on film, here is a brief explanation of his work. However, I must tell you that one of his pictures is worth much more than a thousand words. Dr. Emoto says that he had always wondered if there were methods of discerning the different "natures" of water. After exploring several avenues, he was inspired to freeze water molecules and then observe them under a microscope. Sure enough, it worked and he began zooming in on thousands of droplets of water, obtained from sources all over the world, to capture their molecular structure on film. What he found and documented is truly amazing, pure water when crystallized becomes pure crystal—with intricate, beautiful, symmetrically configured atoms and molecules. Contaminated water showed deformed, collapsed and warped structures. His photos of water crystals obtained from the tap water of cities all over the world is significantly different than that taken from pure, glacial, spring or sacred sources.

Dr. Emoto writes: "During the photographing, we observed the crystallization process a few thousand times. Then, strangely, we came to feel and see the crystal trying to become a 'beautiful crystal figure' of water, and that crystal pictures carry wonderful messages... We came to understand that these crystal pictures show 'different faces' of water. Water, basically, is trying hard, bravely, to be 'Clear water! I want to be clear water!' We felt such expression coming out from the crystals of water."

What's even more interesting than the differences between piped municipal water and fresh glacial spring water is that Dr. Emoto states we can change the structure of water molecules with our thoughts! When they taped a negative word like "hate" or "kill" to the container holding pure water, its molecules skewed, blurred, significantly darkened, and became asymmetrical in nature. When they taped positive words like "love" and "peace," the molecules took on the most beautiful, delicate and complex patterns—and the same happened when they prayed over the water.

If—as Dr. Emoto's research confirms—water is so easily affected by negative and positive energy, then it only makes sense to cultivate a conscious relationship with the water you drink and use in your daily life.

This may be more important than you think. At conception, water accounts for about 95% of the fertilized egg—in other words, it is almost all water. When we reach maturity, our bodies are 70% water. So it stands to reason that water, along with sunlight and air, influences our lives more than any other factor. We live surrounded by various kinds and aspects of water every day of our life.

Dr. Emoto's work makes it easier to comprehend what goes on with water, and all of life, at an energetic level. Water has a mind of its own—a Divine Mind—that **must** flow. It is its imperative, just as your blood must flow through your heart while you are alive.

WATER—NECESSARY FOR LIFE

As was stated earlier, water, sunlight and air are three things that are necessary to sustain the life of a human being.

Unfortunately, studies show that 75% of Americans are clinically dehydrated. It's no wonder if you consider the foods that are being eaten. A typically consumed fast food meal at Kentucky Fried Chicken—a drum stick and thigh, a buttermilk biscuit, corn and cole slaw—contains 0 oz. of water. The same goes for the following combo at Burger King—a chicken sandwich, french fries, a strawberry shake and an apple turnover. On the other hand, a single apple contains 3 oz. of water and a salad with lettuce, cucumber, celery, avocado, and green peppers contains 1-1/4 cups of water. A diet of fresh, whole fruits and vegetables contains large amounts of water. Given the typical fast food diet, it is even more important to replenish the fluids in our bodies—not with soft drinks or other beverages, but with pure, clean water.

> *"Water is responsible for and involved in nearly every life process."*
>
> ~ Arthur M. Baker, M.A., author of *Awakening Our Self Healing Body*

SOFT DRINKS ARE REALLY HARD CORE

Next time you feel thirsty and are tempted to grab a soft drink, think about what it would feel like to take a bath or shower in it, or any other sugary beverage—*not all that cleansing and refreshing*! The cells inside of our bodies are very similar to the cells on the outside of our bodies. They need to be bathed and cleansed as well. Sugary beverages can't do this—*but water can.* In fact, water can *cleanse* better than any other substance on earth.

Water has solvent and diluting properties. It breaks down particles in the body and dilutes waste better than any other medium. Not only that, but it is one of the most *economical* substances on the planet. It is almost everywhere and is virtually free!

No other beverage is as beneficial to the body as water. And some beverages are absolutely *not* beneficial to the body. As stated above, soft drinks are very poor substitutes for water when thirst quenching is the objective. The corrosive properties of carbonated drinks, in general, are well documented and partial juice drinks often contain more sugar than juice. Drinks can only relieve thirst to the proportion that they contain water.

MORE REASONS TO DRINK WATER

Lack of water is the #1 trigger of daytime fatigue. If you find yourself lagging in energy, and you've had plenty of rest, drink water before you reach for something to eat. A lot of hunger pangs are really thirst signals. Chances are that you're dehydrated and your body is working hard to carry on its normal functions without being able to cleanse itself. Some of the body's thirst signals are headache, pain (local dehydration), dizziness, dry mouth, constipation, dry skin and fatigue. Built-up toxins are very fatiguing to our bodies. We need to continually flush them out of our systems.

Drinking water first thing in the morning cleanses the body. Just as you wash off in the morning by taking a shower, your internal organs benefit from an inner shower or bath. Develop the habit of drinking a full 8 oz. glass of water flavored with some lemon or lime for a refreshing start to your day.

The amount of water needed daily varies from individual to individual, depending on their diet and activity. But, on average, the body loses about 10 glasses of water per day. Five and a half glasses are lost through urination, a full two glasses through breathing, and in a healthy body, at least two glasses through perspiration. One-half cup is eliminated through the stool. To counteract these losses, and to keep your body well hydrated, it is important to replace the fluid. So aim for drinking at least 10 to 12 glasses of water during a day of normal activity. The exception to this rule is if you are a raw food vegan or fruitarian. In that case, you are getting a good amount of water in your food. So you can adjust the amount of water you consume according to your own individual feelings and needs.

A CLOSER LOOK

Water allows our organs and body systems to perform their necessary work. The circulatory system, one of the most important and vital systems, depends on water to function. Water is the medium of exchange for nutrients and waste, serves as the lubricant for all moving parts during exercise, and regulates body heat. All of the chemical reactions that occur in the body depend on water.

Here is how much our various systems depend on water…

- In our **circulatory system**, the red blood cells are 60% water. They carry oxygen and nutrients to the cells of the body and carry waste products away from the cells. The heart, which is 70% water, is responsible for pumping 1,250 gallons of blood throughout the body daily.

- In our **immune system**, the white blood cells, which fight infections in the body, are made up of 10% water. White blood cells must be hydrated to flow freely and fight off disease.

- In our **digestive system**, saliva is 99% water. The enzymes in saliva break down carbohydrates in the mouth before they enter the rest of our digestive system. The proper digestion of carbohydrates keeps us healthy, as well as free of hunger and cravings. Our gastric juices are also 99% water. These juices, found in the stomach, contain the enzymes that break down most of the food that enters our bodies—including proteins. Excess proteins can putrefy our system if these juices are not working properly.

- Our pancreatic juices are also 99% water. **The pancreas** excretes enzymes that digest food, and it also produces insulin. Thus, having ample amounts of water is very important to those who have diabetes. Liver bile fluids that help to break down fat are 99% water. **The liver**, the largest organ, which performs **500 different tasks** within the body, is composed largely of water. The liver is the body's major filtering organ, without which we would die within 8 to 24 hours.

- In our **excretory system**, the kidneys are 80% water. The kidneys are our other major filtering organs. All of our blood passes through the kidneys every five minutes, where it is purified.

- A part of our **nervous system**, the brain is 85% water. It weighs approximately 3-1/2 pounds, but without water it would be only about 10 oz. Drinking water leads to good memory, improved thinking skills, and overall strong brain power. Conversely, headaches, fatigue and memory loss can be caused by a dehydrated brain. In addition, our nerves are composed of 75% water. Nerves are the electronic messengers of the body. To these, water has a soothing effect. Crankiness, anger and hyperactivity can be calmed by drinking water. Many ADD symptoms may also be alleviated simply through drinking water.

- In our **respiratory system**, the lungs are made up of 75% water. The lungs, in addition to supplying the body with oxygen, are one of the major excretory organs of the body. Through exhalation, the lungs help to get rid of one-third of the body's waste.

So think of these very important illustrative facts the next time you feel that you'd like to do something kind and honoring for yourself. Then drink a nice tall glass of water and feel proud for taking care of yourself.

FILTERED WATER

Some people, like me, purchase water filters to ensure the safety of the water we drink. But, fortunately, as the University of Missouri points out, only about 1% of the 61,000 public water systems nationwide fail to meet the EPA's standards under the Safe Drinking Water Act, and far fewer are affected by bacterial outbreaks. Actually, the vast majority of problems with water are purely aesthetic; most people just want their water to look and taste better. So by all means don't panic and stop drinking water altogether if you don't have a water filter, and don't want to pay for bottled water. It is far better to drink tap water than to not drink any water at all.

But consider purchasing a water filter. There are affordable types such as the *Consumer Reports* pick—the *Pur Ultimate Filter* ($40 to $50)—which screws directly into standard faucets.

Listed below are some other water filters that are on the market today.

Pitchers

Pitchers are the easiest way to filter water. You simply turn on your faucet and allow the tap water to flow through the pitcher's filter by the pull of gravity. However, the process takes longer than most people would like. It takes about 15 minutes to filter half a gallon of water. Also, the amount of filtered water you can make is limited by the size of the carafe. The larger the pitcher, the heavier it will be when full. Pitchers range in size from about eight cups to a gallon.

Faucet Mounts

Faucet-mounted water filters treat water closer to the source. They typically have a lever that allows you to select between filtered water for drinking, or unfiltered tap water for other uses. These models are easy to install, and cost about as much as a pitcher or slightly more. Filter cartridges have to be changed every one to three months to reduce clogging and maintain water flow. Faucet mounts are handy if you want to use filtered water for coffee or ice cubes.

Undersink Water Filters

These models are best if you want to keep your filtration system out of sight. Undersink models filter water faster than faucet mounts. Professional installation is recommended, though an experienced do-it-yourselfer could probably manage. Filter cartridges last longer in the undersink models, and generally need to be changed every six months or so.

Whole House Water Filters

As implied, these filters attach to your home's water main to provide filtered water throughout the house. The units themselves are inexpensive, but experts recommend hiring a plumber to install the system. Filters last six months or more.

Reverse Osmosis Water Filters

These systems used to be popular, but since then advances have been made among other filter types, and reverse osmosis water filters are not recommended for most people. Part of the problem is that this process—which pulls water through a membrane—wastes about five gallons of water for every gallon of purified water produced. Also, the filtering process is very slow compared to other methods. Nonetheless, reverse osmosis water filtering is very effective, and can filter out more obscure pollutants like arsenic. They are also adept at capturing dissolved minerals such as iron. That makes them a good choice for well owners who may have these problems with their water. Reverse osmosis water filter systems fit under the sink and require professional installation.

Distillation

Other filtering systems include distillation, which involves boiling water, allowing it to cool, and then filtering the collected sedimentation. The sediment filters help remove large particles like sand and silt.

BOTTLED WATER

World-wide, the bottled water industry has exploded in recent years—with annual sales of more than $35 billion—and the market is still growing strong. Why? Because bottled water has become synonymous with high social status and healthy living. Also, the message is clear; bottled water is "good water" and tap water is second rate. Whether you're in a health food store, a supermarket, eating in a restaurant, working out at a fitness center, or just stopping at a mini-mart for a quick refresher, you'll likely feel tempted to purchase bottled water.

Bottled water is the fastest-growing segment in the beverage industry. Millions don't even blink an eye when paying 240 to over 10,000 times more per gallon for bottled water than for tap water. I confess, I'm one of them. As I write this, I'm sitting at my computer with a bottle of Penta—"ultra purified drinking water"—in front of me. Its label says this water has a unique molecular structure that has been proven to hydrate cells more effectively, and that's not all. It also explains it's known to improve cellular function by increasing alkalinity, aiding detoxification, and supporting production of repair proteins. Now I know most any pure water will do all of those things, but actually I buy it because I like the taste. And I'd have to say, I am a water connoisseur. I've drunk hundreds of brands of water from all over the world in a wide variety of types—including spring, purified, carbonated, oxygenated, mineral, distilled, vitamin-enriched and flavored. But that's mostly because I travel a lot. However, I can easily taste a difference between most tap waters and bottle water, as well as the water from bottle to bottle. My personal preference is reverse-osmosis filtered tap water.

Is Bottled Better?

Here are some of the Natural Resource Defense Council's (NRDC's) findings about the quality of 103 out of the 700 brands of bottled water sold in the US…

The NDRC found that most bottled water is of good quality. But some contain contamination; it should not automatically be assumed to be purer or safer than tap water.

1. The Council reported that government bottled-water regulations and programs have some serious deficiencies—a big city has to test its tap water 100 times or more each month for coliform bacteria—and many times a day on average. Yet bottled water (even at enormous bottling plants) must be tested for coliform bacteria only once a week under FDA rules. There are no FDA standards requiring bottled water to be disinfected or treated to remove bacteria or parasites. (The FDA has stated that bottled water regulation carries a low priority.)

2. Phthalate—a toxic chemical produced in plastic-making that tests show can leach from plastic into water under common conditions—is regulated by EPA in tap water but the FDA does not require this for bottled water. (Check the bottom of your water bottle. You'll find a recycle symbol with a number inside—although typically this number is 1, it's best if this number is 5—which is 5PP polypropylene—a high grade plastic that is less likely to leach chemicals or harmful substances into the water. Other plastics that are not known to leach are #2 HDPE and #4 LDPE. "Single use" plastic bottles made of polyethylene terephthalate [#1 PET or PETE] are not recommended for repeat use because of the risk of bacterial contamination from infrequent and insufficient washing.) Most at risk from the chemicals leached into water by plastics are people with developing endocrine systems: pregnant women and newborns, followed by young children, and women who might get pregnant.

3. Voluntary bottled-water industry controls are commendable, but an inadequate substitute for strong government rules and programs.

4. Bottled water marketing can be misleading. Some bottled water comes from sources that are vastly different from what the

labels might lead the consumers to believe. One brand was sold as spring water, but its label showed a lake and mountains in the background.

5. The long-term solution to drinking water problems is to fix tap-water—not switch to bottled water. The NRDC urges us not to give up on tap-water safety because of environmental concerns (manufacturing, transporting and disposal of bottles affects air, water, our already overflowing landfills and other parts of the environment), public health concerns, and equity concerns (some people just can't afford it).

The NRDC recommendations:

*   Fix tap-water quality. Don't give up and just rely on bottled water.

*   Establish the same public's right to know laws for bottled water as now required for tap.

*   The FDA should set up a website and phone-accessible hotline information system for bottled water.

*   FDA rules on bottled water should be overhauled with annual inspections of all bottling facilities.

*   Institute a "penny-per-bottle" fee to assure bottle water safety.

*   Establish "certified safe" bottled water.

DISTILLED WATER

Distilled water is the purest water. It is excellent for detoxification and fasting programs and for helping clean out the cells, organs, and fluids of the body because it can help carry away harmful substances.

The distillation process involves vaporizing water into steam and then cooling it in a separate chamber or through coils. When vaporized, the steam rises leaving the impurities behind. It then passes into a cooling chamber where it condenses into liquid once again. *Distillation is extremely effective at eliminating most impurities.*

The disadvantages of distillation are the costs involved, the energy needed, as well as the slow output. One other concern voiced by some is that since all of the minerals are removed in the distillation process, drinking distilled water may "leach out" minerals such as fluoride, magnesium and calcium from the body.

LIVING WATER

I have friends who bypass the tap, filtered, bottled water issue completely and just drink "living water," which is the water that comes from organically grown, raw, fresh squeezed or juiced fruits and vegetables and they are never thirsty. Of course, they eat very little, if any, cooked or processed food. So I would not recommend drinking just "living water" to people who eat a primarily cooked-food diet. But if you'd like to try drinking living water in addition to your normal water intake, here is a chart that shows the approximate water content of some favorite fruits and vegetables.

Fruit	Water	Fruit	Water
Apples	85%	Melons	95%
Apricots	85%	Nectarines	85%
Bananas	80%	Oranges	87%
Blueberries	80%	Papaya	87%
Cherries	80%	Peaches	88%
Cranberries	90%	Pears	85%
Grapefruit	80%	Pineapples	85%
Grapes	85%	Raspberries	85%
Kiwi	70%	Strawberries	90%
Lemons/Limes	90%	Tangerines	90%
Mangoes	75%		

Vegetables	Water	Vegetables	Water
Avocados	80%	Cucumbers	95%
Beets	85%	Fennel	85%
Broccoli	85%	Lettuce	95%
Cabbage	85%	Peppers	85%
Carrots	85%	Spinach	80%
Celery	95%	Tomatoes	85%

* Coconut water is another excellent source of living water at 99%.

SOMETHING TO CHEW ON

 Do you drink bottled water or tap?

If your tap water tasted as delicious and was proven to be as pure and clean as your favorite bottled water, would you drink it? The NRDC suggests that the long-term solution to having an ever-available source of pure drinking water is to fix the nation's tap-water supplies. But until that happens and stronger regulations are in effect regarding bottled water, they caution that it's best to observe the rule of "buyer beware."

SOUL-FULL EXERCISE #24

Find out how your favorite bottled drinking-water holds up against your well-water or municipality's tap water. Compare the figures. To get the data, ask your water utility (the company that sends you your water bill) for a copy of their annual water quality report and also contact the offices of your bottled water company.

RESOURCES

The Natural Resource Defense Council

www.nrdc.org

Websites with information about bottled water:

www.bottledwaterblues.com

www.bottledwaterweb.com

Websites about water filters:

www.waterfiltercomparisons.net

www.consumersearch.com/www/kitchen/waterfilters/fullstory.html#into

CHAPTER TWENTY-FIVE

The Soul–Less 7

(AKA, The 7 Energy Stealers)

"My Soul is dark with stormy riot, directly related to diet."
~ Samuel Haffenstein

IT'S THE STORY OF MILLIONS of people across the globe. You get up in the morning feeling as though you could use a few hours more sleep and that it's nearly impossible to dive enthusiastically into your day. But after a cup of strong coffee or tea and "a little something" (most often sweet), you make it to mid-morning at which point your energy takes a nosedive. Realizing you'll never make it to lunch without eating something, you grab another quick snack. Then later, a couple of hours after lunch, you find that you're even more exhausted. So you have a candy bar or another snack of some sort which "holds you over" until dinner. That night, you feel as though the only thing you have to look forward to is passing out until you wake up the next day to start it all over again. What happened to all that energy you used to have?

The reasons why people experience fatigue are many. However, if you fit the above description, most likely you are consuming some, if not all, of what I call the Soul-Less 7, or the 7 Energy Stealers.

I believe the best approach for diet advice is to relate to what you can do, rather than what you shouldn't do. However, I am going to break my own rule this time and offer some insight that I've gleaned from studying many of the world's Spiritual traditions. For those of you who are committed to realizing your full Divine potential, the following guidelines for consumption are fairly consistently prescribed for the sincere seeker—who wants to live in a more peaceful, centered way.

Avoiding consumption of these seven things will make it infinitely easier for you to live a consistently balanced life, to focus on your Soul, and to advance Spiritually:

"What I emphasize is for people to make choices based not on fear, but on what really gives them a sense of fulfillment."

~ Pauline Rose Chance

THE SOUL-LESS 7

Meat

Drugs

Alcohol

Tobacco

Excess Salt

Excess Sugar

Strong Tea and Coffee

Now you may feel like shutting this book and relegating it to a place in the far back of your bookshelf after reviewing this list. So I'd like to remind you that I am not dictating any path or advocating any one way to best attain your own individual Soul-Full experience with food and with life. Nor do I think feeling deprived makes for a happier, healthier existence. I just ask you to read on and see that there are very practical and tangible ways to discern whether or not the choices you're now making are the most Soul-Full ones for you. My goal is to impart information that I've found most helpful, while urging you to take what you will and leave what you don't resonate with. To that end, let me put the ball back into your court as far as these seven things to avoid. Because you don't have to take my word for it. Instead you can try energy testing.

WHAT IS ENERGY TESTING?

"I have many times arranged to meet a client at the supermarket for the purpose of energy testing to see which foods elicit a positive response and which do not."
~ Donna Eden, author of *Energy Healing*

There's a way for you to get tangible guidance from yourself about anything—it's called Kinesiology, a type of energy testing. I've found it particularly helpful whenever I have a question about a certain food's value for me. Kinesiology is a well-established science that originated in the 1960s through the work of a chiropractor, Dr. George Goodheart. It is widely used today by many notable scientists, researchers and healers as a reliable test method. The technique is simple and anyone, not just trained professionals, can learn how to do it with a bit of practice. I don't believe it's infallible, but using it instead of relying solely on outside sources for your information and validation, can be a step toward gaining a deeper connection to the Wisdom within you.

To begin, all that is necessary is for you to see that your body is a streaming fountain of highly complex, exquisitely coordinated energy systems. These energetic parts of you are, in fact, powerful, yet at the same time subtle and intangible—not entirely evident to your five senses. Since you can't physically see, hear, feel, touch or taste them, the logical mind has a tendency to diminish their value. That's unfortunate, because if you solely rely on what your five senses can discern, you won't notice that all of your environment, your thoughts and emotions affect your energy. .

You were born with not only a unique personality, but also a unique distinguishing energy that is found in every cell, system and organ of your body. That's why no one else, no matter how "expert" they are, can tell you specifically what you must do to thrive. We are all created perfectly and uniquely to achieve our own specific Soul's purpose in life.

Although the innate intelligence and capacity of your energetic body is almost incomprehensible in its scope, it is not entirely obscure—it does have physical components. For instance, you have an estimated 72,000 electrical pathways that extend from the base of your brain down your spinal cord. That's your nervous system, and it's how your brain stays in continuous communication with every part of your being. It's an astounding 37 mile-long antenna that is 100% electrical in nature. It sends signals to all parts of your body, including your muscles, but its scope is not limited to just your body. It can very astutely feel your outer world as well as your inner world. When something is introduced anywhere in your environment, your body immediately registers its vibrational impact through your nervous system.

Simply stated, your body has within it *and surrounding it* an electrical network or grid. When you are testing something to see its value for you using kinesiology, you are accessing this grid to connect with your energy body's (your Soul's) wisdom. Here's how it works. If a negative energy (that is, any physical object or energy vibration that does not maintain or enhance health and balance) is introduced into your energy field, your muscles, when having physical pressure applied, will not be able to hold their strength. That's because your ability to hold muscle power is directly linked to the balance of your electrical system. In other words, if pressure is applied to your extended arm while your field is affected by a negative (energy), your arm will not be able to resist the pressure. It will weaken and fall to your side. If pressure is applied while you are being affected by a positive (energy), you will be able to easily resist the pressure and hold your arm in position. This energetic/muscular relationship is a natural part of the human system. It is not mystical or magical in the least.

Using Kinesiology, you can test not only for environmental stressors, but also how you uniquely interpret certain input from the outside world. So you really don't need elaborate medical tests to tell you what is, and what is not, good for your body when built right into you is all the "equipment" you need to discern which energies are beneficial for you and which are not.

HOW TO DO KINESIOLOGY

Some people refer to Kinesiology as "muscle testing" or "energy testing". Here are three different ways you can use it to determine what foods (and vitamins, supplements or stimulants) you should and should not take into your body. Experiment with them all and see which one you like best.

"Life is the sum of all your choices."

~ Albert Camus

PartnerTesting

For the first approach, you need to have a partner. Before testing, always be certain that you are both well-hydrated. Water is an energy conductor, so whenever possible drink a full 8 oz. glass of water before you begin.

1. First align with each other's energy by standing in front of one another, as each of you are taking a deep breath. With the exhalation, focus inward and release expectations.

2. **The person being tested**: Stand straight, hands at your side. Then raise the arm of your dominant hand straight out from your side, parallel to the floor, fingers pointing away from your body.

3. **The tester**: Place one of your hands on top of the out-stretched arm of the person you are testing—just below the elbow—and ask your partner to continue to hold his or her arm out firm, elbow straight. Then, push down, telling him or her to resist. You can say something like: "Now don't let me push your arm down."

Neither person should be straining. This is not a competition, nor is it about muscle strength. The person being tested, if in good health, should be able to easily resist the pressure asserted by the tester.

4. Now that you've established a baseline muscle strength and an ability to resist, you can introduce various foods or other substances you'd like to test into the energy field. To do this, **the person being tested** should hold the item—say a pack of cigarettes or a package of sugar—over their heart or solar plexus (abdomen) with the hand of the arm not being tested.

5. **Tester**: Once again, press down on your partner's outstretched arm after asking him or her to resist.

If the substance is beneficial for you, there should be no problem resisting. But that won't be the case if something is introduced into your energy field that's unhealthy or toxic for you. If so, when your arm is pushed, instead of being able to resist, you'll find that the arm will be weak, and perhaps even flops down to your side like an old fish.

You can also do energy testing on your own. Here are two solo methods adapted and reprinted with permission from the *Perelandra Microbial Balancing Program Manual* by Machaelle Small Wright. No arm pumpers needed!

First Solo Method: The Circuit Fingers

  If you are right-handed, place your left hand palm up. Connect the tip of your left thumb with the tip of the left little finger. (Not your index finger. I'm talking about your thumb and little finger.)

  If you are left-handed, place your right hand palm up. Connect the tip of your right thumb with the tip of your right little finger. By connecting your thumb and little finger, you have just closed a major electrical circuit in your hand, and it is this circuit you will use for testing.

Before going on, look at the position you have just formed with your hand. If your thumb is touching the tip of your index finger, laugh at yourself for not being able to follow directions, and change the position so you touch the tip of the thumb with the tip of the little finger. Most likely this will not feel at all comfortable to you. This is because you normally don't put your fingers in this position and they might feel a little stiff. If you are feeling awkwardness, you've got the first step of the test position! In time, the hand and fingers will adjust to being put in this position and it will feel fine.

Circuit fingers can touch tip to tip, finger pad to finger pad, or thumb resting on top of the little finger's nail. I rest my thumb on top of my little finger. And I suggest this position for anyone with long nails. You're not required to impale yourselves for this.

When you have the circuit fingers in position, they form a circle. If you straighten your other three fingers a bit, you'll get them out of the way and you'll see the circle.

The Test Fingers and Testing Position

To test the circuit (the means by which you will apply pressure), place the test fingers, thumb and index finger of your other hand, inside the circle you have created by connecting your circuit thumb and little finger. The test fingers (thumb/index finger) should be right under the circuit fingers (thumb/little finger), touching them, with your test thumb resting against the underside of your circuit thumb and your test index finger resting against the underside of your circuit little finger. Don't try to make a circle with your test fingers. They are just placed inside the circuit fingers that do form a circle. It will look like you have two "sticks" inserted inside a circle.

Positive Response

Keeping this position, ask yourself a simple question in which you already know the answer to be "yes." ("Is my name _____?") Once you've asked the question, press your circuit fingers together, keeping them in the circular position. Using the same amount of pressure, try to press apart or separate the circuit fingers with your test fingers. Press the lower thumb against the upper thumb, and the lower index finger against the upper little finger.

The action of your test fingers will look like scissors separating as you apply pressure to your circuit fingers. All you are doing is using these two testing fingers to apply pressure to the outer two circuit fingers. Don't try to pull your test fingers vertically up through your circuit fingers.

If the answer to your question is positive (if your name is what you think it is!), you will not be able to easily push apart the circuit fingers. The electrical circuit will hold, your muscles will maintain their strength, and your circuit fingers will not separate. You will feel the strength in that circuit.

TIP—Resting your forearms: If you are having a little trouble feeling anything, do your testing with your forearms resting in your lap. This way, you won't be using your muscles to hold your arms up while you are trying to test.

Calibrating the Finger pressure

Be sure the amount of pressure holding the circuit fingers together is equal to the amount of your testing fingers pressing against them. Also, do not use a pumping action (pressing against your circuit fingers several times in rapid succession) when applying pressure to your circuit fingers. Use an equal and continuous pressure.

Play with this a bit. Ask a few more questions that have positive answers. Now I know it is going to seem that if you already know the answer to be "yes," you are probably "throwing" the test. Well, you are. This is your tool for calibrating your fingers for feeling the strong positive. You are asking yourself a question that has a positive answer. If your circuit fingers are separating, you are applying too much pressure with your testing fingers. Or you are not putting enough pressure into holding your circuit fingers together. You need to keep asking the question and play with the testing until you feel pressure in all four fingers and the pressure in your testing fingers is not separating your circuit fingers. You don't have to break or strain your fingers for this; just use enough pressure to make them feel alive, connected and alert. When this happens, now you have a clear positive kinesiology response.

Negative Response

Once you have a clear sense of the positive response, ask yourself a question that has a negative answer. Again, press your circuit fingers together and, using equal pressure, press against the circuit fingers with the test fingers. This time, if the testing-fingers' pressure is equal to the circuit-fingers' pressure, the electrical circuit will break, and the circuit fingers will weaken and separate. Because the electrical circuit is broken, the muscles in the circuit fingers do not have the power to hold the fingers together. Conversely, in a positive state, the electrical circuit holds, and the muscles have the power to keep the two fingers together.

Calibrating and equalizing the pressure used by the circuit fingers and the testing fingers for negative responses: Play with negative questions and continue adjusting the pressure between your circuit and test fingers until you get a clear negative response.

When you're feeling a solid separation, return to positive questions. Once again, get a good feeling for the strength between your circuit fingers when the electricity is in a positive state. Then ask a negative question and feel the weakness when the electricity is in a negative state. Practice your testing by alternating the questions.

In the beginning, you may feel only a slight difference between the two. With practice, that difference will become more pronounced. For now, it is just a matter of trusting what you have learned—and practicing.

Different Styles in How the Fingers Separate

How much your circuit fingers separate depends on your personal style. Some people's fingers separate a lot. Others barely separate at all. (Mine separate about a quarter of an inch.) Some people's fingers won't separate at all, but they'll definitely feel the fingers weaken when pressure is applied during a "no" answer. Let your personal style develop naturally.

The Testing Calibration

Especially in the beginning, and even sometimes after you have been doing kinesiology successfully for a while, you may lose the strong feeling of the positive response and the weakness of the negative. You've just lost the equal pressure between your circuit and testing fingers and one set is overpowering the other.

When this happens, just back away from whatever you are trying to test and do a testing calibration. Ask yourself a question that you know has a positive answer and test for the response. Adjust the pressure between your testing and circuit fingers until you feel a strong, positive response. Play with this a bit and get a good feel for the strength of the positive responses.

Then switch to questions that have a negative response and play around with the pressure until you feel a clear breaking of the circuit.

After this, alternate your questions between positive and negative a few times and test the answer. In no time, you'll have the "kinesiology feel" back and you can resume testing where you left off.

Don't forget the overall concept behind kinesiology. What enhances our body, mind and Soul makes us strong. Together, our body, mind and Soul create a holistic environment that, when balanced, is strong and solid. If something enters that environment and negates or challenges the balance, the environment is weakened. That strength or weakness registers in the electrical system, and it can be discerned through a muscle-testing technique—kinesiology.

Second Solo Method: The Pointing Finger

Here's a third method of kinesiology, one also recommended by Machaelle Small Wright (author of the *Perelandra Microbial Balancing Program Manual*). It uses the pointing finger of your test hand and your leg. If you have a physical impairment, this may be easier for you to use.

Place the pointing finger of your test hand on top of the center of your thigh. This finger should lay flat on the leg. Your other fingers may be in whatever position is comfortable. Place the pointing finger of the other hand in a face-up position under the first knuckle of the test finger. Make sure you are using the knuckle section, not just the tip of the finger (the first knuckle of each pointing finger should be in contact). The electrical circuit that you are using runs down the center of the leg and you are connecting it with the circuit in your finger. To test: Ask the question, press your test finger down on the leg, then try to lift up the finger of the test hand with the same amount of pressure that you use to hold the finger down on your leg. If the circuit breaks easily, the answer is negative; if the circuit holds and it is difficult to lift the finger, the answer is positive.

So you see that there are ways of independently testing any substance's value for you, even if you are often alone. Of course, you can forgo the energy testing altogether and just ask your Inner Wisdom what's best for you, remembering that you are not a body, but a Soul, and so much greater than the sum of your physical parts! You can ask yourself internally at any time if any action you are about to take is in your best interest, aligns you with balance, and most effectively expresses your Highest Self.

SOMETHING TO CHEW ON

Your Soul is not only your deepest Wisdom, but is also simultaneously a link to all of the knowledge in the Universe. So why wouldn't you use it to gather reliable information? It's already "running the show" whether you acknowledge that fact or not.

Recognize now that our bodies can serve our Souls quite efficiently. And if you fear that thought consider this—if you cut your finger, it's this Intelligence that clots your blood, forms the scab, and creates brand-new skin cells. You never have to remind your Soul to fill and empty your lungs, pump your heart, or make your digestive system run. You do all of this without any need to think about it at all! Cultivating an active appreciation for this part of you, by relinquishing control to it, is a very wise thing to do. It is the part of you that also knows exactly what strengthens and weakens your physical body's energy.

SOUL-FULL EXERCISE #25

After a bit of practice at home, take an energy testing "field trip" to the supermarket with a friend, or alone if it is easier for you. Use one or more of the kinesiology techniques described above to test your body's energetic reaction to all of your favorite foods. For a study in contrasts, test foods that you know are whole and nutritious as well as all of the Soul-Less 7.

CHAPTER TWENTY-SIX

Breathe Deep

"Breath is the bridge which connects life to consciousness, which unites your body to your thoughts."
~ Thich Nhat Hanh

YOU MAY NOT THINK that a section on breathing belongs in a book about eating Soul-Fully, but the air you breathe is in fact your most vital nutrient. The human body can last up to 90 days without food, 60 to 90 hours without water, but only a few minutes without oxygen.

So often we think we are hungry, tired or thirsty when we really are *oxygen deprived*. We don't want food or water; we want to breathe!

I take "a breather," so to speak, one day each week. Every Monday, I fast and I am silent. I do this because I feel I need a break since my life's calling requires me to be with and speak to so many people the other six days of the week. I know that I cannot be authentically still, present and connected to my Soul, nor offer any sound advice, if I do not have time to settle myself and re-energize. So Mondays are reserved just for me and my Soul. I stay still, regroup and deliberately deep breathe. The entire day I surround myself in stillness as I simply watch my breath—the best way I know of to connect with the Soul.

BREATHING—*YOUR* SOUL CONNECTION

"Nowhere can man find a quieter or more untroubled retreat than in his own Soul."

~ Marcus Aurelius

Through my work with many clients the world over, I've found that far and away the most prevalent and universal craving is the hunger to know one's Soul. So when I begin working with a new client, usually one of the first things I do is help them get better acquainted with their breath and see it as their connection to their Divine inner self. I tell the client that they came into this life with their first breath and that they'll leave it with their last breath. In between that first breath and their last, they'll breathe millions of breaths, entirely unaware of having ever breathed most of them—those many breaths will have just "breathed themselves" through their body.

It's miraculous, really, when you think about it. Our breathing continues on and on while we give it little thought. The very thing that keeps us alive is just effortless, which is the #1 quality of our Soul—our effortless Being.

You can deny your Soul, dismiss it, try to drown it out, or cover it up with all manner of activity or consumption. Even so, its small, still, peaceful voice will always speak to you of its innate fullness and wholeness. It never dies—it is Eternal.

However, when you are in the habit of denying that you have a Soul to honor, the Presence of your Inner Self will feel more like an ever-present, nagging voice—a persistent reminder of the emptiness and lack of alignment that you feel. But if you take the time to deliberately stop and listen to it, you will find it is your call home—the way to know your own unique, tailor-made Spiritual path—and if you follow it, you will find it suits you perfectly.

DEVELOPING A BREATH AWARENESS

If a client of mine realizes that they would like to stop living the madness of Self-denial and instead get in touch with their Soul, I often have them complement their Self-Inquiry with the practice of getting familiar with their breath. The key is to breathe *consciously*.

When you were a baby, you knew exactly how to breathe right. (That's when you were closest to your "birth right"—to your access to Heaven, to God, to your Soul.) You breathed in and each breath went effortlessly right down to your belly. With each inhale, your tummy puffed out—and with each exhale, it gently fell. This is the type of breathing you'll want to develop.

I remember lying in the bed next to my first-born daughter, Heather, when she was less than two hours old. I was watching her breathe and having the miraculous realization that if I had cared to I would have been able to have counted every single breath she'd breathed up until that moment, and it would have only numbered in the thousands. I recall thinking about the many breaths she'd breathe during her entire lifetime, and with how many people and in how many situations. And I remember realizing something that was just as profound to me as the experience of her birth—which is knowing that no matter how many changes she'd experience in her life, one thing would be with her through it all—*her breath*.

We each breathe about 12 to 18 breaths in a minute, which comes to about 17,000 to 26,000 breaths a day, over 6,205,000 breaths a year—and, on average, more than 450 million breaths in a lifetime! How many of your breaths have you been aware of? The more conscious you are of your breathing, the more cognizant you will be of your Soul. Why? Because, although your breath is invisible and intangible—just like your Soul—it is also so evidently such a large and vital part of you. That's why a breathing practice is the basis of so many of the Eastern Spiritual traditions. They've been on to something for a long time!

THE SOUL BREATH

Just as a bellows can fan a fire, deep breathing can ignite the "fire" of your Soul—which is comprised of Light. This may sound a bit obscure or airy fairy, but it's true according to quantum physics. Our timeless Self—our Eternal Soul—travels (or vibrates seemingly still—experiencing "the peace within"—its greatest "talent!") at the speed of Light. That's why we can't see it visibly while we are energetically operating at a lower frequency or identifying solely with a physical "I'm a body" perception. So to know your Soul—or the Soul in anything (such as your food!)—all you have to do is shift your perspective. Conscious breathing is one method of changing the "lense" you're "looking" through.

The way to use Soul breathing to connect yourself to your Soul is to inhale gently all the way down into your *tan tien* (a Taoist Qi Gong name for the area that lies an inch or two below your navel). As you inhale, put your attention on this area of your abdomen and sense your breath-energy filling it up. Feel how your belly naturally expands. Then to experience this even better, you may want to put your hands on your belly to help focus your breath there. As you exhale, sense all of the tension and toxins being exhaled with your breath as your abdomen naturally falls and contracts.

While you do this, notice the vital warmth or vibration of the breath-energy that still remains in your abdomen even after you exhale. Feel it being absorbed deep into your cells as you exhale waste products upward and out through your nose or mouth. It's not necessary to use any force or effort in doing this practice. Use only your awareness and intention. Breathing this way promotes a natural state of fullness and completion. See the Belly Breathing Meditation, this chapter's Soul-Full Exercise, below to take this further.

SOMETHING TO CHEW ON

Watch yourself whenever you feel hungry today. Does your belly really need food, or perhaps just a deep breath of fresh air? As mentioned earlier in the book, many people eat in an effort to soothe themselves when they feel stress. But there is a much more effective and healthy way to experience calm and achieve an overall sense of satisfaction that eating can never afford you (when you're not truly physically needing to eat). You can deeply and deliberately breathe.

So next time you realize you're not *really* hungry, remember to relax and breathe with your eyes closed and focus your attention on having a "soft belly" as they say in the Buddhist tradition (which means relaxed stomach). This will help you not only to de-stress and center yourself, but also to turn off the mechanisms in your body that increase your appetite and cause you to gain weight.

And when you're stressed, observe your body—see that your breathing probably quickens, becomes shallow, and races high in the chest. Conversely, notice that when you are relaxed, you naturally breathe low and deep into your abdomen. Shallow, quick breaths cause your adrenal glands to work over-time to pump out the hormones necessary to manage your increased anxiety. All this unnecessary activity and stress not only increases muscle tension but also floods the bloodstream with toxins. And what's the end result of this type of empty belly, one deprived of the replenishing oxygen provided by big, deep belly breaths?—it's an increased appetite which leads to an eventual buildup of abdominal fat.

Ironically, as you well may know, the very weight-loss plans which are supposed to help you to lose weight—such as strict diets and demanding physical training—also cause stress. This can lead to compulsive binge eating and further weight gain.

Note: Remember while doing any sort of physical exercise or training with weight-loss in mind—Breathe Deep!

"When I see patients whose lives seem out of balance, whose energy levels fluctuate wildly, who eat erratically and have unstable relationships, I usually recommend breathing exercises and meditation as methods to restore balance."

~ Andrew Weil, MD

"No matter
what looms
ahead, you
can eat today,
enjoy the
sunlight today,
mix good
cheer with
friends today,
enjoy it and
bless God for it."

~ Henry
Beecher Ward

SOUL-FULL EXERCISE #26

Belly Breathing Meditation

Sitting comfortably and focusing on the breath is actually a form of meditation. Even though this may not burn as many calories as say running or swimming, practicing deep breathing allows you to filter out toxic chemicals directly related to the thickening of your waistline.

The Preparation

Preparing to meditate is like preparing for a good meal. It sets the tone for the experience.

Find a quiet place, without disturbances such as doorbells, telephones, etc. You may want to play some music—if so, a soft, instrumental, contemplative-type of music is best. If you don't have that kind of music, classical music by Mozart, Bach or Beethoven may work for you. I prefer complete silence myself. You can also ignite a candle as a symbol for the Light of your Soul. Many people burn incense.

All of this may seem a bit flakey or odd to non-meditators at first, but there is good reason to set the tone this way. When you stimulate all five of your senses simultaneously (hearing, sight, touch, taste, sound), it automatically puts you into a state of presence quite effortlessly. Meditation music, incense, and soft-lighting also help to activate the right brain. As you may know, our brain is divided into two parts—the left and the right brain. The left brain is responsible for all logical thought-processes like calculating, analyzing and anything requiring a structural approach. The right brain is responsible for our creative ability, emotion, music, art, etc. The better our capacity to align and ignite both hemispheres, the more harmoniously and efficiently our brain works and the more full our life experiences will naturally feel.

(By the way, it's best not to meditate after eating a meal; eating can make you feel tired and less available to your meditative experience.)

Once you've set the stage, make yourself comfortable. There's no specific meditation position required, but how you position yourself should help you to relax and go inside. However, it shouldn't be a stance that is conducive to having you fall asleep. I find it best to sit in an upright position, with my spine as straight as possible. You might sit on the floor in the lotus position, for instance. (If you do, consider placing a pillow under your tailbone for added support.)

Counting Your Breaths

While focusing your mind on your breath, inhale deeply as you count to 10. Next, exhale out completely to the count of 10. Now let your breathing follow its natural pattern. Just count your breaths as you sit silently, filling your stomach with air first, and then the lungs, and exhaling from the stomach first and then the lungs. As you focus on this physical process, breathing will naturally bring your attention to the present moment. Your focus will also highlight the flow behind the usual scattered pattern of your thoughts. When you connect to this flow, you'll see there is a purpose—"a rhyme and reason to it all." No one but *you* can let you in on this secret to life, and feeling it for yourself for the first time is incomparable to anything else. It's like tapping into a big, beautiful extended exhale that allows you to finally relax and *then show up to life fully attentive*. With continued practice, you'll find yourself able to let go of the everyday stuff that clutters the mind and more consistently align with and follow the "golden thread" that runs through and connects all of creation. The objective, detached perspective that meditation and deep belly breathing provides is a wonderful way to experience firsthand how far your mind is out of your control most of the time. It may surprise you to realize that all of the thinking you do is not all that necessary and is actually, as *A Course in Miracles* puts it, a "defense against the moment." You may also find it quite revelatory to discover how much of your attention is ordinarily focused on other people, other places and other times—in other words, situations that are entirely beyond your control—rather than on the present. Forgive it all and just Breathe. It lets you see that there is another, more effortless way to experience life.

Try counting your breaths in this way for a period of at least 15 minutes each day. This practice will teach you that "being in the now" is worthwhile. Anyone can do this, and it is an effortless way to cultivate the Divine perspective of a loving observer of yourself, as a being—not a "doing"– in the here-and-now. I feel that simply observing the breath and forgiving any unsettling thoughts that arise about anyone or anything is the most powerful and direct path to transformation.

Reciting a Mantra

Although optional, repeating a mantra can help you to stay focused in meditation and bring you into a unitive state. At the same time, you can stay open to whatever experience comes up appropriately in the course of your silence. Some traditions involve the repetition of mantras, or prayers, while fingering beads—such as with the Islamic and Catholic Rosary or the Hindu and Buddhist Mala.

The most revered of all Hindu mantras is "*Om/Aum*"—considered to be the Sound of Creation. Ghandi's mantra was "*Rama, Rama*"—a Hindu name for God related to the Sanskrit term for "to rejoice." *Om mani padme hum*," a Buddhist mantra, means "The Jewel in the Lotus of the Heart," and it refers to the Divinity in each person—*their Soul*. In Islam, "*Alhamd-Allah, Ya Allah*"— "Oh, Dear God" is a profound prayer. "*Baruch atoh Adonai*"—"Blessed art thou, O Lord" is a popular Hebrew mantra. You can use any of these, or you can make up your own mantra relating to something you specifically desire to focus on— perhaps a prayer of petition, such as "I Am the Light of my Soul" or just simply "Love."

Make it a practice to start every meal with five deep Soul-Full breaths and a mindful prayer or meditative thought about what you'd like this experience of eating to bring to your life—nourishment, connectivity, wellness and perhaps even a thinner you!

I was just thinking
one morning
during meditation
how much alike
hope
and baking powder are:
quietly
getting what is
best in me
to rise,
awakening
the hint of eternity
within.

I always think of that
when I eat biscuits now
and wish
that I could be
more faithful
to the hint of eternity,
the baking powder
in me.

~ Macrina Wiederkehr
in *Seasons of Your Heart*

RESOURCES

Here are some of the best books ever written—the classics, from a variety of traditions—on meditation and the powerful experiences that can be attained from contemplation. I've also included some contemporary titles.

Meditation by Eknath Easwaran; meditation teacher from India;
     published in 1978
The Cloud of Unknowing by an anonymous 14th century
     Christian writer from England
The Life Divine by Sri Aurobindo, published in 1939
Autobiography of a Yogi by Paramahansa Yogananda;
     Hindu tradition, published in 1945
Mindfulness Meditation by Jon Kabat-Zinn
Meditation for Beginners by Jack Kornfield
Living Buddha, Living Christ by Thich Nhat Hanh

In addition, you might also want to check out these breath-work books.
The Tao of Natural Breathing: For Health, Well-Being and Inner Growth
     by Dennis Lewis
The Breathing Book: Vitality and Good Health through Essential Breath Work
     by Donna Farhi
Science of Breath: A Practical Guide by Swami Rama,
     Rudolph Ballentine, MD and Alan Hynes, MD

—*CDs*
Getting in the Gap: Making Conscious Contact with God Through Meditation
     by Wayne Dyer (book and CD)
Mindfulness Meditation: Cultivate Mindfulness, Enrich Your life
     by Jon Kabat-Zinn

Stepping Up
to a New Plate

THERE ARE MANY APPROACHES to nutrition, some of them ancient, which give wonderful basic guidelines if you feel inclined to follow any one style or systematic approach to eating. I'll discuss six of them—The Raw Food Diet, The Kosher Diet, The Ayurvedic Tridosha System, Food Combining, Alkaline/Acid Balancing, and the Yin/Yang of Foods, and also give some resources which explain them in greater detail. See whether you feel drawn to any one in particular or want to combine aspects of each to create your own unique eating style. Don't be surprised if you notice contradictory information in each of these diets—in researching many eating programs, I found that seems to be the norm in the diet world—which is largely why you are holding this book in your hands. I had to look deeper to find my own balanced, healthy way of eating that is entirely unique to me—and you will too. As you make changes in your diet, stay aware of your body and what works best for you.

Let's first look at an approach that I've touched on briefly already in Chapter 13, "Living Foods"—"The Raw Food Diet".

CHAPTER TWENTY-SEVEN

The Raw Food Diet

"Find the flame, that existence, the Brilliant One within, who can burn beneath the water. No other kind of light will cook the food you need."
  ~ Hafiz, Sufi poet

THERE'S SOMETHING that actor Woody Harrelson, model Carol Alt, Alicia Silverstone, designer Donna Karan, and Chicago-based celebrity chef Charlie Trotter all have in common. They all eat a raw food diet—a way of eating that, due to such noted celebrity proponents, is starting to make its way into the mainstream. But actually this way of eating is far from faddish and has been around since human life on earth began. Raw foods are the foods that have nourished humanity for over 3,950,000 years of the roughly 4,000,000 year-evolution of our species. It is *the* most natural, basic way to eat—following a single, natural path: seed or nut—water, soil and sun—harvest—table.

INTRODUCTION TO THE RAW FOOD DIET

Most raw foodists are vegans, that means they eat absolutely no animal or dairy products. Others, such as Carol Alt, eat raw fish in the form of sushi. The main point is that all raw food is prepared without being "touched by fire." The food is basically unprocessed, or minimally processed, and uncooked. None of the food is heated above 118 degrees, since that is the temperature at which essential enzymes are destroyed and the nutritional value diminished.

Mainstays of the diet include fresh fruits and vegetables, seeds, nuts, grains, beans, dried fruit, seaweeds, and purified water. Some say at least 75% of the diet should be uncooked. Others say 100%. Many people use the terms Raw and Living Foods interchangeably although there is a subtle difference. Living Foods, such as raw fruits and vegetables, have both their "life force" and their food enzymes available. Raw foods, however, even though they have not been heated above 118 degrees, don't necessarily have their food enzymes available. For instance, seeds and nuts have enzyme inhibitors that prevent them from growing into a plant or tree until they have been exposed to water, or sprouted. Once they are sprouted, these enzyme inhibitors dissolve. But unless they are sprouted, nuts and seeds are almost as difficult to digest as cooked ones. (See "How to Soak Nuts and Seeds" in Chapter 13, "Dead and Live Foods.")

I began eating raw food because my Soul was prodding me towards living the most pure and basic way possible. Whenever I eat primarily raw food, I notice that my energy and focus increases and my awareness naturally heightens. I've found it to be a very connecting way of eating. I feel that eating food that's close to its resources of the earth, air, water and fire (the sun) awakens me to the inherent ease of life—as the energy that connects all of these elements flows through me with every bite. I love the sensual experience of eating foods in their natural state, and I love the way eating them makes me feel. Another benefit of eating raw, for the Spiritually inclined, is that there seems to be far less "mind-chatter" when on this diet, most markedly in meditation when you are so tangibly connected to the flow. Everyday graces that normally go unnoticed become very apparent, as often happens when we step away from what is considered routine or "normal" behavior.

Although I have recently become a proponent of a raw food diet, I do reside in Florida where we get lots and lots of fresh, organic produce all year long—not to mention that I live right next door to an organic market. In many parts of the US, and in the world for that matter, it's simply not as easy to get such fresh, whole food year round. My environment is such that raw foods fit well into my lifestyle.

Even if you live in a cold climate and feel the need to eat heartier cooked foods, or if you feel intimidated by the thought of eating only raw food as a steady diet, I still recommend that you try eating only raw foods—that is, fresh fruits, veggies, nuts and seeds—every so often, as it best suits you. Do it just so you can feel the difference between how you perceive yourself, your life, and how you feel in your body when eating cooked foods as opposed to eating them raw.

You don't have to be extreme and go "cold turkey" eliminating cooked food altogether—in fact I don't recommend that approach at all. Just read further on in this chapter, as a beginning. Then if you learn anything new about raw food that prompts you to want to experience it for yourself, begin to gradually add more raw food to your present diet. Even eating one more piece of fresh fruit a day or increasing the size of your typical raw side-salad to a full-meal size portion will allow you to feel a difference in your life.

THE BENEFITS OF EATING RAW

Proponents of the raw food diet say it has numerous health benefits including:

- Reduced disease (and healing of present disease conditions)
- Increased energy
- Improved skin appearance (and reduction in skin cancers)
- Better digestion
- Weight loss
- Reduced cardiovascular problems
- Balanced pH
- Longevity

HOW TO PREPARE RAW FOOD

"My raw cuisine is about discovering the inherent sensuality of each ingredient in its natural state, and then highlighting it in the final dish."
~ Roxanne Klein, owner of Roxanne's Restaurant

It sounds easy. If you want to eat raw food, just pick up an apple and take a bite, or grab a handful of nuts, then chew and swallow. That's what I thought too, when I first started eating raw food. But there are many people who actually prepare raw food in amazing ways. To do so, you have to learn how to use a different set of ingredients than is typical to achieve various textures and degrees of richness. One of my close friends, Peter Cervoni, is a raw food chef. He is classically trained and has worked in many noted restaurants in New York City, such as *Angelica's Kitchen*, preparing raw and vegan fare. The first time I tasted his food, I truly felt I'd died and gone to heaven! There was no feeling of sacrifice or abstention, it was pure gourmet eating—literally! We feasted on guacamole burritos made with avocado guacamole, sprouts, onion, veggies and sauce wrapped in sprouted-wheat dehydrated tortillas and romaine lettuce leaves. There were also falafel balls with cucumber dill dressing, sunseed and portabello-mushroom veggie burgers, and the raw version of pizza! made with a buckwheat, veggie and flax crust topped with pine nut "cheese," red sauce and veggies. And we enjoyed dessert too—chocolate macaroons and coconut crème pie (my favorite!) made with whipped coconut meat and milk and cashew nut crème. Delicious! It was during this experience that I first realized you can actually eat raw and feast.

There's just one drawback to preparing raw food "by the book" with minimal processing—it can be very time-consuming. Everything must be made from scratch. Many people don't have the time or energy (especially before eating the diet!) to make that kind of commitment. So it's not unusual to have the tendency to get lazy and eat nearly the same food every day or to go to the other extreme and become nearly obsessed with food and its preparation. I've gone through phases where I've barely prepared anything and other times when I am the preeminent gourmet. Right now, I am focusing on the "pure basics," since I live alone, am writing a lot, and am focusing on my Spiritual journey. I do just grab the handful of nuts and eat the apple. The most preparing of food I do these days, unless it's a very special occasion, is to prepare an amazing salad. When I do, I put my entire Self into it—heart and Soul. But when I'm just chewing on nuts and seeds or a big beautiful carrot, I love knowing that although my food may not be surrounded with frills, all of my basic needs are absolutely being met, in a most pure and, I feel, Soul-Full way.

I've spoken to many different people at my local organic market who eat primarily a raw food diet and I've eaten with many as well. The variations of foods they eat is endless. Typical would be large vegetable salads made with a mix of lettuce, spinach, sprouts and other greens (key to long-term raw food diets are the greens), plus shredded or cut beets, carrots, celery, onions, radishes, fennel, tomatoes and many other vegetables. Along with that, possibly cold or very slightly warmed soups, and perhaps sides of guacamole or chick-pea hummus with dehydrator "cooked" flax-seed crackers. There is no sign of lack, deprivation or starvation at all in my raw food friends. But I do have to say it is a very individual decision to eat this way and most people

"No matter from which angle we view health and disease, we cannot escape from being entangled in the conclusion that intractable disease is as old as cookery. Disease and cookery originated simultaneously."

~ Dr. Edward Howell, author of *Enzyme Nutrition*

who "go along with it," because a spouse or significant other prompts them to do so, usually fall off the wagon rather quickly. Remember, everyone is unique; each Soul's path is perfect for their own individual evolution to consciousness. What may be right for you *in this moment* may not be helpful or healing for another *right now*. If you choose to eat more raw food or solely raw food, even if no one else you know or love agrees with what you are doing, or wants to eat raw food themselves, that's OK. Just do what you feel is best for you—your radiance will speak for itself.

TWO CAVEATS

First, I personally feel that this diet is actually *best suited to warm climates*, such as Florida, Southern California and other tropical locals. According to many healing traditions, a strict raw diet should not be followed by people living in cold climates. I know that although I eat primarily raw food right now, I feel wonderful when I dine on a big bowl of hot and steamy lentil soup while in Boston visiting my family in the winter.

It does take great commitment, energy and a lot of time to be healthy on this diet. But I would recommend that anyone give it a try, especially if you realize that you've been eating in a less than whole way and feel that your body could use a good cleanse. If that's your case, just remember that on such a pure diet your body will release many toxins that have accumulated in your cells. Some people experience a *detoxification reaction* when they eat raw for any length of time, especially if their previous diet contained a lot of meat, sugar and caffeine. If so, you may experience mild headaches, nausea, and food cravings. Be sure to consult with someone who is experienced in cleansing and can answer any questions about symptoms that you may have.

Something else to keep in mind is that often when people begin to eat raw foods, their digestive fire is weak and raw roughage is not necessarily easy to digest while a body is realigning. Taking digestive enzymes is vital to compensate for a weakened system. Over the years, however, your system will become very strong.

"The fashionable cult of the raw is not a reversion to savagery, but a rebellion against processing, a rejection of the industrial idea of freshness."

~ Felipe Fernandez-Armesto author of *Near a Thousand Tables*

EQUIPMENT YOU MAY NEED FOR A RAW FOOD DIET

- **A good-quality juice extractor**—For juicing fruits and vegetables. This yields delicious elixirs that can be used as soups or beverages.

- **A dehydrator**—Used instead of an oven, this is a piece of equipment that blows air through the food at less than 118 degrees. A dehydrator greatly concentrates flavor, at times delivering products that almost taste roasted.

- **Very good, sharp knives**—You'll be doing a lot of cutting and chopping!

- **A food processor or chopper**—To save you time

- **A high-speed blender**—To transform fruits and vegetables into smooth and silky purees

- **Large, glass jars**—To store foods and sprout seeds

FOODS WITH A WARMING ENERGY

You may have heard that certain yogis can walk for miles barefoot in the snow. And not only barefoot, but also just clothed in a loincloth. Obviously they've got some well-stoked *agni!*—which is the Sanskrit word for (inner) fire.

Until this inner fire is very well built up inside of you, a raw food diet can leave you feeling quite chilly at times, especially if you live in, or are visiting, a colder climate. If this happens to you, here is a list of some warming foods that can be eaten raw that you may want to add to your diet.

- Black and white pepper
- Ginger
- Garlic
- Cayenne
- Walnuts
- Green onion
- Chili peppers
- Nutmeg
- Chives
- Rice wine and vinegar
- Cinnamon
- Green and red pepper
- Caraway
- Mustard greens
- Pine nuts
- Rice milk
- Parsley
- Tumeric
- Squash
- Sunflower seeds
- Chestnut
- Brown sugar
- Clove
- Coconut
- Dates
- Coriander

Note: Pungent greens, like mustard, watercress and arugula, are alternatives to pungent spices.

Other ways to increase your digestive fire are through vigorous exercise such as cycling, rebounding, distance running and swimming. Some raw foodists report that these kinds of activities not only sharply increase their body's warmth but also greatly improve their digestion. There are several Hath yoga postures that are specifically designed to increase the digestive fire. The best ones include the peacock pose, agni sara dhauti, agni sara prananyama, kapalabhati, uddhiyana banda, and my favorite the nauli kriya. In this nauli kriya posture, you place your hands on your knees while you bend forward and on the out-breath pull your abdomen in and up, as if pulling it under your rib cage. Of course this is done on an empty stomach (or after having a bit of a cleansing-type liquid such as warm water with lemon), preferably first thing in the morning. For a more detailed description of any of these postures, ask a certified yoga instructor to demonstrate them for you. All of them are fairly basic and widely known among professionals.

Another option that may seem too easy but that really works is to do a daily warm oil self-massage, Ayurvedic-style (using unrefined sesame seed oil), with a clockwise, circular massage of the stomach area. Just make sure that the temperature of the oil is warm (not hot!) and safe.

AVOIDING AND OVERCOMING PROBLEMS IN THE RAW FOOD DIET

If you choose to adopt the raw food diet, chances are you'll have much greater success if you are aware of some of the pitfalls inherent in this lifestyle from the outset. Here are some of the more common problems that can occur along with ways to overcome them:

- **Physical problems**, for example headaches, nausea, diarrhea, strong body odor, rashes and acne. Be assured that these symptoms are fairly common and due to the detoxification taking place in your body. They are usually short-term. If they are persistent or are overly uncomfortable for you, you can slow down the detox by increasing the percentage of cooked food in your diet or by eating some of the "heavier" raw foods—such as coconut meat, nuts, seeds and avocados. Consult a qualified health professional if any one symptom persists.

- **Cravings**, for undesirable foods, often continue until your body is rid of toxins. You can avoid succumbing to them by substituting suitable raw foods, for example:

    For sugar cravings—Sweet fruits (such as berries and mangos), dried fruits (apricots, dates, figs), carrot or beet juice, and comb honey (use sparingly!) often satisfy.

    For salt cravings—Seaweeds, tomatoes and celery juice are good.

For fatty food cravings—Raw sesame tahini, avocados, soaked nuts, coconut and raw dairy are great substitutes.

- **Incessant Hunger**, even when you feel full, is sometimes *a result of feeling deprivation*. This could be a result of too narrow or restrictive an approach. Expand your diet to include a wide-array of living and raw foods. Get some raw "cookbooks" and experiment. Try filling up all of your senses when you eat and practice caring for your subtle bodies as explained in Chapter 3, "Be Mind-Full." Eat mindfully in a non-stressed environment. And do consider that your body may be telling you something. Listen to its wisdom. Perhaps you need more calories, fats or protein or are deficient in certain vitamins and/or minerals. Pay attention to a consistent call of any kind and honor it.

- **Excess Energy**, is a result of the substantial energy available from the diet that must be burned in some way. Meditation and yoga are helpful to calm your nerves and simple, deep breathing is not only simple but *the* most effective way I know of to center and relax (See Chapter 26, "Breathe Deep"). Regular exercise, such as hiking, cycling and running, are all wonderful ways to balance energy. Finally, change your attitude about waking up in the middle of the night, if you happen to do so. Use the extra time constructively—clean house, read, journal or even write a book!

- **Fatigue.** Conversely some people feel extremely tired as their body detoxifies or if they are not eating in a well-balanced way. Assess your lifestyle objectively to discern whether you are not eating well or are needlessly wasting energy. Carrot juice can be a good short-term pick-me-up, but be careful of sugar addiction as carrots are high in sugar. For long-term fatigue, consult a qualified health-care professional as it may be a symptom of a B-

12 deficiency or other more serious problem. A B-12 deficiency is rare on a well-balanced raw diet, but take a B-12 supplement if you experience symptoms such as tingling in the extremities and persistent fatigue.

- **Excessive weight loss** can be counterbalanced by eating heavier raw foods such as nuts and seeds, avocados and sprouted sesame tahini. Raw goat milk also is reported to put weight on people rather quickly.

- **Feeling cold** is common but usually passes in time and sometimes even reverses. I know some long-time raw foodists who say they always feel hot! Vigorous physical exercise often helps as well as adding more spicy foods to the diet and warm-oil massages. (As explained earlier in the chapter.)

All of these symptoms can be easily avoided or eliminated by paying attention to what your body and your intuition tell you, following many of the nutritional guidelines given in this book in previous chapters, and by eating in a balanced, well-thought-out way. Now you're ready, if you so choose, to explore the raw-world a little bit further by eating those raw foods you like best. Enjoy!

SOMETHING TO CHEW ON

Extremists are not uncommon in raw food circles, and you'll find no lack of very knowledgeable, but also extremely opinionated people when in them. After all, these folks have cultivated a real "fire in their belly" added to by the fact that many of them started eating this way to leave behind very unhealthy lifestyles and/or cure themselves of diseases such as cancer, diverticulitis and allergies—and it worked!—giving them a whole new lease on life.

I personally don't find any outward expression of true individuality extreme, since I live in circles where people quite often leave the well-trodden path. However, I've realized there is a vast difference between *trying* to do or be some "thing"—living yet another label—and genuinely owning a new quality of being for yourself. There's a very apparent inner comfort and noninvasive, respectful air about those who are truly and authentically dancing to a different beat and are entirely comfortable with that. It is much different than the attitude generally possessed by those who are out to prove "their point" to the world.

If you want to find out more about the raw food lifestyle, look to learn from those who exhibit a sense of balance and peace in their lives—they are out there. Many raw food enthusiasts are just that—enthusiastic proponents of a lifestyle they feel is diametrically opposed to the way they've lived (and nearly died from living!) in the past.

With this diet, it is possible to find yourself at either end of the spectrum. You might eat near obsessively, since raw food digests much more quickly than cooked and so you are *genuinely* hungrier more often. Or you may eat next to nothing, since the nutrients of the foods are also digested more efficiently. So it's important to listen to your body to find what truly works for you. Approach this way of eating (and all other ways of eating) with balance and a strong conviction to be true to your own individual voice for wholeness.

One of the body's ways of signaling us that it is being over-worked and stressed by our eating too much cooked or processed food is by producing excess mucus. The body creates this excess mucous as sort of a filter to protect our blood, cells and organs from the toxins of an over-processed diet. Then the surfaces of the digestive tract that are meant to absorb the nutrients in food become covered with a mucus film that begins with our tongue and continues all the way through to the intestines. The more harmful the foods we are prone to eat, the more mucus builds up in our systems.

As I've mentioned earlier, I have friends who eat primarily living foods. The moment they ingest something cooked, their body reacts with a runny nose— mucus! Of course, they can splurge from time to time and still stay healthy by paying attention to such indicators and not straying too far from their chosen living-food path. For instance, do you get a little "cold" every now and then? That's one way the body tries to discharge excess mucus.

After reading the above, if you find yourself wondering how much mucus is in your body, here's one way to determine—try running around the block! If at the end of that run, you have mucus coming out of your nose, you have an excess buildup of mucus in your system. If you can run two times around the block, or vigorously walk or dance, while breathing through your nose for an extended period of time, then you probably have clear lungs. By the way, have you ever noticed how it appears natural, and part of the race, to see professional runners spit up phlegm from time to time in order to clear their lungs? That is not the case when you eat mucus-free or living foods, at least in moderation.

If you have not yet experienced Soul-Full Exercise #13, return to Chapter 13, "Dead and Live Foods," and experiment with it now.

RESOURCES

—BOOKS ON THE RAW FOOD DIET

Conscious Eating by Gabriel Cousens

Rawsome! by Brigitte Mars

Raw in Spirit by Matt Monarch

The Sunfood Diet Success System: 36 Lessons in Health Transformation by David Wolfe

Living Foods for Optimum Health: Staying Healthy in an Unhealthy World by Brian Clement

Eating in the Raw: A Beginner's Guide to Getting Slimmer, Feeling Healthier, and Looking Younger the Raw-Food Way by Carol Alt

Nature's First Law: The Raw-Food Diet by Stephen Arlin

Raw Power!: Building Strength and Muscle Naturally by Stephen Arlin

—BOOKS ON RAW FOOD PREPARATION

Raw Food Real World: 100 Recipes for Getting in the Glow by Mathew Kenney and Sarma Melngailis

Dining in the Raw: Groundbreaking Natural Cuisine that Combines the Techniques of Macrobiotic, Vegan, Allergy-Free, and Raw Food Discipline by Rita Romano

Eating for Beauty by David Wolfe

Eydie Mae's Natural Recipes: For the Live Foods Gourmet by Eydie Mae

Living with Green Power: A Gourmet Collection of Living Food Recipes by Elysa Markowicz

The Raw Gourmet: Simple Recipes for Living Well by Naomi Shannon

Raw: The Uncook Book by Regan Juliano

Recipes for Longer Life by Ann Wigmore

Warming Up to Living Foods by Elysa Markowitz

The Complete Book of Raw: Recipes by some of the World's top raw food chefs.

CHAPTER TWENTY-EIGHT

The Kosher Diet

"The Kosher diet is Spiritual. It doesn't promise to make you lose weight or feel healthy, but it is supposed to refine the Spirit, so we can be a living example of a refined Kosher Soul."
~ Aron Moss

WHEN I FIRST BEGAN MODELING in New York City, I experienced some leaner years, money-wise, and so I took a waitress job at a wonderful Kosher vegan restaurant called Greener Pastures. It was frequented by many notable veggie stars, such as Yoko Ono, as well as by a good many of the Hassidic Jewish residents from the East Side of Manhattan. What a lovely group of people!—the very nicest clientele I had ever worked with in the restaurant business. It was obvious to me that their choice in lifestyle and diet truly added to their experience of living as part of the whole. It was then that I felt compelled to find out about the Kosher Diet.

Kosher doesn't just mean having bagels with lox and cream cheese for breakfast. To the devout Jew, it has much more to do with God's command, "You must carefully preserve the Soul." This approach has traditionally included making healthy, Soul-centered dietary and lifestyle choices. Historically speaking, it has always been common knowledge among Jews that what we eat and drink almost immediately becomes part of our flesh and blood, and that once a food is incorporated into the body, it has not only a physiological but emotional effect upon us. Hence, it is felt that eating Kosher foods heightens Spiritual awareness, allowing us to become more in tune with the Soul within us and within the world around us. It is felt that if a person holds to high standards of eating with kosher food, their emotions will be positively influenced and refined so they will have far less of an inclination to be selfish, impulsive or coarse. Instead they will more easily be able to make proper and holy decisions and be more fluid in their speech and actions.

WHAT IS KOSHER?

The Jewish ritual dietary laws of *kashrut*, include detailed instruction for proper food selection, slaughtering, cooking and eating. These laws are said to have been handed down to Moses on Mount Sinai along with the Ten Commandments. As a covenant with God, kashrut teaches reverence for life. Each category of food is subject to certain of these laws.

Kosher, meanwhile, is a term originally used to denote that which is "fit" and "proper." Most often, it refers to foods that are permitted to be eaten by people who observe Jewish dietary law.

Foods may be rendered non-kosher for a variety of reasons including the species of animal, improper slaughtering or processing procedures, mixing of meat and dairy ingredients, use of ingredients derived from non-kosher sources, or preparation of food with non-kosher utensils and equipment.

A Kosher kitchen must include separate sets of cookware and dishes for meats and milk products. Kosher goods, whether sold by large companies or corner butchers, must carry the certification of a rabbinical organization that has overseen the production and can vouch for its purity.

"My mind can't wrap itself around what the Soul knows… ultimately we must be attuned to the world's deeper rhythms and meanings— those that can't be easily seen or measured, only felt."

~ Rabbi Zalman Schachter-Shalomi

Here is a summary of rules for Kosher cooking:

- Meat and dairy are cooked and eaten separately, using separate utensils, including dishes and flatware. All utensils are washed separately as well.

- All meat is slaughtered by trained, certified kosher slaughterers; the blood is then removed according to Jewish law.

- Foods that are neither meat nor dairy (such as vegetables, grains, etc.) are called *parve*. They may be eaten with meat or dairy, but to maintain their parve status they must be cooked using designated utensils and cookware.

- Fish is parve and does not require special koshering. Only fish with fins and scales are kosher. All other seafood is prohibited.

- Eggs with bloodspots are discarded.

- Liver is "Koshered" by salting and broiling.

- All processed-food products, including wine and cheese, require kosher certification.

- Produce must be well washed and checked for insects.

- Passover requires its own set of meat, dairy and parve utensils, as well as Passover certified foods.

- When following these rules, the cooks know that both family and guests are eating food prepared in accordance with Jewish law, ensuring their Spiritual, as well as physical, well-being.

VEGGIE KOSHER

Now you may wonder why there are so many specific rules for the slaughter of animals. In their book, *The Hadassah Jewish Family Book of Health and Wellness*, Robin E. Berman, Arthur Kurzweil and Dale L. Mintz provide the answer. They write that so many rules exist surrounding butchering because originally Jews were vegetarians. However, by the time of Noah, humanity had greatly degenerated and people had sunk so low that they may even have eaten a limb torn from a living animal. So as a concession to people's weakness, permission to eat meat was given, but the kosher laws were given to provide guidelines. The laws say that a Jew's first preference should be vegetarianism; however, if one does eat meat, it should be kosher, which will serve as a reminder that the animal being eaten is a creation of God. So a move towards vegetarianism is actually a return to Jewish traditions and values, and some feel it can help revitalize Judaism.

THE ESSENES

Around the 2nd century BC to the 2nd century AD, a majority of the Jews—more specifically, the more mainstream Pharisees and Sadducees—were adhering to kosher law as given to Moses on Mt. Sinai. In addition, there was another ascetic Jewish sect that mostly lived on the western shore of the Dead Sea away from the towns in simple cloistered communities. They are identified by many scholars as the Essenes, the Qumran community that wrote the documents popularly called *The Dead Sea Scrolls*. They numbered about 4,000 members. The Essenes practiced the seventh day Sabbath, believed in reincarnation, shared material possessions, and most important, practiced non-violence to all living creatures—it is believed that they were vegetarians.

The piety of the Essenes toward God was renown. Their highly regimented life centered on prayer, rigorous work, and the study of Scriptures. Their meals were solemn community affairs, which included regular prayer sessions, especially on the Sabbath.

Living by agriculture and being strongly connected to the earth, the Essenes came to believe that there were hidden virtues in food. Contained in the Dead Sea Scrolls is much advice on eating and fasting as a Spiritual practice as well as a way of healing.

WHY KEEP KOSHER?

Rabbi Kalman Packouz offers two simple reasons why Jews have kept Kosher for thousands of years, and why it is valuable to do so today. First, Jews believe that there is a God who created the world, sustains it, and supervises it. Secondly, God entered into a covenant with the Jewish people, and gave them the Torah. The Kosher laws are part of that covenant.

FIT FOR A QUEEN

I feel that the Jewish tradition, in its observance of Kosher law, Shabbat and the various other holy days, has Soul-Full eating down pat. For instance, imagine if you were told that your home would be visited by the Queen. How would you prepare it? That is precisely how a Jew is meant to greet the holy day of Shabbat, starting each Friday at sundown, and ending each Saturday at sundown. This practice is known in sacred Jewish literature as the "Sabbath Queen." Since the Queen is honored each week, she is considered and treated as much like an old friend as an honored guest, so the Shabbat atmosphere is meant to be both elegant and relaxed.

One of the many ways to celebrate Shabbat is for a family to share three meals together. The first meal, on Friday night, begins when the female figurehead of the household lights the Shabbat candles precisely 18 minutes before sundown. As the Shabbat candles are lit, the tranquil mood is meant to turn the thought of all present from the mundane to the the Spiritual. There are a series of family blessings that are recited before dinner, which is often eaten on the finest china. After the meal, many families enjoy

"As Kosher consumers, it is our duty to realize that our kitchens are actually frontiers of mitzvah [meritorious or charitable] opportunities, including making sure that the food we share is both kosher and healthy."

~ Rabbi Moshe Goldberger

adding to the beauty and celebration of Shabbat by singing songs. Communion at its best!

A NEW KIND OF KOSHER

Kosher law states that no food should be eaten from plates or utensils that have ever been tainted by *trafe* or unkosher food. As a result, disposable plastic, take-out containers such as Styrofoam cups and dishes, and soft-drink bottles and cans, are ideal in the classical kosher sense. From an ecological stance, however, this is disastrous. In his book, *Jewish with Feeling*, Rabbi Zalman Schachter-Shalomi suggests that a new "eco-kashrut" (or eco-kosher) way of thinking be adopted, "one which would combine the ancient ways of thoughtful consumption and avoidance of cruelty and violence with the new awareness of the wider repercussions of our actions."

He says, "What could be more kosher than a potato latke or kugel?" Yet then he raises awareness by citing a passage from author Michael Pollan's book, *The Botany of Desire*: "the typical potato grower stands in the middle of a bright green circle of plants that have been doused with so much pesticide that their leaves wear a dull-white chemical bloom and the soil they're rooted in is a lifeless gray powder." He goes on to question genetic engineering, irradiated foods, and fish taken from dangerously depleted stocks as well.

The Rabbi suggests that Jews adopt his notion of eco-kashrut, a concept that adapts the very traditional Jewish way of asking consumption-related questions to the issues of our day. It is different from traditional kashrut in three ways:

- **First**—Eco-kashrut is concerned not only with the origin of the things consumed—what animal the meat came from, say, or the dishes it was cooked in or consumed from—but also the results of the consumption, such as the environmental impact and human toll of our actions.

"The Torah prescribes a holy diet. You are what you eat. Kosher is God's diet for spirituality. Jewish mysticism teaches that non-kosher food blocks the Spiritual potential of the Soul."

~ Rabbi Shraga Simmons

- **Second**—The consumer is asked to consider all of the multiple interactions a food goes through and the interlocking costs and repercussions that result from eating it.

- **Third**—An eco-kashrut practice is a matter of individual conscience, rather than a matter of mandate. It is meant to be an evolving practice, as over the years our understanding of the laws of Nature grows and the friendliness of our technology improves. Scientists will keep us informed, and ethicists or rabbis trained in the practice of eco-kashrut can help us sort out the results of our actions. But the day-to-day weighing of conflicting considerations—personal as well as social, environmental, and technological—is up to each of us.

What a wonderful way to connect to oneself and the whole simultaneously! Acting in a manner that is ecologically sound may not appear to have much of an impact on an individual basis. However, if we look at the impact of an entire group of people adopting the same practices—such as those that are congruent with honoring the earth—we see that it will have a substantial influence.

SOMETHING TO CHEW ON

Although Kosher is primarily associated with Judaism, Kosher law is adhered to, in varying forms and by varying names, by some Muslims and Seventh-Day Adventists. Jews are thought to account for 29% of Kosher consumers today, while Muslims and a few other religious groups account for an additional 19%. The remaining consumers who buy Kosher products do so for reasons that have more to do with personal preference and health reasons rather than religious beliefs.

Whether you are Jewish or not, try adhering to the original intention of the kosher diet, for a time, which is to eat with honor—that is, not only eat in a way that takes care of your health, but shows compassion to animals, protects the environment, conserves resources, considers hungry people, and pursues peace.

CHAPTER TWENTY-NINE

The Ayurvedic Way

"In Ayurveda, we like to look at everything in a holistic way relative to the entire human being, which is body, mind, Spirit and all aspects of our life and behavior. So we start at the physical level with certain dietary changes—foods that can help at the physical level."
~ David Frawley, teacher and practitioner of Ayurvedic medicine

I PRACTICE YOGA, and not just the physical postures of *Hath yoga*, but all of the many other aspects of yoga as well. For instance, with my transformational coaching work and seminars, I practice *Karma yoga*—which is about selfless service—and *Jnana yoga*—which is the process of converting intellectual knowledge into practical wisdom. I meditate several times a day—that's *Dyana yoga*. I also work with other subtle energies through specific breathing exercises—that's *Kundalini yoga*. In addition, I practice devotional prayer and chanting which are *Bhakti yoga* and *Mantra yoga*. Then I put it all together in a daily practical way through *Kriya yoga*, which is based on "moving with active consciousness." In the Hindu tradition, all of these are pathways to the Divine.

There is another way in which I slip easily into a Divine connection—by eating Indian food. This ethnic sensory smorgasbord heightens the awareness of my every sense—from sight to smell—the colors, tastes and aromas of a well-made Indian meal can bring me instantaneously into Nirvana.

Because of my interest in the yogic tradition, I've been to India three times. So I am very familiar with the Indian cuisines, of both the North and the South. Even though the ingredients of the main dishes may vary—for instance, Southern India is primarily vegetarian, while in the North, they eat a variety of meat—Ayurveda is widely practiced countrywide.

According to Ayurveda, each meal should be a feast for all of your senses. When your plate reflects an appealing array of flavors, textures, colors and aromas, your digestive juices will begin to flow freely in anticipation and your body, mind and Soul are fulfilled by the eating experience.

To be technically correct, Ayurveda is actually much more than just a way of eating. The translation for the word Ayurveda actually means "science of life." And this ancient system of medicine, which dates back to the 9th century BC, uses not only diet, but various other therapies—such as yoga and herbal medicine—to restore harmony and balance in the body. But for the purposes of this book, let's look at Ayurveda's Tridosha approach to nutrition.

THE TRIDOSHA DIET SYSTEM

The principles of Ayurveda are based on the belief that every individual has a need for balance and is born with a unique *prakriti* (Sanskrit for *essential nature*). Each person's constitutional blueprint is composed of a varying degree of influence from each of three doshas.

The three doshas are known as *Vata, Pitta* and *Kapha*. They are composed of the five basic elements (water, wind, fire, earth and ether) and are believed to be dynamic forces, with distinct characteristics that shape all things in the Universe.

In humans, the doshas control all physical, mental, emotional and vital functions and responses. They also determine one's ability to connect to the Soul. They are responsible for natural urges and individual preferences, especially with food. They also govern all of the essential functions of the body, such as the maintenance and destruction of body tissue and the elimination of waste.

"Cheerfullness is as natural to the heart of man in strong health as color to his cheek; and wherever there is habitual gloom there must be either bad air, unwholesome food, improperly severe labor or erring habits of life."

~ John Ruskin

In the Aryuvedic view, if there is an imbalance between the doshas, it produces a condition called *vikriti*, meaning "deviation from nature." Vikriti is the result of an over-expression of one dosha (usually the dominant one) and a diminished expression of another. A person acquires such an imbalance through the stressors in life, such as negative emotions, chronic lack of sleep, physical overexertion, or eating the wrong food. To avoid the escalation of these symptoms into diseases such as chronic fatigue, mental disorders and obesity, you would maintain the doshas, or restore them to their proper balance.

During times of *vikriti*, or imbalance, the diet can be used to either increase or decrease any of the three doshas until balance is restored.

Ayurvedic healers generally design diets for their clients based on various factors such as gender, age, the strength of the body tissues and digestive fires (which they detect through the pulse), the doshic tendencies that need balancing, appearance of the tongue, skin and eyes, and the level of *arma* or toxins in the body. The place where a person resides and the season are also determining factors.

Note: It's unlikely that you have purely a Vata, Pitta or Kapha constitution. Most of us possess a portion of all three doshas and typically a combination of two doshas defines your dominant physiological and personality traits.

THE FIVE ELEMENTS OF AYURVEDA

Ether Air Water Fire Earth
These manifest in the human body/mind as doshas.

There are three doshas or principles/groupings.

Vata	**Pitta**	**Kapha**
air and ether	fire and water	earth and water
dry	heavy	oily

THE VATA DOSHA

"Tell me what you eat and I'll tell you who you are."

~ Jean Anthelme Brillat-Savari, author of *Physiology of Taste*

Vata, translated as "wind," is derived from the air and ether elements. This energy regulates all movement in the body including the flow of blood, our breathing, and all movements of our muscles and tissues—including the heart and nerve tissues and the contractions of the digestive tract. People who are predominantly Vata usually have a thin build with noticeable veins and muscle tissue, and they often have problems with dry skin. Vata people have alert minds, and they demonstrate great enthusiasm, creativity, imagination and vivaciousness. They grasp new concepts easily, but forget them just as easily. Vatas are quick, both mentally and physically, although they often quickly tire. They have little willpower and lack a strong sense of stability and poise, which often makes them act anxious or timid. Vatas tend to have irregular eating and sleeping patterns. They prefer sweet, salty and sour tastes, and avoid bitter or dry foods. For optimum health, Vata people should eat certain foods and avoid others. (See chart in the subsequent "Discovering Your Dosha" section of this chapter.)

When Vata people are out of balance, they often have skin troubles, insomnia, fatigue, poor or irregular appetite, arthritis, increased physical sensitivity, constipation or bowel disorders, cold hands and feet, anxiety and worry. The Vata constitution is characterized by swift change, and as a result, it goes out of balance more easily than the other doshas.

THE PITTA DOSHA

Pitta energy is derived from the element of fire, and it is the force which regulates the metabolism, digestion, body temperature and appetite—the overall homeostasis of an individual. People who are predominantly Pitta have large appetites, strong digestion, and sensitivity to the heat or sun. They typically have blonde, red or light-brown hair, freckles or ruddy skin. They are of medium build and strength. The basic theme of this constitution is intensity. They are intelligent, ambitious, enterprising, articulate, outspoken, warm and loving. Pitta people like cold drinks and bitter food.

And unlike Vata types, Pittas experience intense hunger and cannot skip meals. They can often be characterized by strong feelings and traits such as vanity, pride, intolerance, stubbornness, anger and jealousy. Pitta people are most likely to be at their best late at night rather than in the morning or in the heat of the day. Grief, pressure, fear and excess physical-exertion often have great effect on them.

When out of balance, Pitta types experience rashes, heartburn, inflammation, peptic ulcers, irritability, vision problems, and compulsive behaviors such as alcoholism and eating disorders.

THE KAPHA DOSHA

The Kapha energy is derived from the elements of water and earth, and it controls the structures of the body. It gives strength and physical form to cells and tissues. Kapha energy controls the immune system, vigor, strength, growth and resistance. Kapha people usually have solid, well-built bodies and display great physical strength and endurance. Kaphas digest slowly and have moderate hunger, though they find comfort in eating. They like bitter and astringent foods best, and although they often crave sweet and salty foods, their systems do not work well after consuming these. They do not perform well after eating fatty or oily foods either. They are also not usually very thirsty, and do not require as much water as everyone else. Exercise is important for Kapha people to stay in shape, and they often feel lethargic after long naps. They tend to be obese more often than Vata or Pitta types. Contentment, tolerance, patience and stability are the most common psychological traits of Kapha people. They are slow to anger, forgiving, happy with the status quo, and respectful of the feelings of others. On the flip side, they can be greedy and possessive. Intellectually, they can often be slow to grasp a concept, but can remember it for a long time after.

When they are out of balance, Kapha types may experience colds and flu, allergies, depression, sinus congestion, asthma, lethargy and joint problems. They can easily be thrown into imbalance by cold and damp weather.

THE THREE DOSHAS GO TO A PARTY

To give you a clearer picture of these three different doshas as they manifest in people, let's walk into a party where these three types are gathered. Although, as I previously stated, it's unusual for a person to be strictly one dosha type, let's assume for the sake of illustration that only one dosha is predominant in each of these individuals and the others are minimal.

Bobby—The Vata

Bobby is a Vata, through and through. He's a fast talker, and he walks into the room and quickly grabs the hand of the first person he encounters, shaking it profusely. Mary notices his hands are cold and his skin feels rough and dry. But Bobby's very engaging, even though he seems to jump around a lot in the conversation changing the topic often and not going too deeply into any one subject. That's okay. Before she knows it, he's off to mingle with another group of people. He delights everyone with his expansive imagination and the way he illustrates all of his stories with sweeping hand gestures and other quick moves.

When it's time to eat, Bobby makes a B-line for the buffet table. However, once he gets there, this Vata can't decide what to eat. He picks at a few items, focusing mainly on desserts since he's satisfied his salt-craving earlier with chips and salsa. As Bobby grazes, he talks away with George, who is next to him in line, mentioning in the course of the conversation that no matter what he eats, he usually doesn't gain any weight. For the remainder of the evening, he flits from one group to another, since it's important for him to meet as many people as he possibly can and take part in every conversation. At the end of the night, Bobby says his many good-byes without mentioning anyone's name, because he can't remember any of them.

Claudette—The Pitta

In walks Claudette; she's a typical Pitta. Claudette's really up for this party since she's been in much of the day. Even though friends had invited her to go with them to the beach, she'd opted not to go. It was way too hot for her, since she's so sensitive to heat.

Now at the party, Claudette realizes she still feels hot, so she immediately heads to the kitchen to find herself a cold drink and settles on a huge glass of lemonade. She stopped drinking alcohol several years ago, since she had a tendency to overindulge. Everyone is happy to see her, so she chats with the other guests for a while. However, soon she spies a painting across the room and quickly hones in on it. Her appreciation is so intense that she draws the attention of several other guests who walk over to her and the painting to get a better look. Meanwhile Claudette's looking at it very closely, because she forgot to bring her glasses. The group around Claudette listens to her tell stories about her childhood in Ireland, and the many places that this painting reminds her of so much.

Midway through the conversation, Claudette realizes that she is STARVING. So she drops everything to head to the buffet table, where she fills her plate high. Claudette mentions to her good friend, Pat, that she has to avoid certain foods lately, since she's been experiencing so many digestive problems. She says, "I chalk it all up to stress. It's been tough since Matt broke up with me." Pat asks her why she thinks that happened, to which Claudette tosses back her flaming red hair and replies, "Well, his version of the story is that I'm too strong-willed, angry and full of pride—not to mention jealous. Ha! Oh well, his loss."

She's the last one to leave the party.

Matt—The Kapha

Matt has an entirely different persona from Bobby and Claudette; he's a Kapha. He arrives late, when the party is already in full swing. He holds back for a while assessing the situation before diving into the fun. Matt immediately notices Bobby and decides to stay clear of him—"Too jumpy," Matt thinks. Then he spies a few other long- time friends and walks over to them. He claps one of them on the back nearly knocking him over, and then grabs the hand of another friend with his own massive paw. "Hey, big guy," these friends shout in unison. Matt *is* a big presence, but it's his even-tempered, calm demeanor that everyone loves. "You can always rely on Matt" is the word among his friends. They know Matt's slow to anger and easy to forgive, but he never seems to forget anything. His memory is excellent. So once he shows up, his buddies take up with one of their favorite pastimes and begin riffling trivia questions at him. They listen with rapt attention as Matt rattles off sports scores and statistics from 10 years ago.

When it's time to eat, everyone makes way for Matt, who piles his plate high with bratwurst, sauerkraut and pickles. Later Matt complains that he thinks he overdid it. At the end of the night, Matt says good-bye to his pals and realizes he had a really good time—even though he didn't meet one new person!

DISCOVERING YOUR DOSHA

Use the chart below to determine your dosha. Check the description in the Vata, Pitta or Kapha column that best describes your body traits and personal tendencies. Then total your check marks in each column. The column with the highest total indicates your primary dosha. Remember that everyone has all three doshas in varying degrees.

BODY

	Vata	Pitta	Kapha
Appetite	variable	sharp or strong	low or constant
Body Frame	thin	medium	large
Eyes	unsteady, small	focused, reddish	white, wide
Finger Nails	thin and/or cracking	pink, soft medium	thick white, wide
Forehead Size	small	medium	large
Lips	thin, dry, cracking	soft, medium	smooth, large
Resting Pulse	80 to 100	70 to 80	60 to 70
Stool	gas, hard, small	burns, loose	solid, moderate
Voice	low, weak	sharp or high	silent or slow
Weight	bony and low	muscular, medium	gains easily
Which bothers you?	cold and dry	sun and heat	cold and damp
BODY TOTALS			

MIND

	Vata	Pitta	Kapha
Beliefs	changing, radical	goals, leader	constant, loyal
Dreams	flying or anxious	color, fighting	romantic, few
Emotions	worry, enthused	angry, warm	attached, calm
Habits	nature and travel	politics, sports	flowers, water
Memory	short, quick	clear, sharp	slow, remembers
Mind	adaptable, quick	critical, penetrates	lethargic, slow
Sleep	light	moderate	heavy
Speech	talkative, quick	argues, moderate	silent, slow
Temperament	fearful, nervous	impatient, irritable	easygoing
MIND TOTALS			

Adapted from the Dosha Quiz, www.ayurveda-foryou.com.

"Ayurveda is a Sanskrit word which literally means 'science of life'."

~Albert Camus

MY DOSHA (TYPE) IS: 1st) _____

2nd) _____

3rd) _____

PULSE DIAGNOSIS

Here's the way that I learned to determine my Ayurvedic body type. It's a bit more complicated, but you can use it to confirm the results you found by taking the dosha quiz.

1. Note the speed of your pulse while you are at rest. Is it…

Slow?	Moderate?	Fast?
60-70 minute	70-80 minute	80-100 minute

Pulse	Type
Slow	Kapha
Moderate	Pitta
Fast	Vata

2. Check the pulse in the tip of your ring, middle and index fingers. Note which finger has the strongest pulse. (This may take a bit of practice, but be patient—you'll get it!)

Ring-Kapha   **Middle**-Pitta   **Index**-Vata

3. Note the type of "movement" of the pulse:
   a. **Kapha**—strong, regular, warm, broad (like an elephant)
   b. **Pitta**—jumping, regular, hot (like a frog)
   c. **Vata**—weak, cool, thin, irregular (like a snake)

FOOD AND THE DOSHAS

So you've determined your body type—now what?

Based upon which type of energy is predominant in your system, there are guidelines as to what kinds of foods are most easily digested and used by your body. The Ayurvedic diet recommends foods for each dosha based on the taste and quality of food.

In Ayurvedic nutrition, there are six different tastes and six major qualities. The tastes and qualities that have attributes similar to a dosha increase that dosha, while tastes and qualities dissimilar to the characteristics of a dosha decrease that dosha. Including foods in your diet that have some of each taste and quality minimizes cravings and balances the appetite and digestion. Below I cover the six tastes and the six major food qualities, and their effect on the different doshas.

The Six Tastes

Bitter—The bitter taste is found in spinach, romaine lettuce, endive, chicory, chard, kale and tonic water. The bitter taste decreases both kapha and pitta, but increases vata.

Pungent—The pungent taste is found in chili peppers, cayenne, ginger, and other hot-tasting spices. The pungent taste decreases kapha, but increases pitta and vata.

Astringent—The astringent taste is found in beans, lentils, cabbage, apples and pears. The astringent taste decreases kapha and pitta, but increases vata.

Salty—The salty taste is found in any food to which salt has been added. The salty taste increases kapha and pitta, but decreases vata.

Sour—The sour taste is found in lemons, limes, vinegar, yogurt, cheese and plums. The sour taste increases kapha and pitta, but decreases vata.

Sweet—The sweet taste is found in table sugar, honey, rice, pasta, milk, cream, butter, wheat and bread. The sweet taste increases kapha, but decreases pitta and vata.

The Six Major Food Qualities

Heavy—Heavy foods include bread, pasta, cheese and yogurt. The heavy quality decreases vata and pitta, but increases kapha.

Light—Light foods include millet, buckwheat, rye, barley, corn, spinach, lettuce, pears and apples. The light quality decreases kapha, but increases vata and pitta.

Oily—Oily foods include dairy products, meat, fatty foods, and cooking oils. The oily quality decreases vata and pitta, but increases kapha.

Dry—Dry foods include beans, potatoes, barley and corn. The dry quality decreases kapha, but increases vata and pitta.

Hot—The hot quality describes hot beverages and warm, cooked foods. The hot quality decreases vata and kapha, but increases pitta.

Cold—The cold quality describes cold beverages and raw foods. The cold quality decreases pitta, but increases kapha and vata.

PUTTING IT ALL TOGETHER

According to the Tridosha diet, you would eat a diet suited to your dosha to experience optimum health. And during times of vikriti, or imbalance, the diet can be used to either decrease or increase the three doshas until balance is restored. By selecting foods appropriate for your dosha, you can maintain or restore your proper balance. Here are a few dietary and lifestyle suggestions for balancing the different doshes.

To Balance Vata

If you've discovered that you're a Vata, then consistency is very important for you. Your constitution is characterized by swift change and so you are easily thrown out of balance. Above all else, you will benefit from sticking to a daily routine. Try to have consistent meal times and regular sleeping patterns. It's to your advantage to eat plenty of heavy, hearty foods, such as stews, breads and warm desserts. Anything salty, sour or sweet is perfect for you, and dishes that are heavy, oily and hot in quality are great. You do well with a meat-based diet and you can handle lots of dairy products. You feel best when eating well-cooked foods and drinking lots of warm fluids, like herbal teas. On the other hand, foods with bitter, pungent or astringent tastes and those that are light, dry and cold in quality, like raw fruits and vegetables and cold beverages, are not your most satisfying food choices. According to Ayurveda, if you want to feel your best, these other foods should comprise only a small part of your Vata-balancing diet.

Vata Eating Raw

If you're a Vata type who feels committed to eating mostly raw food, like me, here are some ways to help your digestion:

- Have one-dish meals, such as blended salads (one bowl-salads with the ingredients chopped into small pieces.) and raw soups or stews (sprouts and/or avocados with raw vegetable blended soup poured over them.)

- Use spices to enhance and strengthen your digestion—ginger, peppers (hot/black), nutmeg, etc. The spice will counteract the cold constitution of the Vata type.

- Warm the food up a bit. Anything below 118 degrees F won't cook it.

- Eat oily dressings or oily foods like avocados. This increases the time the foods take to digest, thereby improving digestion. Oil strongly increases Vata.

I can attest to the fact that people with a Vata constitution can eat a raw food diet, since I often do this myself. But it can be challenging, and you have to be informed and make intelligent choices. If this is your situation, pay close attention to your feelings. It's also much, much easier if you live in a warm climate.

To Balance Pitta

If you're a Pitta type, you tend to work excessively when you get stressed or out of balance. It's important for you to avoid over-scheduling and to be sure to balance your work and commitments with sufficient recreation and leisure. To the best of your ability, avoid skipping meals, and try not to overeat.

Pittas are well-suited to a vegetarian diet, so if you fall into this category, you'll benefit tremendously from eating fruits, raw vegetables and drinking cold beverages. Emphasize foods with a bitter, sweet or astringent taste, as well as those that are heavy, oily and cold in quality. You may also add starchy vegetables, grains and beans to your diet. Meanwhile, do your best to eliminate spicy, pungent, salty and sour tastes as well as foods that are light, dry, hot in quality, and overcooked.

To Balance Kapha

If you've discovered that you're a Kapha type, you already know that you tend to gain weight easily and have difficulty shedding unwanted pounds. Regular exercise is crucial for you to help with your weight management. It's best for Kaphas to eat only when they're hungry. Also, if this is your dosha, you should consider doing a 24-hour liquid fast (more on that in Chapter 34, "Getting on the Fast Track") as often as once a week.

No matter how much it "hurts," you should avoid ice cream, butter, milk, rich and sugary desserts and anything heavy, oily or cold in quality. Also, stay away from meat and fried foods. You can tolerate meat, but you should eat it only occasionally. Instead, choose things that have a bitter, pungent or astringent taste. And eat lots of dishes with a light, dry and warm quality, more specifically vegetables. All vegetables are suited to you, so try eating large amounts of raw vegetables, fruits and beans. To stimulate your digestion, eat a little bit of ginger each day. You can also improve your digestion by drinking hot ginger tea.

GOOD FOOD–GOOD MOOD

The Effects of Food on the Mind and Emotions

In Ayurveda, foods are also classified by the effect they have on the non-physical aspects of the physiology—mind, heart, senses and Spirit. Food choices are divided into three categories or *gunas*—sattvic, rajasic and tamasic.

If you eat *sattvic* foods, you will feel an uplifting, stabilizing influence. Foods that are *rajasic* may stimulate or aggravate some aspects of your mind, heart or senses, and *tamasic* foods are considered to be an absolute deterrent to Spiritual growth because they breed lethargy and confusion.

Through my work with thousands of clients as a Spiritual Teacher, I've discovered something interesting: *people, consciously or unconsciously, gravitate towards a diet that reflects their own mental, emotional and Spiritual state of consciousness.*

You can often discern the temperament of a person from which of these three types of foods they prefer. Here's a more detailed description of each.

Sattvic Foods

Sattvic foods promote a cheery, clear, peaceful, strong and harmonious state of being. They are easy to digest and add energy to the body when consumed—while small in bulk, they're great in nourishment. Sattvic food choices are juicy and attractive in form, soft to touch, and pleasant to taste. This group includes all fruits and vegetables, grains, grasses, beans, milk, honey, almonds, dates, and small amounts of rice or prepared bread. When living on a diet made up of sattvic foods, the alkaline/acid balance in the body is 80/20, which is a very good, health-promoting acid balance. (More on this in Chapter 31, "The Acid/Alkaline Balance.")

It is my experience, from working with many people on a Spiritual level, that adding sattvic foods to the diet is extremely helpful. But regardless of whether you are seeking Spiritual growth or not, you can benefit by including some of the sattvic foods to each meal you eat. They can help you gain mental clarity, emotional balance and a deeper sense of serenity, as well as help you align your senses with your heart, mind and Soul. To get the full benefit of sattvic foods, prepare and eat them whole and fresh and with lots of love.

Rajasic Foods

Rajasic foods stimulate the nervous system. They are bitter, sour, salty, pungent, hot and dry. They increase sexual appetite, sensuality, greed, jealousy, anger and egotism. According to Ayurveda, you can tell a rajasic man or woman because they are always planning ways to satisfy their insatiable palate. Since this is impossible, their stomach is usually completely full of pungent things.

Since rajasic foods are stimulating, eating them will cause you to be energetic and active. However, this can often lead to an imbalance in your system, manifesting as restlessness and agitation. If you consume rajasic foods for a long enough period of time, they can cause disease. Examples of rajasic foods are coffee, tea, tobacco, fried bread, eggs, fresh meats, onions, garlic, salt and spices. This group of foods causes the body's alkaline/acid balance to be about 50/50 or 60/40.

Tamasic Foods

Tamasic foods are all dead foods: leftovers; stale, spoiled and processed foods; as well as alcohol, other fermented products and all drugs. They include preservatives and chemicals. Any meat products which are not freshly killed (which means pretty much anything that is bought pre-packaged in a supermarket) are also included in this group. They take energy away from our bodies in the digestive process rather than giving us energy. This diet brings out the worst characteristics in humans, including demoralization and lethargy.

They increase pessimism, ignorance, lack of common sense, greed, criminal tendencies and doubt. They keep us from being in harmony with our world and environment. Tamasic foods also cause diseases and greatly decrease life-expectancy.

I've worked as a life coach in the prison system helping inmates rehabilitate, and unfortunately much of the food fed to them is tamasic. Adding whole, sattvic foods to their diets would greatly benefit them, most especially those prone to addiction.

"The body and mind are interconnected and interdependent."

~ Sri Swami Satchidananda

ONE MORE CONSIDERATION

We're almost finished discussing everything you need to know to make an informed decision as to whether or not you want to incorporate Ayurvedic principles into your Soul-Full approach to eating. There's just one more factor to consider. In the Ayurvedic view, one of the doshas is dominant at specific times during the day, a theory called the "Master Cycles of Vata, Pitta and Kapha." In the first cycle, Kapha predominates from 6 a.m. to 10 a.m. Pitta predominates from 10 a.m. to 2 p.m. and Vata predominates from 2 p.m. to 6 p.m. In the second cycle, Kapha predominates from 6 p.m. to 10 p.m., Pitta predominates from 10 p.m. to 2 a.m., and Vata predominates from 2 a.m. to 6 a.m.

Because the Pitta dosha is responsible for digestion and metabolism, the ideal time for a large meal is during the period from 10 a.m. to 2 p.m. when Pitta is dominant. As a result, all people, regardless of their dominant dosha, should take their largest meal sometime around 12 noon.

QUICK REFERENCE CHART | FOODS THAT BALANCE YOUR DOSHAS

Now that you know your body constitution, select the right diet to maintain your Tridosha balance.

VEGETABLES

Vata		Pitta		Kapha	
Unbalancing	Balancing	Unbalancing	Balancing	Unbalancing	Balancing
Raw	Cooked	Pungent	Sweet & Bitter	Sweet & Juicy	Pungent & Bitter
Broccoli	Asparagus	Beets	Asparagus	Cucumber	Asparagus
Brussels Sprouts	Beets	Carrots	Broccoli	Potatoes (sweet)	Beets
Cabbage	Carrots	Eggplant	Brussels Sprouts	Tomatoes	Broccoli
Cauliflower	Cucumber	Garlic	Cauliflower	Zucchini	Brussell Sprouts
Celery	Garlic	Onions	Celery		Cabbage
Eggplant	Green Beans	Peppers (hot)	Cucumber		Cauliflower
Leafy Greens*	Okra	Radishes	Green Beans		Celery
Lettuce*	Onion	Spinach	Leafy Greens		Eggplant
Onions (raw)	Potato (sweet)	Tomatoes	Lettuce		Garlic
Parsley*	Radishes		Mushrooms		Leafy Greens
Peas	Zucchini		Okra		Lettuce
Peppers			Peas		Mushrooms
Potatoes (white)			Parsley		Okra
Spinach*			Peppers (green)		Onions
Sprouts*			Potatoes		Parsley
Tomatoes			Sprouts		Peas
			Zucchini		Peppers
					Potatoes (white)
					Radishes
					Spinach
					Sprouts

*These Vegetables are okay in moderation with oil dressing.

FRUITS

Vata		Pitta		Kapha	
Unbalancing	Balancing	Unbalancing	Balancing	Unbalancing	Balancing
Dried	Sweet	Sour	Sweet	Sweet & Sour	
Apples	Apricots	Apricots	Apples	Avocado	Apples
Cranberries	Avocado	Berries	Avocado	Bananas	Apricots
Pears	Bananas	Bananas	Coconuts	Coconuts	Berries
Persimmon	Berries	Cherries	Figs	Figs (fresh)	Cherries
Pomegranates	Cherries	Cranberries	Grapes (dark)	Grapefruits	Cranberries
Watermelons	Coconuts	Grapefruit	Mangoes	Grapes	Figs (dry)
	Figs (fresh)	Grapes (green)	Oranges (sweet)	Lemons	Mangoes
	Grapefruit	Lemons	Pears	Melons	Peaches
	Grapes	Oranges (sour)	Pineapples/sweet	Oranges	Pears
	Lemons	Papayas	Plums/sweet	Papayas	Persimmons
	Mangoes	Peaches	Pomegranates	Pineapples	Pomegranates
	Melons (sweet)	Pineapples/sour	Prunes	Plums	Prunes
	Oranges	Persimmons	Raisins		Raisins
	Papayas	Plums (sour)			
	Peaches				
	Pineapples				
	Plums				

GRAINS

Vata		Pitta		Kapha	
Unbalancing	Balancing	Unbalancing	Balancing	Unbalancing	Balancing
Barley	Oats (cooked)	Buckwheat	Barley	Oats (cooked)	Barley
Buckwheat	Rice	Corn	Oats (cooked)	Rice (brown)	Corn
Corn	Wheat	Millet	Rice (basmati)	Rice (white)	Millet
Millet		Oats (dry)	Rice (white)	Wheat	Oats (dry)
Rye		Rice (brown)	Wheat		Rice, Basmati
		Rye			(small amount)
					Rye

LEGUMES

Vata		Pitta		Kapha	
Unbalancing	Balancing	Unbalancing	Balancing	Unbalancing	Balancing
All Legumes	Mung Beans	Lentils	All Other	Lentils	All Other
	Tofu		Legumes OK		Legumes OK
	Lentils				
	(black & red)				

NUTS

Vata		Pitta		Kapha	
Unbalancing	Balancing	Unbalancing	Balancing	Unbalancing	Balancing
All nuts OK in small quantities		No nuts except coconut		No nuts at all	

SEEDS

Vata		Pitta		Kapha	
Unbalancing	Balancing	Unbalancing	Balancing	Unbalancing	Balancing
All seeds OK in moderation		Only Sunflower & Pumpkin		Only Sunflower & Pumpkin	

SWEETENERS

Vata		Pitta		Kapha	
Unbalancing	Balancing	Unbalancing	Balancing	Unbalancing	Balancing
All sweeteners are OK except white sugar		All sweeteners are OK except molasses and honey		No sweeteners except raw honey	

CONDIMENTS

Vata		Pitta		Kapha	
Unbalancing	Balancing	Unbalancing	Balancing	Unbalancing	Balancing
All spices are good		No spices except: **		All spices are good except salt	

DAIRY

Vata		Pitta		Kapha	
Unbalancing	Balancing	Unbalancing	Balancing	Unbalancing	Balancing
All dairy products are OK (in moderation)		Buttermilk Cheese Sour Cream Yogurt	Butter (unsalted) Cottage Cheese Ghee Milk	No dairy except ghee & goat milk	

OILS

Vata		Pitta		Kapha	
<u>Unbalancing</u>	<u>Balancing</u>	<u>Unbalancing</u>	<u>Balancing</u>	<u>Unbalancing</u>	<u>Balancing</u>
	All oils are good	Almond	Coconut	No oils except almond, corn,	
		Corn	Olive	or sunflower in small amounts	
		Safflower	Sunflower		
		Sesame	Soy		

**Except coriander, cinnamon, cardamom, fennel, turmeric & small amounts of black pepper
Adapted from ayurveda-foryou.com.

As you can see from the above charts, when you follow the Ayurvedic approach to eating, you won't have to want for variety. As stated earlier, according to Ayurveda, every meal should be a feast for all of your senses. A diet exclusive in nature is incomplete by definition, and so cannot balance all aspects of your physiology. A plate that contains a variety of foods will allow your body, mind, heart and Soul to be completely fulfilled by the eating experience.

Although it may seem a bit complicated at first, I like the Tridosha System. It requires that you be attuned to both your internal needs and the external play of nature. You need to look at the whole picture of your life. And, as you know by now, I feel this approach is an important part of any diet.

SOMETHING TO CHEW ON

Hindu legend holds that Lord Brahma, the God of Creation, began to teach various Spiritual leaders ways to ease the burdens of humankind, after recognizing the intense suffering on earth. For thousands of years, these ways were transmitted orally. They were eventually recorded in the Vedic texts; that is how we know of the three doshas today.

SOUL-FULL EXERCISE #29

Using the chart and pulse reading technique, find out your prominent dosha. Then experiment with the Ayurvedic way of eating. Try at least a few new foods each week, or prepare familiar foods in new ways. That way, your taste buds and digestive system will be continually exposed to new stimuli. You'll also want to eat a wide variety of foods to insure a balance of nutrition. Today resolve to make your meals an adventure!

RESOURCES

Find out more about the Tridosha way of eating. The following books can help.

Ageless Body, Timeless Mind by Deepak Chopra, MD

Perfect Health by Deepak Chopra, MD

Perfect Weight by Deepak Chopra, MD

Freedom from Disease by Hari Sharma, MD

Ayurvedic Secrets to Longevity and Total Health by Anselmo Peter
     and James S. Brooks

The Ayurvedic Cookbook by Amadea Morningstar, with Umila Desai

Ayurvedic Cooking for Westerners by Amadea Morningstar

The George Mateljan Foundation is a non-profit organization with no commercial interests. Its mission is "to offer a healthier way of eating that's enjoyable, affordable, quick and easy to fit anyone's personal needs and lifestyle." To access recipes and information about Ayurvedic cooking type in the word "Ayurveda" once you're on the site.

www.whfoods.com

Ayurveda for You is a comprehensive site that offers not only some of the basic, fundamental principles of Ayurveda but more detailed information.

www.ayurveda-foryou.com

The Ayurveda Holistic Community offers positive personal, educational, social, environmental and Spiritual growth based on Ayurveda.

www.ayurvedahc.com

CHAPTER THIRTY

The Wisdom of Food Combining

"Food and drink are relied upon to nurture life. But if one does not know that the nature of substances may be opposed to each other, and one consumes them altogether indiscriminately, the vital organs will be thrown out of harmony..."
~ Doctor Chia Ming in a letter to the
Emperor of the Ming Dynasty 1368 AD

AS ILLUSTRATED BY THE ABOVE QUOTE, the belief that there are proper and improper ways of combining food has been around for a long time—the Jewish Torah purports it, with the Kosher law of not having flesh and dairy at the same meal, and Moses is quoted in Exodus as saying, "The Lord shall give you in the evening flesh to eat, and in the morning bread to the full." Now this approach to eating is once again gaining substantial momentum.

The idea behind food combining is elementary. In fact, when I was a teacher, I taught this concept in my 7th and 8th grade science classes. In a very dramatic experiment, I'd illustrate the caustic nature of acid by adding several objects—such as a small cracker, a piece of hard candy and a gum eraser—into a beaker of it. The items would be eaten away. (Acid's nature is the very reason you may have reached for bicarbonate of soda [a strong alkaline], when you've suffered from an upset nervous stomach.) Then in a second beaker, I would add

"The simplest rule
of food combining
is to eat foods
or combinations
of foods that
in our direct
experience
are easiest
to digest."

~ Gabriel
Cousens, MD,
in his book
Spiritual Nutrition

an equal measure of an alkaline to an equal measure of acid and voila, I'd have a solution as neutral as plain water. Next, I'd illustrate the nature of this mixture to the class by putting the same type items into the beaker again with no caustic reaction.

So say you're hungry and you want to grab a turkey sandwich. In the food combining world, this is a no-no. Why?

Well, your stomach secretes various enzymes to digest the food you eat and to digest an animal protein, such as turkey, the enzyme pepsin is necessary. This enzyme can only do its work inside of your stomach in a highly acidic medium, which presents a problem if you eat a carbohydrate, such as bread, at the same meal. The moment you put a carbohydrate into your mouth, your salivary glands start secreting ptyalin—a digestive enzyme that helps digest carbohydrates—as well as other alkaline juices. When the carbohydrate gets swallowed, it requires an alkaline medium to complete the digestive process. It's not too difficult to figure out what happens when the alkaline juices needed to digest the carbohydrates combine with the acidic juices needed to digest the proteins—they promptly neutralize one another—leaving a weak, watery solution in the stomach that can digest neither carbohydrates or proteins properly. Instead, the proteins putrefy and carbohydrates ferment, causing all kinds of problems—such as gas, heartburn, cramps, constipation and even colitis with habitual abuse.

You may feel that you have an iron-clad constitution and that food-combining isn't something that's necessary for you to know about. But I wanted to include it in this book because I feel that being aware of this system can help you notice some very subtle, or not so subtle ways, that your body might be reacting to the *way* you eat food (i.e. the combinations) and not necessarily just to *what* you're eating.

Once you're aware of how to combine foods properly, you may be able to eat foods that you love, but have avoided, because you've been thinking, "That just doesn't agree with me." It may very well be the combination of food you've tried that aggravated you, much more than that food itself.

In addition, it is believed that many so-called "allergies" are also the result of improper food combining. The symptoms appear after the bloodstream picks up the toxins from the improperly combined, undigested foods and carries them throughout the body. This can cause rashes, headaches, nausea and other symptoms that are commonly branded as allergies. In fact, it has been found that many of the same foods that cause distress when improperly combined have absolutely no ill side effects when eaten alone or when properly combined.

There are many methods of food combining that have been touted in recent years. I find most of them confusing, so I am going to focus on the two approaches that I've found easiest to apply in my own life.

MY COMMON SENSE APPROACH

I personally don't adhere to a strict food-combining regime. I find it imprisoning to be so consumed with the method of my food consumption. However, I do like being familiar with the basics, and loosely adhering to the principles does make a difference for me—the result is that what I eat just "sits" better in my system.

I wholeheartedly agree with Gabriel Cousens, MD, who wrote in his book Spiritual Nutrition that "The simplest rule of food combining is to eat foods or combinations of foods that in our direct experience are easiest to digest." That means to eat foods that feel comfortable to your own system and to find out what suits you and your body.

Awareness is the key in a Soul-Full approach to eating. Becoming more aware of how you feel when you eat different foods is a big part of making a strong, aware connection to yourself. Because even when you're following an entirely wholesome, fresh, additive-free diet, you may find yourself feeling uncomfortable after eating certain things. Each of us is an individual; therefore, pay attention to your own body. Honor its signals. Heartburn, gas, diarrhea and other digestion-related problems are signs that your food combinations and/or choices might need some refining to best suit your needs.

BASIC RULES OF FOOD COMBINING

- **Eat proteins and starches at separate meals**–For example, you might have chicken breast or a soy-veggie burger with a salad for lunch, and eat a vegetable stir-fry with rice for dinner.

- **Eat carbohydrates and proteins at separate meals**— Carbohydrates require an alkaline medium for digestion, and proteins require an acid medium for digestion. If you frequently find yourself with bloating or an upset stomach after a meal, try eating a combination of proteins—say a cheese omelet for one meal, and all carbohydrates—such as a large vegetable salad and garlic bread—for another.

- **Eat proteins and fats at separate meals**—Some fats require hours for digestion, so as a general rule fats are best eaten alone. Examples of such fat containing foods are macadamia and cashew nuts and pumpkin seeds.

- **Eat sugars (fruits) separate from both proteins and starches**— Fruits undergo little digestion in the stomach, so they are held up if eaten with foods which require more digestion there.

- **Do not eat raw, fresh or dried fruits after any cooked food.** Raw and dried fruits digest much more quickly and will ferment in the digestive system when held back by the more slowly digesting cooked food.

- **Do not combine vegetables, proteins or starches with fruits**. The exceptions to this rule are nuts and citrus—which are a fair combination—and lettuce, celery and fruit—which are a very good combination since they all have a high water content. Also, lettuce, celery and fruit are very easily digested and move though the body at approximately the same rate.

- **Do not combine acid fruits with sweet fruits**. Acid fruits such as pineapples, citrus and pomegranates do not digest well when eaten with sweeter fruits such as bananas.

- **Eat tomatoes with greens and non-starchy vegetables and protein**. This is a very good salad combination.

- **Always eat melons alone**. Their high water content makes them digest the quickest of all foods.

"Don't take food combining to the extreme, but tap into its wisdom to feel better and experience smoother digestion."

~ Maureen Whitehouse

FOOD COMBINING SIMPLIFIED

One food at a meal is the most ideal for the easiest and best digestion.

A combination of several foods at a meal should be according to the chart on the following page.

FOOD COMBINING CHART

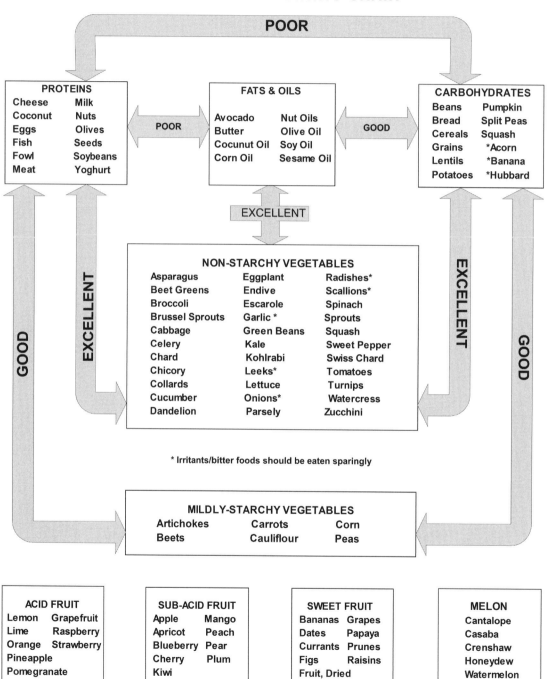

POOR

PROTEINS
Cheese	Milk
Coconut	Nuts
Eggs	Olives
Fish	Seeds
Fowl	Soybeans
Meat	Yoghurt

POOR

FATS & OILS
Avocado	Nut Oils
Butter	Olive Oil
Cocunut Oil	Soy Oil
Corn Oil	Sesame Oil

GOOD

CARBOHYDRATES
Beans	Pumpkin
Bread	Split Peas
Cereals	Squash
Grains	*Acorn
Lentils	*Banana
Potatoes	*Hubbard

EXCELLENT

NON-STARCHY VEGETABLES
Asparagus	Eggplant	Radishes*
Beet Greens	Endive	Scallions*
Broccoli	Escarole	Spinach
Brussel Sprouts	Garlic *	Sprouts
Cabbage	Green Beans	Squash
Celery	Kale	Sweet Pepper
Chard	Kohlrabi	Swiss Chard
Chicory	Leeks*	Tomatoes
Collards	Lettuce	Turnips
Cucumber	Onions*	Watercress
Dandelion	Parsely	Zucchini

GOOD — EXCELLENT — EXCELLENT — GOOD

* Irritants/bitter foods should be eaten sparingly

MILDLY-STARCHY VEGETABLES
Artichokes	Carrots	Corn
Beets	Cauliflour	Peas

ACID FRUIT
Lemon	Grapefruit
Lime	Raspberry
Orange	Strawberry
Pineapple	
Pomegranate	

SUB-ACID FRUIT
Apple	Mango
Apricot	Peach
Blueberry	Pear
Cherry	Plum
Kiwi	

SWEET FRUIT
Bananas	Grapes
Dates	Papaya
Currants	Prunes
Figs	Raisins
Fruit, Dried	

MELON
Cantalope
Casaba
Crenshaw
Honeydew
Watermelon

Adapted from alderbrooke.com

"The next time you have a tangerine to eat, please put it in the palm of your hand and look at it in a way that makes the tangerine real. You do not need a lot of time to do it, just two to three seconds. Looking at it, you can see a beautiful blossom with sunshine and rain, and you can see a tiny fruit forming... You can see the color changing from green to orange and you can see the tangerine sweetening. Looking at a tangerine this way, you will see that everything in the cosmos is in it—sunshine, rain, clouds, trees, leaves, everything. Peeling the tangerine, smelling it and tasting it, you can be very happy."
~ Thich Nhat Hanh

SEQUENTIAL FOOD COMBINING

There's another method of food combining that I feel is helpful to know about and try, even if just for a day or two, to get a better feeling for how your unique digestive system processes food. It's called *Sequential Food Combining*. Here's how it works. You eat different foods, one variety at a time, in sequence (at one meal). This way, according to the theory, each of the different foods will form its own layer in your stomach. When Layer One is digested and leaves the stomach, then Layer Two can take its place, and so on. Therefore, each layer digests separately, without mixing and without disturbing the adjacent layers. A basic principle here is that for the most efficient healthful digestion, you should eat the most watery foods first. For instance, you could eat vegetables before a piece of fish. I know people who live by this way of eating, and because of it, they've freed themselves of such diet-related problems and/or diseases as obesity, colitis, chronic fatigue syndrome, and even cancer. If nothing more, it's a great way to get to know your body and cleanse your system.

DIGESTION TIME OF VARIOUS FOODS

Approximate Times to Digest Various Foods When Eaten Alone, or Sequentially:

Water
When the stomach is empty, water leaves immediately and goes into the intestines.

Juice
Fruit, vegetable and vegetable broth
—*15 to 20 minutes*

Fruit
Watermelon
—*20 minutes*
Other melons:
Cantaloupe, Honeydew, Cranshaw, etc
—*30 minutes*
Oranges, grapefruit, grapes
—*30 minutes*
Apples, pears, peaches, cherries
—*40 minutes*

Vegetables
Raw
Raw tossed-salad vegetables: tomato, lettuce, cucumber, celery, red or green pepper, and other succulent vegetables
—*30 to 40 minutes*

Steamed or Cooked Vegetables
Leafy vegetables: escarole, spinach, kale, collards
—*40 minutes*
Zucchini, broccoli, cauliflower, string beans, yellow squash, corn on cob
—*45 minutes*
Root vegetables: carrots, beets, parsnips, turnips
—*50 minutes*

Semi-Concentrated Carbohydrates—Starches
Jerusalem artichokes, acorn and butternut squashes, corn, potatoes, sweet potatoes, yam, chestnuts
—*60 minutes*

Concentrated Carbohydrates—Grains
Brown rice, millet, buckwheat, cornmeal, oats
—*90 minutes*
Legumes and Beans: (Concentrated Carbohydrate and Protein) lentils, limas, chick peas, peas, kidney beans
—*90 minutes*
Soy beans
—*120 minutes!*

Nuts and Seeds
Nuts: almonds, filberts, peanuts (raw), cashews, brazils, walnuts, pecans
—*2-1/2 to 3 hours!*
Seeds: sunflower, pumpkin, sesame
—*approx. 2 hours!*

Dairy
Skim milk, cottage or low-fat pot cheese or ricotta
—*approx. 90 minutes*
Whole-milk cottage cheese
—*120 minutes!*
Whole-milk hard cheese
—*4 to 5 hours!*

Animal Protein
Egg yolk
—*30 minutes*
Whole egg,
—*45 minutes*
Fish: cod, scrod, flounder, sole
—*30 minutes*
Fish: salmon, trout, herring (fatty fish)
—*45-60 minutes*
Chicken
—*1-1/2 to 2 hours (without skin)!*
Turkey
—*2 to 2-1/4 hours (without skin)!*
Beef, lamb
—*3 to 4 hours!*
Pork
—*4-1/2 to 5 hours!*

Note 1: Raw animal proteins have much faster digestion times than the above times for cooked/heated animal proteins.

Note 2: The digestion times given are under an ideal situation of eating only one food, chewing well, and having efficient digestion, as is the case after a fast. They are digestion times for optimally healthy persons, with good eating habits.

Digestion times are much longer on a conventional diet, and for persons with non-optimized digestive systems, or persons lacking in energy, and for meals with many ingredients put together haphazardly and not in the optimum sequential order.

SOURCE:
Ideal Health Through Sequential Eating by Stanley S. Bass; *www.drbass.com*

So remember, symptoms such as gas, bloating, constipation, heartburn or stomachaches can be an indication that the foods you have eaten are not combining well. Listen to your body and find out what the right diet is for you. Apply the food-combining principles described above when they are useful to you.

SOMETHING TO CHEW ON

My advice? Don't take food combining to the extreme, but tap into its wisdom to feel better and experience smoother digestion.

Think of children at birthday parties. It's not the one who eats a little bit of cake or ice cream who gets a tummy ache—it's the one who overindulges. Even the theoretically worst combinations of food can often be easily tolerated if eaten in moderation. And even if you decided to eat a mono-diet (in which you ate only one type of food such as fruit), you could find yourself with digestive difficulties if you ate too much of it. I present these food-combining ideas to be a rough guideline. Allow yourself to be your own scientist, and discover what foods combine best for you.

SOUL-FULL EXERCISE #30

Try implementing the idea of food combining into your life, following your own inner guidance.

For the next week, pay attention to the foods you eat and the way you feel after eating. Do you have any symptoms of discomfort? If so, try combining the foods you eat with greater awareness.

RESOURCES

The Complete Book of Food Combining by Kathryn Marsden
Food Combining: A Step-by-Step Guide by Kathryn Marsden
Food Combining Made Easy by Herbert M. Shelton
Food Combining and Digestion by Steve Meyerowitz
Ideal Health through Sequential Eating (Perfection in Food Combining)
    by Stanley S. Bass

CHAPTER THIRTY-ONE

The Acid/ Alkaline Balance

"Like the oceans and fresh bodies of water which are dying because of pollution, if our body fluids become polluted, an acidic acid/base imbalance develops, which kills us too."
~ Gabriel Cousens, MD

I HAD NO IDEA that a body could be acidic. Then one day a friend asked me to put a piece of litmus paper on my tongue so that he could test my body's pH. I thought it was a weird request, but I complied. My reading came in at 6.4—just a tad below the optimum "normal" range. Needless to say, I had to find out more.

Now, several years later, it's common for me to note whether or not a food has an acid or alkalizing promoting tendency on the body before I eat it. Here's why...

The pH level (acid—alkaline measurement) of our internal fluids affects every cell in our bodies, and research points to the fact that extended acid imbalances of any kind can overwhelm your body. That's because just as the body regulates its temperature in a rigid manner, so does it strive to maintain a very narrow pH range—especially in the blood. As a matter of fact, your body will go to such great lengths to maintain a blood pH of about 7.365 that it will even create stress on other tissues or body systems to do so. If your body becomes chronically acidic, it won't be long before the function of all of your cellular activities will be disturbed. This not only can greatly interfere with your lifestyle but might even cause you to ultimately experience dis-ease of your body, mind and Spirit.

If the pH of your body gets out of balance (too acidic), you could experience low energy, excess weight, poor digestion, fatigue, aches and pains, and more serious disorders—some even say cancers.

In his book, *Alkalize or Die*, Dr. Theodore Baroody says, "The countless names of illnesses do not really matter. What does matter is that they all come from the same root cause… too much tissue acid waste in the body!"

"Acid is pain—alkaline turns off pain."

~ Gary Null,
author of
*Kiss Your
Fat Goodbye*

WHAT'S GOING ON HERE?

Our body's pH level is normally slightly alkaline, with a range of 7.36 to 7.44. So the theory behind the alkaline approach to eating is that our diet should also be slightly alkaline. A diet that is too high in acid foods—such as sugar, caffeine, processed foods and meat—will disrupt the balance. It can also deplete the body of essential alkalizing minerals such as potassium, sodium, magnesium and calcium, which weakens our system. If you are a low-key type, who eats in a well-balanced, whole way, you're most likely alkaline enough without needing to consider this approach to eating. But if you lead a stressful life and consume large amounts of sugar, protein, processed foods and caffeine, then you may want to learn more about alkalizing your system.

If you're wondering whether you're acidic, consider this list of symptoms associated with excess acidity:

- Nervousness, stress, irritability, anxiousness and agitation
- Colds, flus, nasal congestion and infections
- Excess mucous
- Bladder and kidney conditions, including kidney stones
- Immune deficiency, low energy, chronic fatigue
- Neuritis, joint pain, arthritis, hives, headaches, leg cramps and spasms

- Hormone concerns
- Osteoporosis*, joint pain, aching muscles and lactic-acid buildup
- Weak nails and dry skin
- Cysts—such as ovarian cysts, polycystic ovaries, benign breast cysts
- Weight gain, obesity and diabetes
- You feel better after a detox diet.
- Premature aging

* The body borrows calcium from the bones to balance the pH. In a recent University of California study that was cited in the *American Journal of Clinical Nutrition*, the pH levels of over 9,000 women were tested. Those who had chronic acidosis proved to be at a greater risk for bone loss than those with normal pH levels.

Testing Your pH

If you have any of the above symptoms, then you may want to physically test your pH. Most medical professionals test the acidity or alkalinity of the body tissues by analyzing the blood. But there are also ways to measure urine pH, and the pH of your saliva, using a strip of litmus paper—just as I first did. Most proponents of the alkaline diet look at the pH of all three components—blood, saliva and urine—in addition to assessing health symptoms.

What Is pH?

The term *pH* means "potential of hydrogen," and it is a measure of the acidity or alkalinity of a solution. The scale on which it is measured ranges between 0 and 14—the lower the pH, the more acidic the solution, and the higher the pH, the more alkaline (or base) the solution. When a solution is neither acid nor alkaline, it has a pH of 7—which is neutral.

The body continually strives to equalize its pH. When this balance is compromised in any way, problems can occur.

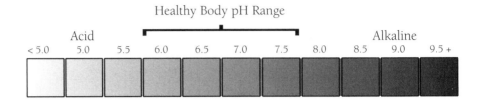

It's important to understand that we are not talking about stomach acid or the pH of the stomach. We are talking about the pH of the body's fluids and tissues, which is an entirely different matter.

Using pH Test Strips

You can use pH test strips to determine your pH factor quickly and easily in the privacy of your own home. The best time to test your pH is about one hour before a meal or two hours after a meal If you get a saliva-test reading between 6.5 and 7.5 at any time during the day (between meals), then your body is functioning within a healthy range. A healthy urinary pH reading is between 6.0 to 6.5 in the morning, and between 6.5 and 7.0 in the evening. While you're discerning your pH levels, it's optimum to test your pH two days a week.

Urine pH

The urine tests you have taken at your doctor's office test for a wide-range of things, but the urine test you can do at home for yourself can only tell you how well your body is excreting acids and assimilating minerals—most especially calcium, magnesium, sodium and potassium. But that's enough. These essential minerals act as "buffers" in the body, so a proper balance here shows your tendency towards vital, good health. On the other hand, when your body ingests or produces too much acidity or alkalinity that cannot be buffered, it must excrete the excess—which it does through the urine. If your average urine pH reading is below 6.5, this is an indication that your body's buffering system is overwhelmed, and you should pay attention to lowering your acid levels.

Saliva pH

Saliva testing is the most convenient way of testing your pH; although it may not be as extensive or accurate as the pH testing that can be done by a competent health-care professional, it is adequate. Between 6.5 and 7.5 is considered to be a healthy range, but a more typical reading is between 7.36 and 7.44. If your saliva pH is too low (below 6.5), this indicates that your body may be producing too many acids or having trouble secreting excess acids.

AN ACIDIC WORLD

This world is a very acidic place to live. So many people, all over the world, are ingesting meals that are far too high in acid-producing animal products like meat, eggs and dairy, acid-producing processed foods like white flour and sugar, and acid-producing beverages like coffee and soft drinks. Also, they're using artificial chemical sweeteners like NutraSweet, Equal or aspartame—which are extremely acid-forming. Far too few people eat foods that are alkaline-producing like fresh vegetables. And if that's not bad enough, to overcome their basic toxicity, they often use drugs—which are acid-forming.

It's time we choose to see progress as getting back to basics and eating simply and wisely, referring to our Soul-Full feelings to guide us. Considering the Acid/Alkaline balance will help.

"The body continually strives to equalize its pH."

~ Maureen Whitehouse

MAINTAINING A BALANCED pH LEVEL IN YOUR BODY

Foods that are high in sodium, potassium, calcium and magnesium, such as fruits and vegetables, help to preserve the alkalinity of the body. When the body has a proper acid/alkaline balance, it is most immune to disease.

Here's a handy reference chart to help you to maintain pH balance:

FOODS THAT AFFECT pH LEVELS	
Alkaline Forming	*Acid Forming*
Fruits	Grains
Vegetables	Fish
Coconuts	Meats, including poultry
Almonds	Legumes, including soybeans
Lima beans	Eggs
Sprouted grains and seeds	Sugar and syrup (except honey)
	Most Nuts

To maintain proper alkaline levels, eat 80% alkaline-forming foods and 20% acid-forming foods.

In his book, *How to Get Well*, Paavo Airola writes that the body's natural and optimum ratio of alkaline to acid is 80/20.

MORE ON ACIDIC AND ALKALINE FOODS

Note that acidic foods are not the same as citrus fruits, such as lemons and oranges. These foods are oxidized into carbon dioxide and water by our system and act as cleansing agents to the body. They are actually considered alkaline foods because they bring alkaline-forming minerals into the body. However, animal products are acid-forming, as are *most* grains and vegetarian forms of protein, such as nuts and seeds (unless soaked in water). However, almonds and brazil nuts are alkaline forming. Yogurt and milk are considered alkaline, but only if they're unpasteurized. Cheese and butter are acidic. Oil is neutral. Sugar and fats are acidic.

For further details, study the chart below from Dr. Darrell L. Wolfe, founder of The Wolfe Clinic.

Alkalizing Foods

VEGETABLES	FRUITS	OTHER
Garlic	Apple	Apple Cider Vinegar
Asparagus	Apricot	Bee Pollen
Fermented Veggies	Avocado	Lecithin Granules
Watercress	Banana (high glycemic)	Probiotic Cultures
Beets	Cantaloupe	Green Juices
Broccoli	Cherries	Veggies Juices
Brussel sprouts	Currants	Fresh Fruit Juice
Cabbage	Dates/Figs	Organic Milk
Carrot	Grapes	(unpasteurized)
Cauliflower	Grapefruit	Mineral Water
Celery	Lime	Alkaline Antioxidant Water
Chard	Honeydew Melon	Green Tea
Chlorella	Nectarine	Herbal Tea
Collard Greens	Orange	Dandelion Tea
Cucumber	Lemon	Ginseng Tea
Eggplant	Most All Berries	Banchi Tea
Kale	Peach	Kombucha
Kohlrabi	Pear	
Lettuce	Pineapple	**SWEETENERS**
Mushrooms	Tangerine	Stevia
Mustard Greens	Tomato	Raw Agave Nectar
Dulce	Tropical Fruits	
Dandelions	Watermelon	**SPICES/SEASONINGS**
Edible Flowers		Cinnamon
Onions	**PROTEIN**	Curry
Parsnips (high glycemic)	Eggs	Ginger
Peas	Whey Protein Powder	Mustard
Peppers	Cottage Cheese	Chili Pepper
Pumpkin	Chicken Breast	Sea Salt
Rutabaga	Yogurt	Miso
Sea Veggies	Almonds	Tamari
Spirulina	Chestnuts	All Herbs
Sprouts	Tofu (fermented)	
Squashes	Flax Seeds	**ORIENTAL VEGETABLES**
Alfalfa	Pumpkin Seeds	Maitake
Barley Grass	Tempeh (fermented)	Daikon
Wheat Grass	Squash Seeds	Dandelion Root
Wild Greens	Sunflower Seeds	Shitake
Nightshade Veggies	Millet	Kombu
	Sprouted Seeds	Reishi
	Nuts	Nori
		Umeboshi
		Wakame
		Sea Veggies

Acidifying Foods

FATS & OILS
Avocado Oil
Canola Oil
Corn Oil
Hemp Seed Oil
Flax Oil
Lard
Olive Oil
Safflower Oil
Sesame Oil
Sunflower Oil

FRUITS
Cranberries

GRAINS
Rice Cakes
Wheat Cakes
Amaranth
Barley
Buckwheat
Corn
Oats (rolled)
Quinoi
Rice (all)
Rye
Spelt
Kamut
Wheat
Hemp Seed Flour

DAIRY
Cheese, Cow
Cheese, Goat
Cheese, Processed
Cheese, Sheep
Milk
Butter

NUTS & BUTTERS
Cashews
Brazil Nuts
Peanuts
Peanut Butter
Pecans
Tahini
Walnuts

ANIMAL PROTEIN
Beef
Carp
Clams
Fish
Lamb
Lobster
Mussels
Oyster
Pork
Rabbit
Salmon
Shrimp
Scallops
Tuna
Turkey
Venison

PASTA (WHITE)
Noodles
Macaroni
Spaghetti

OTHER
Distilled Vinegar
Wheat Germ
Potatoes

DRUGS & CHEMICALS
Chemicals
Drugs, Medicinal
Drugs, Psychedelic
Pesticides
Herbicides

ALCOHOL
Beer
Spirits
Hard Liquor
Wine

BEANS & LEGUMES
Black Beans
Chick Peas
Green Peas
Kidney Beans
Lentils
Lima Beans
Pinto Beans
Red Beans
Soy Beans
Soy Milk
White Beans
Rice Milk
Almond Milk

ALKALIZING GREEN DRINKS

Drinking green juice made with dark leafy greens such as kale, parsley, collard greens, cilantro and dandelion mixed with the juice of cucumber, apple and/or celery is a very effective way to both alkalize and cleanse the body. Also E3 Live blue-green algae is very alkalizing, with five times more chlorophyll than wheatgrass. For more information about therapeutic green drinks, see Chapter 34, "Getting on the Fast Track," (Juice Fasting).

LOVE—THE ULTIMATE pH-BALANCE ANSWER

I travel a lot, and I've eaten meals with many people, in countries all over the world. No matter how "different" we appear to be, we are basically all the same. That is, we're all people who need nurturance and love in order to thrive, otherwise we feel as though we are barely surviving—no matter what level of success and opulence we've achieved.

Through my Transformational Coaching work, I've made many amazing discoveries, which is actually a good part of the reason you're holding this book in your hands. One of the discoveries is that *the most effective way of maintaining a perfect pH-balance is to be "in" love.*

The energy of love promotes an overall feeling of well-being, which is very alkalizing; whereas the emotion of fear is very acidic. Sometimes I work with clients who are physically ill, and I help them to release fear, perhaps disguised in the form of anger, guilt, judgment, doubt or confusion. Quite often, their physical symptoms lessen or are completely alleviated in direct proportion to their newfound ability to love and forgive themselves and others.

When you forgive, you become free of stagnant, helpless, victimizing ways of thinking. As a result, you can embrace a more positive, peaceful and empowering outlook on life. It's only when you adopt this liberating stance that you feel inclined to make whole and self-honoring choices, and your diet will reflect that naturally—even if you don't know any diet or nutrition "rules."

Again, the core teaching of this book is: *Eat with love, what's grown with love, prepared with love, and served with love.* You have to be in a loving state to do that. A commitment to fast from the experience of fear would serve you well!

SOMETHING TO CHEW ON

If you live in an urban area or suburb, you live in a highly acidic environment. It's vitally important for you to pay loving attention to yourself to counteract the acid-effects of the polluted air you breathe and the chemicalized food and water you ingest. Unless you are practicing such mindfulness, you could find yourself experiencing stress on every level—physically, emotionally, vitally and mentally. This causes the body to overproduce acid waste and upset your body's delicate pH balance.

SOUL-FULL EXERCISE #31

Test your pH using the above instructions (you can buy the pH test strips at most pharmacies). If your pH is acidic, try nurturing yourself for one week, by eating wholesome, lovingly prepared alkaline foods that are chemical-free and blessed! Drink lots of pure water and *Breathe*. Take walks in the fresh air and sun or under the moonlight (which is highly alkalizing!).

Feel gratitude for all of the good things in your life. Then test your pH again. See how taking the time to love yourself, and your life, can make all the difference.

RESOURCES

Alkalize or Die by Dr. Theodore A. Baroody
Sick and Tired? by Robert O. Young PhD, DSc
The Acid—Alkaline Diet by Christopher Vasey
The pH Miracle by Dr. Robert O. Young, PhD, DSc

CHAPTER THIRTY-TWO

The Yin/Yang Energies of Food

"Without correcting individual dietary habits, personal health and happiness will not be achieved, and without correcting society's dietary habits, environmental harmony and global peace will not be realized."
~ Mishio Kushi, the Father of Macrobiotics

WHEN I WAS MODELING in New York City, I explored many diets to keep myself "runway-thin"—one of which was Macrobiotics. I was drawn to it because a model I'd worked with, Eva Voorheeze, mentioned to me that this was her key to diet success. At the time, Eva was experiencing great popularity—adorning the cover of *Vogue* and the like.

My motivation to follow a Macrobiotic path was in no way Spiritually inclined; it was purely success-oriented. However, as I explored it further (eventually studying with Mishio Kushi, a chief proponent of Macrobiotics in the US), I realized a whole new way of relating to food. It was my first taste of seeing food in a Soul-Full way.

Macrobiotics is based on the idea that everything is composed, in varying degrees, of two opposing forces—*yin* and *yang*. And if you look at the world with awareness, they become evident to you in the natural order of things—for example, the day turns to night, the sun sets and the moon rises, summer turns to winter, we inhale and exhale, we begin life young and grow old, etc. These are the physical laws of the Universe, and when you respect their simple eloquence, you naturally feel free.

So you can see that Macrobiotics is not just a diet, but also a philosophy and a way of life.

Looking closely at the term *Macrobiotics*, "Macro" means great and "bio" means life, and its basic premise is to attain balance by tuning into the grand but subtle forces that govern all life. It is through this connectivity, along with the right foods and lifestyle, that Macrobiotic people believe you can cure any illness.

Here's a bit of history… although Mishio Kushi is responsible for popularizing Macrobiotics in the East, it was his teacher, George Oshawa, who developed the diet after coming down with tuberculosis at age 15. Oshawa's mother and two younger siblings had already died of the disease when his doctor pronounced this diagnosis for George. So, for him, it could have been taken as a death sentence. But Oshawa was determined to beat the verdict. He began to fervently study ancient Eastern healing and Spiritual concepts and soon after developed his own unique interpretation which he began to impart to others.

> *"The key to health is restoring balance."*
>
> ~ Gary Null, author of *Kiss Your Fat Goodbye.*

WHAT IS YIN AND WHAT IS YANG?

Yin and yang energy are actually one force—like two sides of the same coin. Yin is expansive, so it has the tendency to fill up space. This energy grows big, quickly. Its qualities are cool and dark—like space. Yang energy, on the other hand, is contractive. It has the tendency to be more compact and grow slowly. The longer something takes to grow, the more yang it will be.

Yin Foods	In Between	Yang Foods
Expand as they grow	Cereals/Grains	Condense as they grow
Cold		Hot
Watery		Dry
Sweet		Salty
Feminine		Masculine
Fruits		Roots

Macrobiotics teaches that the more in balance the yin and yang aspects of your food selections are the more healthy and happy you will be.

The standard Macrobiotic diet is just good, wholesome food—primarily whole grains, a variety of vegetables, beans (including soy), sea vegetables, soups, various condiments and even desserts. Just as in the other Soul-based diets I've mentioned earlier, there is little room in this one for highly refined sugar, or chemicalized and processed foods. Plus there are no animal foods permitted (with the exception of fish)—so no meat, dairy or eggs.

If you're unsure of what foods exhibit what qualities, here's a chart to help you discern the yin and the yang of some typically Macrobiotic food selections:

The Yin and Yang of Typical Macrobiotic Foods			
Moderately Yin	**Very Yin**	**Moderately Yang**	**Very Yang**
Tofu	Tea	Whole Grains	Butter
Local Fruit	Alcohol	Garlic	Meat
Natural Sweeteners	Artificial Colors Flavors and Sweeteners	Legumes	Fish
Soy	Chocolate	Miso	Eggs
Soy Milk	Coffee	Nuts	Hard Cheese
Sprouted Grains	Most Dairy	Onions	
Tempe	Non-local Fruit	Peanut Butter	
Veggie/Fruit Juices	Refined Foods	Root Veggies	
Vegetables	Soft Drinks	Seeds	
Veggie Oils	Hot Spices	Sourdough Bread	

Note: Macrobiotics recommends avoiding (or consuming only occasionally) all extremely ying and yang foods to maintain proper yin/yang balance.

A BALANCED WAY

Since Macrobiotics is all about balance, its philosophy is that nothing is taken to the extreme. (Well, I suppose that many people could have a hard time seeing anything as more extreme than eating primarily whole grains/brown rice and fresh vegetables *every single day*!) The main belief is that we are all a "growing, changing and learning work-in-progress." We learn through mistakes every bit as well as through failure. The only problem is when we get stuck in guilt-ridden emotions and fear.

So loving this process of eating well—and also loving and accepting yourself when you don't—is the way to liberation. I love that philosophy and I also love the way this approach to eating naturally leads you towards the experience of seeing yourself as "The Master." According to Macrobiotic theory, once you feel you've balanced your system, you will also have acquired a balanced enough mind to make your own healthy decisions as to what you want to eat.

One diet can't be the same for everyone, and no Macrobiotic principles are ever considered to be set in stone, since even your own reference for perfect balance can change! That is because true balance is dynamic, not neutral, and everything in your body and in your surroundings will always be in a continual state of change. So to be truly balanced requires you to be adaptable and accepting. For example, as I said earlier, what I feel inclined to eat in winter in New England is not the same as the foods I gravitate towards in Florida in the summer time, and what someone would munch on as a lanky 14-year-old boy won't be the same as what's satisfying to him as a burly 42-year-old man.

THE STANDARD MACROBIOTIC DIET

Here are some easy-to-remember, basic guidelines for a Macrobiotic diet:

- *50% whole grains/cereals—rice, buckwheat, oats, millet, barley, corn
- 25% vegetables
- 25% beans, lentils, fruits, sea vegetables, nuts

Add more water—yin
Bake or dehydrate—yang

> "Beyond Yin and Yang is Mind, recognizing no boundaries between food and its consumer."
>
> ~ Paul Pitchford, author of *Healing with Whole Foods*

* In her book, *The Hip Chick's Guide to Macrobiotics*, Jessica Porter writes that after years of eating Macrobiotic, she realized that a diet consisting of 50% grains is very yang—and sometime felt too heavy for her. So she suggests women—who are yin—try eating 50-60% vegetables (more yin) and 20-25% grains (more yang) if they feel a diet consisting of 50% grains is too much.

THE POWER OF WHOLE GRAINS

If you're going to follow a Macrobiotic diet, you had better like grains, and not just whole-grain breads and pastas, but the whole grain intact—like brown rice, buckwheat and oats. Macrobiotics believe that the wholeness of the grain is directly connected not only to physical wholeness, but to mental, emotional, vital and Spiritual wholeness as well. Hence, eating at least a bowlful a day of these well-balanced little nuggets from nature is essential.

I understand where Macrobiotic people are coming from with their love for whole grains. When I was a little girl, we spent a lot of time in the farm country of Pennsylvania. From time to time, I'd take off from my family, all by myself, and walk into the middle of our neighbor's field—just to sit.

What a lesson in consciousness! I'd look up to see each graceful plant reaching towards the sun, strong and steady enough to support thousands of seeds, yet flexible enough to bend with the wind in unison—"amber waves of grain." That field was alive and sitting in it enlivened my connection to something infinitely wiser and grander than myself.

All over the planet, grains have been unearthed in numerous archeological digs, and when left intact in the hull after harvest, they've lasted for centuries and even millennia. It's evident that they have great endurance and the power to survive. Not only that, consider what even just a handful of such small seeds can grow!

Now imagine yourself eating this kind of energy, on a daily basis. Macrobiotic teachings say that if you make this one change to your diet, it will improve your overall state of health and well-being so much that it will compel you to want balance in your life.

A CORNUCOPIA OF GRAIN OPTIONS

Maybe you're just familiar with the more typical grains, such as rice, wheat, rye and oats. Below are a few others you may want to try. That way, you can add not only taste but also lots of variety to your diet if you feel inclined to try the Macrobiotic way.

Spelt

This grain comes from the same family as wheat, but it contains up to 30% more protein. It also contains more fiber. It possesses mucopolysaccharides, special carbohydrates that stimulate the immune system. Eat it whole—cooked like you would rice or oatmeal. You can also buy it ground as flour. When spelt is cooked in breads, it has a wonderful aroma, and many feel it beats the taste of traditional wheat breads. It's also available in many health food stores as a pasta.

"Yin and Yang are in continual transformation. Nothing is constant, even for a moment. A state of ultimate health occurs when the moment-by-moment transformation of the body and mind are harmonious."

~ Paul Pitchford, author of *Healing with Whole Foods*

Kamut

I often see Kamut labeled as an ancient grain. Although its history is a bit unclear, Kamut is thought to have been derived from a grain used by peasant farmers perhaps in Egypt. Kamut is higher in nutrients than traditional, modern wheat, and particularly appealing for those people who have wheat allergies because they seem to tolerate this grain well.

Quinoa

This grain was originally grown in the South American Andes, and it was eaten by cultures as ancient as the Incas. Quinoa is one of the best protein sources in the plant kingdom, and it's very alkalizing as well. This grain is a big hit among my almost raw-food friends when they splurge on something cooked. I personally love this food and eat it mixed with fruits in the morning or as a side dish with veggies. It's delicious and definitely worth a try.

Amaranth

This member of the wheat family has a nutty taste and chewy texture. It's another ancient grain that can usually be tolerated well by those with wheat sensitivities. Use it to make porridge and to add texture and flavor to recipes.

Millet

Millet has been a dietary staple in Egypt, China, India and Africa for centuries. It has a wonderful texture and can be eaten as a breakfast cereal, side dish or used in soups. I make veggie-burgers with it. It's considered a tonic for the pancreas, stomach and spleen.

Teff

A staple of the Ethiopian diet—Teff is the tiniest grain there is. It's high in calcium and other minerals. It makes a delicious porridge.

THE BENEFITS OF MACROBIOTICS

Practicing Macrobiotics has many benefits, not the least of which is attaining an overall peaceful approach to life. In today's world, so many decisions and choices that people make are prompted by a hurried approach fueled by fast food minds. Basic foods promote awareness of our basic essential nature—which is brilliance. Clearing out the clutter in your diet allows you to experience this.

Physically, the benefits are countless—your outer appearance will reflect your inner harmony. A happy and well-nourished body glows. And as an added benefit, this lightness of being will be most evident in your weight. Pounds drop easily when you give the excess baggage that the emotional disconnect of eating unconsciously requires. You will always feel the need to add more padding and armor as long as you feel you are in constant battle with life. But the more you eat naturally, the more you know all is well, and many times this also enables sickness and ailments to drop by the wayside.

And the most important benefit? The more you eat in sync with the Universe, the more intuitively connected you will feel. Being in the rhythm opens up your line of communication to the Divine.

RAW FOODS AND THE MACROBIOTIC DIET

There's a bit of a conflict between the Raw Food diet and the Macrobiotic diet. As Macrobiotic people see it, raw foods have their place in our diet. However, because raw food is very yin, you can only eat *a small portion* if you want to strictly adhere to a Macrobiotic approach. But again, fortunately for us Soul-Full eaters who are making our own way through this often very contradictory world of diet and nutrition, *everything is allowed in Macrobiotics*. That's because more than anything, this way of eating is about experiencing freedom.

So you can focus on raw foods for detoxifying your body, especially if you've been an extremely yang meat-eater. But the way a true Macrobiotic sees it, your own body will seek balance naturally. So it won't be too long after eating a very yin, raw food diet that you'll be searching out the yang selections. So why not practice moderation from the start and just eliminate the meat and dairy and eat some whole-grain rice (a great detoxifier, though moderately yang) from time to time, along with some other grains and cooked vegetables? That way, you'll avoid altogether the inevitable dramatic swing back to extremely yang foods like meat and dairy.

Another point that Macrobiotic eaters make about raw foods is that the nutrients found in some vegetables can interfere with the thyroid's absorption of iodine and that light cooking eliminates this possibility. So again I say, take what you will from each of these wonderful approaches to eating and eat what you feel most drawn to include in your diet. As you hone your inner compass, trust that you will always come back home to center.

SOMETHING TO CHEW ON

The journey from yin to yang (or the other way around, yang to yin) is very evident in food—soft bread becomes stale and hard, firm pears become soft and ripe. Fresh items soon decay and this rotten compost then becomes the rich soil—alive with nutrients and minerals that support new growth. This becomes that. Eating with balance in mind can allow your whole perspective to widen.

SOUL-FULL EXERCISE #32

If you feel drawn to the Macrobiotic way, you will have to become intimately familiar with whole grains. They are the principal food in this diet. Here's a way to explore it.

For the next 30 days, eat whole grains at one meal (two would be even better!) along with whatever else you would normally eat. Unless, of course, you eat primarily fast food type foods. In that case, you'll most likely be making some additional dietary changes, such as adding more vegetables and fruits to your diet. One batch of cooked whole grains will stay fresh for two or three days, so you don't have to cook every day.

Over the next 30 days, you should notice some big changes in your body. Unless you have a particular intolerance or allergy, you cannot go wrong with grains. Perhaps your skin will glow or your mind will feel clearer. Perhaps your body's discharges will feel different. And don't forget to chew! In Macrobiotics, chewing each bite 50 to 100 times is recommended. I find 50 times is sufficient (to learn more, read the next chapter). There's nothing more complicated to this way of eating than that—just chew the grains and see how you feel.

RESOURCES

Macro-Biotic Diet by Mishio Kushi and Aveline Kushi

The Macrobiotic Way by Mishio Kushi

Pocket Guide to Macrobiotics by Carl Ferre

An Introduction to Macrobiotics: A Beginner's Guide to the Natural Way of Health by Carolyn Heidenry

Basic Macrobiotics, 2nd edition, by Herman Aihara

The Hip Chick's Guide to Macrobiotics by Jessica Porter

The International Macrobiotic Directory

This directory lists resources in all states across the US, including land addresses, email addresses, websites and telephone numbers. *www.strengthenhealth.org*

Foundation for the Macrobiotic Way

www.enjoy-life.com

Macrobiotic Association of Great Britain

www.macrobiotic.co.uk

Online International Macrobiotic Directory

www.macrobioticdirectory.com

The George Oshawa Macrobiotic Foundation

www.gomfmacrobiotic.com

CHAPTER THIRTY-THREE

Chew, Chew, Chew (on This)

"... a man who swallows it [his food], affecting not to know what he is eating... I suspect his taste in higher matters."
~ Charles Lamb, English critic, poet and essayist

A LARGE PART OF EATING'S SENSORY EXPERIENCE takes place in our mouths, via our taste buds. This is also where the physical process of digestion begins, so it is imperative that we chew our food well. Chewing food thoroughly is a habit that not only promotes our greater enjoyment, but also better health.

A CHEW STORY

When I was young, I'd go with my mother to pick up clothes at the tailor from time to time. I remember walking into the corner shop and watching the old tailor, his 85-year-old body still limber and wiry, as he worked over heaps of fabric and among spools of multicolored thread. His name was Aram and he had migrated from Armenia decades before. During one visit, we caught Aram as he was about to take a bite of the sandwich he was eating for lunch. He jumped up and greeted us profusely. As my mother handed him a pile of clothes needing tailoring, she asked him, "Aram, what is the secret to your wonderful health?"

He smiled and answered, "When I was a young boy, there was a war in my country. My parents sent me off to a boarding school in England. It was an all-boys school isolated in the English countryside, and their supervisor was very strict. At meal times, we were made to chew every bite of food fifty times. The teachers stood by our tables and watched us to be certain that we did. I was at the school eight years, and by the time I left to go back home, chewing fifty times had become a habit—one that never left me. I believe this is the secret to my good health."

And indeed, despite the fact that Aram had labored away in his small, dark shop day after day, his old body was defined by muscles and his smile was still warm and radiant after 85 years—the picture of health.

Aram's approach may seem like an awful lot of chewing. However, as you just read in the previous chapter, chewing each bite *50 to 100 times* is the norm in the Macrobiotic diet. Aram actually got off easy!

I personally can't see myself chewing everything 100 times. However, I do practice chewing each bite 50 times and even that is enough to completely dissolve nearly anything I've ever eaten. Most often, my last 10 chews are more like me just swishing around saliva. But I must say that eating primarily whole foods helps. It's much easier to chew a bite of carrot *50 to 100* times than to chew a "melt in your mouth" doughnut that many times.

WHY CHEW MORE?

If you're like most people, who eat on the run or are prone to gobbling down their meals, putting just this one Soul-Full tip to practice can make a big difference in how much you'll benefit from your food.

While so much chewing may seem inconvenient, it's impossible to absorb all of the nutrients and goodness in food without chewing well. As I've already touched on in the acid-alkaline chapter of this book, the

"In Jewish teachings… it is taught that when a person eats… he should have in mind that the taste of the food is also an expression of the Divine in the food, and that by eating it, he is incorporating this spark of the Divine into his body."

~ Aryeh Kaplan, author of *Jewish Meditation*

digestion of carbohydrates—such as grains, and vegetables—begins in the mouth. There our glands secrete ptylin (amylase), an enzyme that mixes in with our food as we chew. If the food we eat doesn't get broken down well in the mouth, then the other enzymes that the food meets up with along the way in your digestive track can't do their job as effectively.

If that happens repeatedly, guess what?—you'll feel more hungry, no matter how much you eat. This is because you're not really nourishing your body as effectively as you could with more enzymes—provided you ate less, but chewed more.

When you chew, you are also doing something else that is equally, if not more important. You're breaking down the food you eat into tiny pieces, which releases more fully the vitamins, minerals and energy inherent in every bite. In addition, un-chewed food can sit in the stomach for a very long time, causing gas, bloating and all kinds of unpleasant physical symptoms. So you're likely to avoid these problems with proper chewing. Many people think that they have digestive disorders in their stomach, when in fact their inability to digest foods begins in their mouth.

As far as the balancing of your acid-alkaline levels is concerned, chewing 50 times is an easy way to adhere to that path. Your saliva is alkaline, so the process of chewing naturally alkalizes your food right in your mouth.

Finally, when you chew whole foods well, the food actually tastes better too. Part of this is due to the fact that you are really taking the time to taste your food. Also, it's because the glucose of grains, vegetables and fruits gets released. What better way to get your sweet tooth satisfied?

YOUR PEARLY WHITES

Let's face it, you can't chew a thing without your teeth, yet according to T.C. Fry, in his article titled, *The Myth of American Health*, 98.5% of the US population has dental problems. What we eat has a direct effect on the health of our teeth. Although your teeth are undeniably strong—with a weight-bearing capacity four times greater than an equal amount of reinforced concrete!—they are also made up of incredibly light calcium phosphate crystals which are formed into a diamond-like pattern. Although they are extremely hard they are living tissues that register many of the imbalances and extremes our bodies experience. This makes them a good indicator of your overall health.

If you have had many dental problems—think back to when they arose, your general health at the time, and what kinds of foods you were typically eating. Chances are that your dental problems arose at the times when you were under the most stress (and therefore your body was most acidic) and/or when your diet was most imbalanced. Mine appeared mostly in junior high school, when it was not uncommon for the dentist to discover 12 to 15 cavities during each dental appointment. Looking back, that was a very stressful time of my life and I was eating a very typical modern "junior-high-type" sugary diet.

It's no surprise to me then that one of the ways anthropologists date human fossils is by looking at their teeth. The more modern the fossil, the more tooth decay! Interestingly enough, most paleontologists agree that tooth decay coincides with the discovery of fire and the advent of agriculture. Fossilized teeth show no premature wear or decay when they date back to the time when indigenous foods were eaten raw.

TAKING CARE OF YOUR IVORIES

Both teeth and bones are living tissues that are constantly being replaced and rebuilt. The best way to support the process is by eating a healthy diet rich in the minerals provided by fresh fruits (not too many acidic) and vegetables (primarily leafy greens—which are very alkaline).

One way to insure that your mouth is an optimal environment for healthy teeth is to chew on greens. Chewing green leaves not only helps provide alkalinity but an optimum calcium-phosphorous balance. In nature, primates load their mouths with greens and then chew and compress the pulpy matter into the teeth and gums for 30 to 45 minutes without swallowing, similar to the way a ball player chews tobacco. This is called "wadging." I stumbled upon this as a great way to reap the benefits of wheatgrass (something I discovered purported in *The Gospel of the Essenes*) since I don't really enjoy drinking wheatgrass juice. Now, from time to time, I just put a wad of the grass in my mouth and chew for up to an hour.

Something else I've begun to do is to have all of the mercury-amalgam fillings removed from my mouth (it's been a long process—since there were so many). I've been seeing a holistic dentist to make sure that the removal and replacement of the fillings is done properly. Mercury is one of the most toxic substances known and it really should not be in our mouths. Many people are unaware that they suffer the ill effects of mercury poisoning, as it leaches from their teeth. Nor are they aware that the presence of mercury in the mouth can sap your vital nerve energy. Replacement fillings are made with gold or porcelain.

"Happiness for me is largely a matter of digestion."

~ Lin Yutang

SOMETHING TO REALLY CHEW ON

*If you've ever had a problem feeling satisfied no matter how much you eat, look at **the way you eat**.* Are you the "grab-and-gobble" type, who barely chews more than three times for each bite? If so, no wonder you've felt as though you were starving. You've been starving your body of nutrients and so it's been craving something more—maybe it just so happens to be *more* chewing.

SOUL-FULL EXERCISE #33

You guessed it!—today you chew each and every bite 50 times. And if you don't like that, you can chew 100 times (just kidding).

While you are chewing away, you'll have plenty of time to notice how different this eating experience is from your typical one. Also, see how much easier it is to feel when you are full when chewing 50 times.

CHAPTER THIRTY-FOUR

Getting on the Fast Track

*"There's an unseen sweetness in the stomach's emptiness.
We are lutes. When the sound box is filled, no music can
come forth."*
~ Jalaluddin Rumi

"NO, I'M NOT GOING TO DIE MOM." That was my response to my mother's continual pleas of "Eat something" the first time I tried juice fasting. After six days of no food, I was feeling great—but the idea of my not eating for over a week was nearly killing her!

Alright, she did grow up in a big Italian household, where four-to-five course meals of pasta, antipasta, spaghetti, meatballs and cannolis were the norm. So the thought of my wasting away to nothing before her eyes was very real to my mother. But I didn't waste away, far from it! This 10-day fast energized me beyond anything I'd ever previously experienced—my eyes sparkled, my hair was silkier, my smile brighter. I felt rejuvenated and alive and very, very clear-minded. And on top of all of that, my Spirit was soaring—liberated from its routine captivity in the three-meals-a-day normal routine. I was in-spir(it)ed!

Those are just some of the many benefits you can receive when you allow your system to cleanse by taking a break from the normal digestive routine.

HOUSECLEANING OF THE BODY

You've probably heard the adage, "Your body is a temple." Well, I'd like you to think for a moment of your body as a house—one that needs regular cleaning, and even a more thorough "spring cleaning" from time to time in order for you to feel your best. If you would like to get back to your optimum level of health and well-being, there is no more effective way than to make fasting and detoxifying a routine part of your life.

The truth is that we live in an impure world. Chemical pollutants are found everywhere, and just by virtue of being alive and breathing, you ingest them. Your body's cells store these along with toxins from overindulgences and body waste. Over time, these build up in your system and can affect your various organs, especially those that are responsible for cleansing and eliminating waste from your body—such as the liver, kidneys and colon.

The physical symptoms of a toxic buildup are so commonplace that, unless you cleanse your body regularly, you most likely experience at least one or two of them often. They include skin blemishes, rashes, headache, nausea, loss of memory, inability to focus, fatigue, chronic sinus congestion, constipation, depression, irritability, insomnia, a coated tongue, aches and pains, gas, stomach disorders, susceptibility to colds and flus… you get the picture. Meanwhile, turn on the television, and in 10 minutes, you'll see a commercial featuring some pharmaceutical product you can take to alleviate one of these symptoms. However, there is a much better way—*you can cleanse your body*! Detoxing will enhance your physical, mental and Spiritual outlook on life.

FASTING BASICS TO GET YOU STARTED

I usually fast one day a week. Most often it is on Monday, because I also practice Silence on that day as well. Refraining from speaking and eating on Mondays allows me to reconnect to myself. It gives me the Spiritual insight and balance I feel I need to be present with the many clients I speak with each week during coaching calls and in seminars.

A one-day food fast is not all that complicated—you just refrain from eating. I usually have one or two large glasses of fresh alkalizing green-juice and lots of pure water throughout the day. Sometimes I have just water.

For longer fasts, I do pay more attention to the process, as extended cleanses are a bit of an art. You may think your body is quite clean. However, if you live on this planet, many toxins will be released from your cells when you do an extended fast.

I recommend juice fasting, but there are many different levels of fasting—both more and less intensive than the traditional juice fast. For someone who normally eats a diet heavily laden with meat and other processed foods, a fast might consist of raw vegetables and fruits only. For someone who already follows a vegetarian diet, a juice fast would probably work best. The trick is, once again, to find out what works best for you; to feel what your body needs and what it's ready for. If you feel that, given your present eating habits, you may not be ready for a complete juice fast, you can take a progressive approach—first eat a vegetarian diet, then another time, eat raw fruits and vegetables only, then during a different fast, just drink juice.

Note: In general, pregnant and breastfeeding women should not fast, nor should anyone who is 10 pounds or more underweight. If you have any medical problems or are taking any medications, it is best to conduct your fast under the supervision of a health professional.

As you see, technically, fasting can be defined as any diet that allows the body to detoxify itself—any diet that is less heavy than what you normally eat. But for our purposes, whenever I speak about fasting in this chapter, I mainly mean refraining from all solid foods.

Theoretically, a fast can last as long as you'd like. Generally, during a juice fast, you will lose your appetite after the first three days. Your body will let you know when to break the fast, and you will suddenly feel very hungry. Also, you'll notice that the white coating on the surface of your tongue will go away. A fast should generally last at least three days but could be as short as one day if that's all you can fit in, or feel comfortable with, for now. If you have any concerns about fasting, and particularly if you're planning to fast for a very long time, over two weeks, I suggest you seek the advice and assistance of a health professional who is familiar with fasting.

Still, despite what many people think, fasting is a *very* safe and effective way to detoxify the body. It has actually been used as a healing method throughout history. And think about it—what is your pet's natural, self-prescribed healing solution when they are feeling under the weather? *They fast.*

Although fasting is not practiced that widely in mainstream America, where drug therapy and prescriptions are the most common medical treatments, fasting is still widely used in Europe. There are hundreds of fasting clinics across Europe that use juice fasting as the #1 healing method. Under supervision, fasting is suggested as a sure-fire way of quitting smoking, as well as breaking free of alcoholism and other drug addictions. It has also been used in natural cancer treatments, and in the treatment of many other diseases—both here and in other parts of the world.

A CLOSER LOOK AT JUICE FASTING

Juice fasts release toxins more slowly than a strict water fast. Also, fresh fruit and vegetable juices are very healing to the body. They are rich in mineral salts and help neutralize toxins. They are also easily assimilated, require minimal digestion, help stabilize blood-sugar levels, and supply calories and nutrients that will help you to maintain high-energy levels while your body is cleansing. There are fewer and less intense withdrawal reactions too—compared to a water fast—as common allergens are eliminated from your system. Fasting becomes a much more pleasant, and easier to endure experience, when juices are taken.

When to Fast

The best time to begin a juice fast is at the change of seasons or at the full or new moon. That is when the body most powerfully aligns with the earth's subtle energies and cleanses the strongest. The very reason that so many people seem to "come down with something" during seasonal changes is that this is when the body is naturally triggered into detoxifying. For women, another powerful time is at the onset of menses—when a natural cleansing of the body has already been initiated.

What to Juice

You can juice almost any fruit or vegetable that you can eat raw, although there are some that don't taste nearly as good as others. So you can juice whatever fruits or vegetables you like best and naturally gravitate towards. If you're suffering from a physical ailment, there are some vegetables that have specific healing properties. For example, celery juice has a calming effect and supports the nervous system. It's also a diuretic. Fennel juice help promote the release of endorphins—the "feel good" brain chemicals. Lettuce juice calms digestion. There are also juice combinations that help tone the kidneys, clear up sinus congestion, give you beautiful hair, skin and nails, and much more! Finding out about these combinations is definitely worth your while. The juices are not only delicious, and regenerating, but also give you a feeling of empowerment from finding a source for healing that is direct from Mother Nature.

If you want to find out more about healing juices, check out the resources I've listed at the end of this chapter.

"Fasting is Nature's foundational law of all healing and revitalization."

~ David Wolfe

THE CHAKRAS AND JUICE CHOICES

I am familiar with the Hindu chakra system, so I make use of it when preparing for a juice fast. In the chakra system, our bodies are divided into seven energy wheels (chakra means wheel). Each chakra has its own color as well as an energy that is associated with it. Let's take a look at the first two chakras and how I might integrate them into planning for a fast.

At the base of the spine, there is the first chakra—the energy there governs our feelings of safety and security and the color is red. So if I feel I need some support in that area, I drink a juice that's made from a vegetable or fruit that is red in color—like beets or cranberries. The second chakra is bright orange in color, and it governs our relationship to our creativity. It's located in the area around the lower abdomen (in women—around an area of supreme creativity—the ovaries). So if I am feeling any stuck or resistant energy with regard to creativity, or if I find that the organs located in this part of my body need healing, I drink juice from an orange-colored fruit or vegetable—such as oranges, cantaloupe or carrots.

If you feel you resonate with this approach, refer to the quick reference chart below for the chakra colors, the sections of the body that they govern, and some of the vegetables and fruits that are beneficial for each area. Have fun with this and be open to the blessings and healing energy!

	COLOR	ENERGY	LOCATION	FRUIT/VEGGIE
Fruits/Vegetables and The Chakras				
FIRST CHAKRA	red	support, safety/security, money/sex	base of spine, genitals	beets, cherries, berries, cranberries
SECOND CHAKRA	orange	creativity	lower abdomen	carrots, oranges, cantaloupe
THIRD CHAKRA	yellow	power, fire	solar plexus	golden apples lemons, ginger
FOURTH CHAKRA	green	love, receptivity	heart	green grapes, limes, all green veggies
FIFTH CHAKRA	blue	creative expression	throat	blueberries
SIXTH CHAKRA	indigo/purple	intuition	forehead, "third eye"	grapes, plums
SEVENTH CHAKRA	all colors	heightened Spiritual awareness	crown	all fruits and veggies, mixed

WHEATGRASS

Although wheatgrass is indeed a grass and not a fruit or vegetable, I felt I could not omit offering information about this incredible healing nectar. Wheatgrass is known to many in the nutritional and healing world as a "super-food." This is mainly due to the miraculous effect it has had on those with ailments ranging from cancer to psoriasis. Its taste, although pleasant (somewhat like a liquid verdant green meadow!), is equally as powerful as its healing effects. It is not gulped by the glass, but rather more often gingerly sipped in small shots. Ann Wigmore is perhaps the most famous pioneer of wheatgrass juice (more about her in Chapter 40—"Food as Healer") as she brought hundreds, if not thousands, of terminally ill patients back to health with it. Wigmore reported that 15 pounds of wheatgrass (unjuiced) contains the nutritional equivalent of 350 pounds of all other green vegetables. Although it is somewhat new on the health-scene, its healing properties are not newly discovered. *The Gospel of the Essenes*, part of the *Dead Sea Scrolls*— which dates back to the time of Jesus Christ—illustrates the wide-spread use of wheatgrass. It was praised (literally) for containing all of the elements (and the angels) of the earth in perfect balance.

On top of being one of the richest sources of chlorophyll on the planet, wheatgrass has an enormous amount of enzymes, 20 amino acids, an astounding amount of antioxidants, and a long list of vitamins and minerals. It's been called "liquid sunshine." When fasting, be certain to drink it by itself, and in between glasses of other fruits and vegetable juices (unless you are very well acquainted with fasting, and you have a pure diet and your system is relatively clean). In my early days of exploring nutrition, while I was still modeling in New York City (and I suppose highly toxic given my lifestyle and the pollution surrounding me), I once fasted primarily on water and drank only intermittent shots of wheatgrass throughout the day. By the end of the first day, I was nearly paralyzed with fatigue. I remember a friend calling and I could barely lift my arm to answer the phone. Apparently I was detoxing way too quickly. But since then I've had many wonderful experiences with wheatgrass and I highly recommend it to anyone who wants to taste "God's Glory"—the concentrated energy of the elements supercharged with sunlight and nutrients.

"More will be learnt from [a fast] than from all the lands you visited or books you have read."

~ Morris Krok

Every blade of grass has its angel that bends over it and whispers, "Grow, grow."
    ~ The Talmud

WHAT ABOUT JUICERS?

Now that you know what to juice, what do you use to juice it? First, it's important to know that a juicer is not a blender and blended foods are not juices. A whirl-top orange juicer is not the kind of juicer I am referring to either. To make juice suitable for fasting, you have to extract the fluid part of the vegetable or fruit; this is what contains all of the vitamins, minerals and enzymes. To do that, you need a juice extractor.

Be sure to get a good juicer. They not only make juices faster and tastier, but also the right kind will not heat the temperature of the fruit or vegetables too high. Temperatures above 118 degrees kill the produce's essential enzymes. I've listed several sources for juicers in the resources section at the end of this chapter.

Look for a large feed tube so that you don't have to cut your produce into very small pieces before juicing. And select a juicer that ejects pulp into a receptacle, instead of holding it inside of the machine. That way, you can juice continuously and you won't have to stop the juicer to scoop out the refuse.

You may also look at the juicer's other features when deciding which one to buy. Some are very versatile and also act as food processors and even ice-cream makers. But one of the things I find most important to find out is how easy it will be to clean. When you're making juice several times a day, cleaning and chopping vegetables is enough of a chore without the added work of having to tediously clean a juicer.

There are many cheap juicers and also many dissatisfied people who have purchased them—so be a savvy shopper. Your juicer may very well become one of your best friends!

THE THREE MOST POPULAR TYPES OF JUICERS

Centrifugal Juicers (price range—$100 to $150) are the most popular and the most affordable type of juicer. In fact, most juicers available in department stores are centrifugal juice machines, but beware of machines with warranties of less than one year. Centrifugal juicers first grate the fruit or vegetable into a pulp, and then use centrifugal force to push the pulp against a strainer screen by spinning it at a very high RPM. They are great at juicing most any fruit or vegetable, but centrifugal juicers are not capable of efficiently extracting juice from wheatgrass, leafy greens, or herbs.

Single Gear (Masticating) Juicers (price range—around $350) use a single gear or auger that literally chews fruit and vegetable fibers and breaks up the plant cells, resulting in more fiber, enzymes, vitamins and trace minerals. These juicers are generally more efficient than centrifugal juicers because they can extract more juice from the same amount of food (i.e. the pulp comes out dryer). Masticating juicers are very capable at juicing most fruits and vegetables, and they will also extract juice from wheatgrass, spinach, and other leafy greens and herbs. (Note: The Champion Juicer does not juice wheatgrass or greens well.)

Another benefit of masticating juicers is that they operate at slower speeds (RPMs) than centrifugal juicers, resulting in less foam and heat, which means more nutrition in your glass. Masticating juicers are also more versatile than centrifugal juicers; in addition to extracting juices, they can also homogenize foods to make baby foods, pates, sauces, nut butters, banana ice-creams and fruit sorbets. Some of these juicers can even extrude pasta and make rice cakes!

Twin-Gear (Triturating) Juicers (price range—$350 to $750) are the most expensive type of juicers, but they offer the most benefits. These juicers turn at even slower speeds (RPMs), resulting in even less oxidation from foam and less destruction of nutrients from heat. Triturating juicers are the most efficient type of juicer available and can extract larger volumes of juice from fruits, vegetables, wheatgrass, pine needles, spinach, and other greens and herbs.

Twin-gear juicers operate by pressing food between two interlocking roller gears. This juicing process yields a larger volume of juice and extracts more fiber, enzymes, vitamins and trace minerals. Twin-gear juicers do more than just extract juice; they also homogenize to make baby foods, nut butters and fruit sorbets. In addition, many have attachments for making pasta and rice cakes like some of the masticating juicers.

Wheatgrass Juicers (price range—$100 to $300) are made exclusively for extracting the juice from wheatgrass and other leafy greens, as well as some soft fruits like grapes. Wheatgrass juicers are not made for extracting juice from vegetables and most fruits. They are available in both electric and manual models. (**Note:** All of the masticating [except Champion] and twin-gear juicers are capable of extracting juice from wheatgrass.)

Juicing Fasting Tips

Here are some basic guidelines:

- **Use between one and three parts water to each part fresh juice**. Vegetable juice (especially when the less-sweet vegetables are used) can be taken undiluted, but fruit juice, which is high in fructose, is best diluted.

- **Use fresh, organic fruits and vegetables whenever possible**. If organic produce is unavailable to you, be sure to peel the skin off of the items you juice or wash them with a non-toxic produce cleaner (found at most health food stores). See resource section at the end of this chapter for names of cleaning products.

- **It's very important to take an enema or colonic while fasting**. Your body will be getting rid of huge amounts of waste, a lot of which will come through the bowels. During fasting, the normal bowel movements cease to take place, and if you don't take an enema, the excess waste will be reabsorbed into the system and transported to the kidneys, which can be damaged by an overload of toxins.

- **Smoking, drinking, or the use of any other kinds of drugs, both prescription and nonprescription, as well as vitamin supplements, are prohibited during fasting**. If you're on medication for any kind of condition, you should see a health practitioner who can supervise your fast. You should also abstain from sexual activity, in order to save your energy.

- **Your body will need exercise during the fast, to aid in expelling waste and to revitalize new body cells.** Up to three hours of moderate exercise are recommended per day, such as long, brisk walks in the fresh air or swimming in salt or fresh water.

- **Daily baths are also important.** Your body will expel about one-third of its waste through the skin. It's important to keep the skin clean, and the pores wide open in order for excretion to occur as efficiently as possible. Saunas and steam baths can be taken if your heart and circulation are good, and if these facilities are available. Hot and cold showers, followed by a dry brush massage, are also very beneficial.

- **Even if you're drinking a large amount of juice, you may drink as much water as you need if you become thirsty.** Just make sure that all the water is filtered and pure. Distilled water is fine. Avoid chlorinated or fluoridated water.

- **The positive effects of the fast can easily be erased if you go back to an unhealthy diet afterwards.** You can keep your body detoxified and healthy by focusing on a vegetarian, or near-vegetarian diet of mostly raw fruits and vegetables.

- **It's preferable that you press your own juices.** However, if you cannot, find a health food store or juice bar that makes the juice right in front of you so you know that it is as fresh as possible.

- You can add blue-green algae, spirulina, chlorella, natural enzymes, or green food powder to juices to provide more energy.

- Adding ginger and/or garlic to juices increases their ability to cleanse the body.

- You can drink decaffeinated herbal teas, but no caffeinated tea or coffee.

- Get plenty of rest.

- **Breathe deeply, in fresh air and sunshine**. Breathing exercises and yoga are good options.

- **Don't use ice**. Water and juice should be room temperature or slightly warm.

- Keep warm.

- **Nurture yourself** with time for reflection, journaling, quiet, prayer and meditation.

Note: You can continue your normal work routine while fasting unless your line of work is very strenuous. Just be conscious to take short rest and quiet periods throughout the day.

PREPARING TO FAST

It's advisable to prepare yourself for an extended fast through a short cleansing diet. For two or three days, eat nothing but raw fruits and vegetables—one meal a day of fresh fruit, the other meal of a fresh vegetable salad. (If you can handle this, you'll know you can go further with this whole idea.)

To aid in the elimination of toxins, it's advisable to be sure that your bowels are moving during this fasting period. So it is suggested that you begin each day with an enema or colonic.

DAILY FASTING SCHEDULE

- Upon arising—Take an Enema. Then do a dry-brush massage followed by a hot and cold shower.

- 9 am—Drink a cup of herbal tea—warm, not hot, or an 8 oz. glass of water with the juice of one lemon squeezed into it. Choose teas that have effects you may be looking for—such as mint to settle your stomach or chamomile to calm your nerves.

- 11 am—Drink a glass of freshly pressed fruit-juice, diluted 50-50 with noncarbonated spring water.

- 11 am-1 pm—It's time for a walk or mild exercise, and perhaps brief sunbathing. You can also take therapeutic baths or a body massage at this time.

- 1 pm—Drink a glass of freshly made vegetable-juice, green juice or a cup of vegetable broth. (Recipes are below.)

- 1:30—4 pm—Rest.

- 4 pm—Drink a cup of herb tea or fresh coconut water.

- 4:15-7 pm—Here you'll get involved in a walk, therapeutic baths, mild exercise, such as yoga, and/or other treatments such as a body massage (if you have not already done that earlier in the day).

- 7 pm—Drink a glass of diluted vegetable or fruit juice.

- 9 pm—Have a cup of non-caffeinated herbal tea.

Drink plain, lukewarm spring-water any time when thirsty. Your total liquid intake should be between 1-1/2 pints and 1-1/2 quarts.

Note: If you intend to fast for a long period of time or have any health concerns, it is advisable to find a medical professional or other person who is knowledgeable about fasting to supervise you.

> "Green is good. Green is the very center of the rainbow. Green is centering."
> ~ David Wolfe

Green Juice Recipe—"The Thank God!"

Chlorophyll, the pigment in plants that converts sunlight into plant energy, is transferred directly to you when you drink chlorophyll-rich juices from green-leafed vegetables. Just as hemoglobin is the blood in our bodies, chlorophyll is the blood in plants. A significant difference between them is that hemoglobin molecules center on iron, while chlorophyll molecules center on magnesium. Drinking green juice is like getting a transfusion of light directly from the sun to your body. It is extremely high in alkaline minerals. This is my friend Josh's recipe for his favorite juice they sell at the organic market next door to my home.

> A handful of Romaine Lettuce
> A handful of Kale
> A handful of Chard or Collard Greens
> 2-3 stalks of Celery
> 1/2 to 1 Cucumber
> Parsley or Cilantro to taste
> A small amount of garlic, ginger and/or aloe vera can also be added to promote the purification process.

> "If you're green on the inside, you're clean on the inside."
> ~ Dr. Bernard Jensen

Vegetable Broth Recipe*

    2 large potatoes, chopped
    1 cup carrots
    1 cup celery
    1 cup any other vegetable
    Add some garlic, ginger, onions or any other herbs you wish,
    plus natural spices.

Cook all of the vegetables with about 1-1/2 quarts of water slowly, for about a half hour. Strain, cool and serve—or store it in the refrigerator and warm the broth before drinking.

This is a cleansing, alkalizing and mineral-rich drink.

*For those who are not on a strictly raw food fast. In colder climates, drinking this really helps, as your body temperature drops when you're fasting.

BREAKING THE FAST

Breaking the fast is the most important part of the process. How you break a fast will largely determine the value of the fast and the overall degree of rejuvenation that takes place. At the end of the fast, the digestive system will work much more efficiently and will absorb nutrients more easily—so eating should be done slowly and mindfully. Make sure that you eat only those foods that you want to build your system back up with. The end of a fast is a good time to introduce yourself to new eating habits, such as a vegetarian or whole-food lifestyle. Fasting tightens your stomach—so when you go back to your normal diet, you will be able to feel when you are full. This makes it easier not to overeat, because you can discern your body's signals—feeling when it needs food or when it's time to stop eating. You also notice what effects certain foods have on your body, such as which foods make you tired, or give you indigestion, and which foods really seem to benefit your overall health.

The main rules for breaking the fast are:

- Do not overeat!
- When you feel full, stop eating. (You'll feel full on much less food than you think.)
- Eat slowly and chew your food extremely well.
- Take several days to gradually transition back to a normal diet.

Here's how I broke my first 10-day fast:

Day One

I ate one half-apple in the morning and a very small bowl of vegetable salad at lunch, in addition to the usual juice and broth menu I had every day during the fast.

Day Two

I ate a few soaked prunes or figs, with the water for breakfast. Then I ate a small bowl of fresh vegetable salad for lunch. I ate vegetable soup made with sea vegetables at dinner. And then I ate two apples between meals—all this is in addition to the juices and broth.

Day Three

Same as above, but I added a yam or baked potato at lunch. (If you're not going to continue to eat your food raw, you can add a slice of whole-grain bread with the soup at the evening meal.)

After this, you can begin to eat as you wish—adhering to a whole-food-oriented diet.

WHAT TO EXPECT FROM A FAST

When you follow a juice fast similar to the one I've outlined, you most definitely will not have to worry about being malnourished—far from it! In fact, you may never have been so well nourished.

What you can expect from your fast is that you will cultivate an entirely new relationship with food. Your cravings for many of the unhealthy foods that contain salt, sugar, fat chemicals and empty calories will diminish—if not disappear entirely. You will be satisfied with much smaller portions. And you'll be amazed at how delicious food really does taste because you'll be able to taste what you're eating once again. Your body will feel lighter and more fit, your mind will be sharper, and you'll feel more alert, awake and alive.

But most beneficial of all, I feel, is the delicious lightness-of-being you feel that is not available to you any other way. This sweet empty space leaves plenty of room for your Soul to surface, magnifying your sensitivity and sense of connectivity to the beauty inherent in all of life.

By the way, the first time I fasted, my parents noticed my great success (yes, even my Italian mother!) and decided to try fasting too. Soon they were sold on fasting as a way to experience greater health. I've been incorporating fasting into my life for a long time—over 20 years. I personally feel it's a cornerstone of true well-being.

SOMETHING TO (NOT!) CHEW ON

I have many friends who undergo an extended fast once a year—some for as long as 40 days! So now that you know you won't die from fasting, and that it is actually beneficial when you approach it in a healthy manner, why not try a one- or three-day fast—just to test the waters? You can follow the guidelines in this chapter, or also find out more online or by reading some of the books listed in the resources section below. Or if you feel resistant—think about why you're hesitant about not eating for a longer length of time than you have in the past.

SOUL-FULL EXERCISE #34

Before starting a fast, even if it's just a short one, be sure you have all of the necessary ingredients on hand.

Here's a short list of the things you'll need:

- Pure water
- Organic fruits and veggies (or standard fruits and veggies, plus vegetable/fruit cleaner)
- Vegetable brush (to clean veggies)
- Juicer
- Sharp knives
- Natural bristle brush (for a dry-brush massage)
- Cast iron or stainless steel soup pot (if you are making vegetable broth)

RESOURCES

Fasting Can Save Your Life by Dr. Herbert Shelton
Juicing For Life by Cherie Calbom and Maureen Keane
The Juice Lady's Guide to Juicing for Health by Cherie Calbom
Juice Fasting by Paavo Airola
The Wheatgrass Book by Ann Wigmore
Rational Fasting by Professor Arnold Ehret
The Miracle of Fasting by Paul Bragg

Here are some sites I found that address both water and juice fasting. Check them out for yourself and see if you resonate with any of the information they offer.

www.juicefasting.org
www.fasting.com
www.freedomyou.com

—*VEGETABLE WASHES*
An all-natural way to remove wax, soil and agricultural chemicals from produce.

Veggie Wash
www.veggie-wash.com

FIT
www.tryfit.com

Juicers
The juicers listed below are most popular.

Green Star
www.greenstarjuicers.org

Champion
www.greenjuicers.com

Omega
www.omegajuicers.com

Allorganic.net
This is an informative site. For your convenience, they offer a "Juicer's Question Form" through which you input your preferences in a juicer. They reply by sending back their recommendations.
www.allorganic.net

CHAPTER THIRTY-FIVE

Fasting as a Spiritual Practice

"Fasting is a natural part of our walk with God."
~ Matthew 6:16

JESUS DID IT, Moses and Muhammad did it—all before experiencing life-altering, history-making events. Fasting has played an important part in many Spiritual traditions throughout time. Because it has been known to aid the body in the release of the Spirit, religions have called for fasting on specific holy days and at certain times of the year. Although it may have become convoluted at times, the point of religious fasting was not to make the body suffer. As you now know, the body actually becomes stronger and healthier with the practice, while the mind becomes clearer and more centered.

Fasting is used as a Spiritual tool because it lessens the everyday emphasis on our physical bodies and frees the mind to focus on more lofty matters—allowing us to connect with and recognize the Divine. The 40-day fast, subsisting on nothing but water, is mentioned many times in the Bible, and it is still used as a means of transcendence for many.

MAGIC ON THE MOUNTAINTOP

"Spirit cannot radiate fully from the body when overfed."

~ Saint Frances de Sales

I once heard a story about a man who was feeling completely dejected and defeated in his life. He decided to leave his home and everything he owned behind—and made a plan to climb to the top of a nearby mountain to die. After the man made the rigorous climb, he just sat there and waited for the Angel of Death to come find him. However, that didn't happen. So after a few days of eating and drinking nothing, he was still alive, but very thirsty. He took a drink from a nearby spring, then sat back down to wait to die. After a few more days of sitting, with only an occasional drink of water, the man began to feel less depressed. Not only was he sleeping less and less, but he also began to find that he had boundless amounts of energy—which he used to just sit.

After a while, as the energy built up in his body, the man began to feel almost invincible. He began to dream of all he could do with this insight and energy and realized one day that he was no longer depressed. In fact, he could not even remember why he'd felt so defeated to begin with. The man felt so good that he took a long drink of the cool, clear water and sat back down to be still once more. After a month on the mountaintop, the man descended to the village below. He didn't speak much to anyone, but his eyes shone with a newfound light. As he passed, other villagers commented that the man seemed to glow. From that day on, he was known to the others as "The Wiseman." And each year he climbed to the mountaintop, with nothing but the clothes on his back, to sit alone.

Fasting

There's an unseen sweetness
in the stomach's emptiness.
We are lutes.
When the sound box is filled,
no music can come forth.
When the brain and the belly
are burning from fasting,
every moment a new song rises
out of the fire.
The mists clear,
and a new vitality makes you
spring up the steps before you.
Be empty and cry as a reed instrument.
Be empty and write secrets with a reed pen.
When satisfied by food and drink,
an unsightly metal statue
is seated where your Spirit should be.
When fasting, good habits gather like
helpful friends.
Fasting is Solomon's ring.
Don't give in to illusion
and lose your power.
But even when all will and control
have been lost,
they will return when you fast,
like soldiers appearing out of the ground,
or pennants flying in the breeze.
A table descends to your tents,
the Lord's table.
Anticipate seeing it when fasting,
this table is spread with a different food,
far better than the broth of cabbages.

~ Jalaluddin Rumi, 14th century Sufi mystic poet

One of the big reasons that I fast regularly is not for health reasons, but because I find there is no more effective way to tap my Soul. When I fast, my senses naturally heighten and I am easily pulled into a deeper experience of living. To get a better sense of this, think about how wonderful a meal tastes when you're "starving"—how much more enjoyable it is—and you naturally take it in with all of your senses. Then conversely think about how anesthetizing overeating can be and how tired you become after eating a heavy meal. Now imagine how much more fully you can take in a moment when your senses aren't being dulled by the input of any food whatsoever—especially once you have experienced fasting as a Spiritual practice once or twice and see for yourself how "full-filling" it can be. It's wonderful to be able to focus on "the formless," rather than strictly on the world of form for a time.

And what about the hunger pangs? I find that people's hunger is often directly in alignment with their intentions. If you are fine with, and even looking forward to, not eating for a time because you are fasting to further connect with your Spirit, then chances are you'll feel much less hunger. Why? Because you'll be experiencing not deprivation, but a greater fullness from tapping into your Soul.

It may seem strange, but one year I even decided to spend Thanksgiving Day fasting. I think it was the most beautiful Thanksgiving I've ever had. I felt so alive, clear and Spiritually lifted.

I've seen that with fasting, food can be put in the proper perspective, recognized for what it is, first and foremost. That is, a vehicle for connecting to the Divine Source within us—via giving and receiving Love.

SOMETHING TO CHEW ON

As I mentioned earlier, fasting is an ancient practice. Why would it continue to this day, if it were not of tremendous benefit? Here is an excerpt from the Gospel of the Essenes, translated by Edmond Bordeaux Szekely. It relates what Jesus reportedly told his new followers about fasting:

"Renew yourselves and fast. For I tell you truly,
that darkness and its plagues may only be cast out
by fasting and by prayer... when the faculties are
empty, then the whole being listens. There is then
a direct grasp of what is right there before you
and can never be heard with the ear or understood
with the mind. Fasting empties the faculties, frees
you from limitation and from preoccupation.
Fasting begets unity and freedom."

SOUL-FULL EXERCISE #35

To make any fast a truly Spiritual one, it's important to remember that the fast is between you and you, just as Jesus counsels in the Bible when he says, "...show your fasting to no man." Also, remember that a Spiritual fast is never about sacrifice or suffering or showing any other person anything—such as your superior stamina. That would be an ego-driven motivation, which would prevent you from reaping the true, deep benefits of a Spiritual fast. A fast, first and foremost, is about aligning with a Greater Fullness of Being. So while you are fasting, not only treat yourself well by taking care of your personal hygiene, but also add some extra-sensory stimuli to your experience. Find a quiet retreat-like setting where you can sit and contemplate your life, meditate or pray—even if just for a few hours a day. Light a candle to remind yourself of the Light within and to center yourself each day. And remember to drink lots of water and breathe! To prepare for your fast, find some books about the lives of saints and sages, or others who've lived a more contemplative life, and follow some of their daily Spiritual routines, ways of processing life and thinking. Observe and connect to Nature however possible. And always, know that you are Divine.

"The journey into fasting is about becoming a finely-tuned Spiritual instrument. Fasting is mentioned as part of nearly every religion on earth."

~ David Wolfe

RESOURCES

Mystics, Masters, Saints and Sages: Stories of Enlightenment by Robert Ullman
    and Judyth Reichenberg-Ullmann

Mysticism by Evelyn Underhill

Autobiography: The Story of My Experiments with Truth by M. K. Gandhi

The Soul's Religion by Thomas Moore

Following Francis of Assisi by Patti Normile

God's Fool (about Francis of Assisi) by Julien Green

CHAPTER THIRTY-SIX

Thought-*full*ness vs. Thought-*less*ness

A Way to Overcome Emotional Eating

"In Infinity, full is no better than empty.
Nothingness is both empty and full..."
~ The Zohar

"SHE SEES THE GLASS AS HALF FULL, instead of half empty" is clearly a way of saying that a woman is optimistic. Optimism is a wonderful asset and a great character trait that will serve anyone who desires to live a happy life. However, the above statement implies that empty is less desirable than full.

Suppose that you now adopt an entirely new point of view—a perspective called *Soul-Full vision*. It's the ability to see emptiness as full of something you just can't see with your two eyes or sense with your other four senses. Yet it is there nonetheless. For instance, what if you began to see an emptied glass as all full, instead of all empty? That would mean that you have the ability to see *and feel* the fullness of space.

If you cultivate this type of vision, more than just your relationship to eating and food will be dramatically changed. In addition, your entire perception of life will be radically altered forever.

I was speaking to a new friend, Mary, about this chapter as I was writing it and she said, "*Oh what a great topic! The reason I am so overweight today is that two years ago I left work to take care of my mother as she was dying of cancer. I sat by her bedside and ate fourteen hours a day. I was stuffing all of my emotions, and on top of that, I felt that I wasn't doing anything with my life. I wasn't being fulfilled so I began eating things to fill in the void I felt inside.*"

The truth is, the only thing that makes us feel uncomfortable with feelings of emptiness, or of being in a state of unknowing, is the idea that we should know or should fill it up with something in order to stay safe. Well, what if we could all just accept that sometimes we don't know what is happening to us, or around us in life, and sometimes we don't even really know who we are. Is that really so bad? What if we let all labels drop for a while. What then? To the ego that is death, but to the Soul, dropping labels and body identification is liberation… the only way to let our true essence emerge from out of "the box." Dropping labels also helps us move beyond thinking that we are only human and so solely identified with our form.

The fact is we are all human *beings*. Our beings are our formless Selves. We are meant to live a balance of both the form and formless as human beings. Notice what happened to Mary as she identified only with the form of her mother as she was dying of cancer; it made her identify only with her own body as well. The only way to be comfortable with the idea of less as being more is if you know yourself as both form and formless, as human and as being—and then balance the two equally in your life In this way, you can see that even death is just the continuum of life lived in the formless or "empty" state. It really isn't empty at all; it just appears to be so to a body.

Just as Mary did under duress, many people eat emotionally. That is, they don't just eat when they're hungry. They don't see food as a delicious way to fuel their bodies, and to infuse their cells with energy and ample vitality. Instead, they use food for "a filler" in life—much like drugs, alcohol, television or superficial relationships. They eat for companionship (for instance, when experiencing a breakup with a significant other), or to assuage feelings of boredom, grief or depression.

Maybe you are one of these people. If you are, here's some good news for you. When you begin to see eating as a path to higher consciousness, every bite you eat can take you closer to Self-realization and the experience of living a vibrant life. That is, a life full of love and creative expression—a life free of "filler" and loaded down with substance.

LIFTING YOUR FEELINGS

Let me use depression as another vehicle to help you cultivate Soul-Full vision. When seen through the Soul's "eyes," depression is not a clinical disease at all, but instead the result of a series of thoughts—one depressing thought after another.

If you find yourself in such a state of mind, in which the rapid succession of thoughts makes you feel overwhelmed and out of control of your emotions, grabbing a donut definitely will not help. In fact, if you've ever done this, you know that eventually it just adds fuel to the fire. Although initially soothing, the eating can lead you to adding "fat pig" or some other self-debasing thought to your internal tirade.

Instead of eating, at these times, try deliberately stopping whatever it is that you're doing, find a comfortable spot (away from the refrigerator!), and sit down and begin to breathe deeply. You'll soon find that you're able to slow down the flow of your negative thoughts if you begin to deliberately watch your breath.

Once you slow your breathing, begin at that point to look for the space between each thought. At first, while your thoughts are getting away with you, it may be difficult to find any space between them. "Little thoughts" about yourself and your life are just that—little—so you can cram quite a lot of them together. But when the thoughts begin to slow, you can see that they are just like clouds floating by in a vast sky. And when you see this, you can make a choice. Do you want to be the cloud—the heavy emotion, or painful, dramatic thought? Or do you want to identify with the sky—the emptiness and space? If you identify with a vast mind, you see that there is lots of space between each thought—lots of room for the Divine.

The fact is that you don't need more—that is, more drugs, more therapy, or more lovers to get over being depressed. You just have to know how to think with awareness, which means to pay attention to the space between thoughts more than to the thoughts themselves. With time, you'll find—as most contemplatives do—that from the empty space arises peace. This peace is highly supportive; supportive enough, in fact, to bolster Big Fat Fulfilling Thoughts—thoughts full of love, appreciation, inspiration and creativity. These are the types of thoughts which will allow you to move deeper into yourself, beyond all surface fret and hungering, to feel how satisfying life can be when we get out of our minds and into our hearts. The most masterful beings who have walked the earth have been those of transcendent faith which naturally afforded them the ability to see the "unseen." Therefore they had a tranquil nature and calm belief in the helpful allegiance we all have with invisible forces. These forces are real and available to each and every one of us. Have faith and you'll soon start seeing the supportive forces of the Universe in your life.

SOMETHING TO CHEW ON

There is a story about noted psychologist Carl Jung and his visit to the Pueblo Indians. Jung asked the Tribal Chief Ochwiay Biano what his opinion was of the white man. The Chief replied favorably, but added that he couldn't quite understand why the white man always seemed upset as if they were constantly hungry and looking for something. He noticed the result of this was that the white men's faces were covered with many wrinkles and their health was often poor. The Chief added that perhaps the white men were so crazy because they think with their heads, and only crazy people do that. Jung asked in surprise how the Chief thought. The Chief replied that, naturally, he thought with his heart.

SOUL-FULL EXERCISE #36

Stop for a moment, get comfortable, and take three deep centering breaths. Now close your eyes and search the inside of your body as though you have a spotlight moving from your head down to your toes. Imagine that this spotlight is capable of finding any pockets of stuck or resistant energy within you. You may feel this resistance in the form of tightness, restriction or even pain. When you find such an area, begin to deliberately add space to it by using your breath. See it as concentrated energy waiting to be released and breathe space and light into it. Do this to every pocket of resistance within you. When you are finished—whether it takes you 10 minutes or an hour, open your eyes. Wherever you happen to be, stay still and take a good look around you. Perhaps you are outdoors, and you see trees or a street. Possibly you notice clouds and the sun. If you are indoors, maybe you see a floor, walls, a table, some chairs, shelves and/or a couch. What you see doesn't matter. It is what you do not see that you will be focusing on.

Now begin to notice the space that is in and around each of the objects near you. See that without the support of the space, these objects would not be able to exist. They would be dust. There would not even be air to breathe if there was no space to hold it. Now begin to consider which is more important to the experience you are now having—is it the object you are perceiving, or the spaciousness surrounding it and moving in, of and through it? It is my belief that space equals the Divine—because it is beyond any limited concepts or judgments we may hold and unconditionally supportive of us in all we do.

Scientists say that our bodies are made up of 99.9% space as is outer space, and all other objects in space. No matter how unbelievable that may seem, quantum physics tells us that this is the nature of matter. Eat with this recognition in mind—cognizant of the spaciousness of the food you eat and of your being—eventually you'll lose the sense of emptiness. Instead you'll be filled with a profound realization that when you identify with space, your thoughts of littleness must expand. Thoughts of grandeur naturally replace them. Try setting the stage of your next meal with this experience as the background next time you are feeling "empty" or depressed. And as often as possible, realize that the unconditionally supportive, all accepting and encompassing nature of space = love!

"I am happy and content because I think I am."

~ Alain-Rene Lesage

CHAPTER THIRTY-SEVEN

Losing Weight

It's an Inside Job

"The ancestor of every action is a thought."
~ Ralph Waldo Emerson

ALTHOUGH A WEIGHT-LOSS DIET affects how you look on the outside, many of the changes that will allow you to slim down need to happen from deep within you. Losing weight—especially if you have many pounds to take off—can be easily approached from a Soul-Full perspective. It's very Spiritual to lose weight with a whole, balanced approach, because you have to get in touch with the same things that are so important to a Spiritual path. For example, dieting is a powerful way to get in touch with that formidable, brilliant presence within ourselves.

To be effective with weight loss, you must either go deep within to find your sustenance, or go high up to more heavenly realms and loftier thoughts to find the wherewithal to persist. There is no value in centering on what appears to be valuable only to the two eyes looking out of everyone else's faces. It is only the true, Soul-Full, inner "I" that knows your worth and perfection and holds the true tenacity of purpose to reveal that Self to you and to the world. Living life fully is between you and you!

A PATH OF SPIRIT AND SELF-LOVE

"You can enjoy encouragement coming from outside, but you cannot need it to come from outside."

~ Vladimir Zworykin

I often think about people who have large amounts of weight to lose. When this is the case, it can be terribly disheartening to look outside of yourself for confirmation. Even if you lose 30 pounds for instance, which is an enormous victory, you may still have 150 or 200 pounds to go. While you know that you just did something that was very difficult and incredible, much of the rest of the world may not notice. That's when it's time to live and breathe *for you*, and just forgive them, which is actually the most powerful discovery of any valid Spiritual path. This may sound easy, but for many it's actually quite tough to do, and that's the reason why there are so few True Masters. But imagine if you choose to see your victory of losing pounds and inches as a Spiritual victory as well as a path to a higher level of self-care.

As you diligently focus on losing weight, you'll realize that Self-love and forgiveness work to uplift you when you find yourself feeling like there is no love or appreciation coming your way from others. Authentically loving and honoring yourself will give you a certain lightness of being as you discover that True Love is never found outside of yourself. Feeling acceptance from another is often just the catalyst that allows us to open our own hearts to ourselves. The fact is that at a Soul level, below surface appearances, *you are love*. Recognizing this, you'll notice that it doesn't matter how others perceive you and act towards you once you become truly connected to the Light within yourself.

That's all you've ever needed anyway—to stop adding layer upon layer over your Light. As the Bible says, don't try to comfortably hide your light under a bushel—or under a few extra pounds!

It takes a huge amount of Spirit to lose 100+ pounds, or any amount of weight for that matter. And luckily we all have that in us—and more! Spirit is HUGE. Know that you are bigger and brighter than you may be acting at any given moment. To feel full, you must let your Soul free. You must let It run wildly through life—giving and receiving joy with wild abandon—no matter what anyone else thinks! The #1 reason we gain weight is from living for the approval of others—*your hunger comes from missing you!* So many of us are in denial of that and we think that "stuffing" these feelings down further will somehow make these longings go away or subside.

All of your Truth and your Beauty lies within. Look inside. Surface perception without a Soul-Full connection keeps us living superficially. From there, it's impossible to access the miraculous life that comes from living as our Authentic Selves.

THE POWER OF BELIEF

Dr. Deepak Chopra states that "Your body is a 3-D projection of your current state of mind. Your slightest shift of mood is picked up by every cell, which means that you do not think with your brain alone—all 50 trillion cells in your body actively share your thoughts. At the level of the quantum mechanical body, you are a constantly flowing river of intelligence." In other words, your beliefs affect your physical body. Your cells are constantly changing and reforming themselves based upon the thoughts you are thinking—now! When you realize this, you can't help but see that your thoughts actually shape the way you look. Your physical body is nothing more than the thoughts you have consistently thought about it and so now believe. Your mind sculpts your body. So you must ask yourself, honestly, what is it I believe about myself? If you don't like the answer you hear—if your beliefs hinder your desires, then change them—but don't look for any outside validation in the process. Keep all of your wonderful, beautiful, healthy and whole thoughts about yourself to yourself— just for a while, until your Soul's brilliance surfaces for all to see.

SOMETHING TO CHEW ON

Make it a habit to leave a surface existence behind by looking deep inside and behind things. On this note, consider the following story. When I was an actress in commercials, the majority of my work took place behind the scenes while on commercial sets. What I discovered was that those commercials you view in just 30 to 60 seconds actually take hundreds of people and often weeks, if not months, of amazing and talented creative power to get them onto the screen. Movies take years of the same focus and forbearance to produce. Remember that if ever feelings of discouragement threaten to overcome your appreciation of yourself and the recognition of your progress—however long your weight loss takes you is OK.

SOUL-FULL EXERCISE #37

During my Transformational Living Workshops and Coaching Programs, I teach about The E3 Transformational Triad—which is the core body of my work. When put into practice, this Triad releases a person's Soul energy, thus raising their creative life-force to the third power.

I explain that a person can only realize such phenomenal power once they open their *mind, heart and will* to the Divine.

Participants learn to do this by practicing *Miracle Mindedness*, which transforms the way they perceive the world into *embrace. Miracle Matrixing* shows them how to *embody* the Divine Divine by living free of the concept that we are limited to a body. Then, in a third segment, they are taught *Miracle Mastery.* This last process illustrates and offers them insight on how to *expand* the Miraculous out from themselves to others, since in the Miraculous realm of the Soul we can only keep that which we give away.

Using the Triad as a method of losing weight would look like this…

First, you shift your perception to view yourself from the inside out—as a free Soul seeking to express your *inmost* desires. The purpose?—to know yourself as more than just a body that can be limited by your beliefs. What is it you were born to do? In what areas of your life are you tenaciously "hiding your Light under a bushel"? Holding onto excess baggage? Need to forgive the past? Once you discover those answers through introspection—journaling is a wonderful aid to this—you can forgive your past and start anew; making the appropriate changes to the way you have been approaching your life.

Then it's time to Matrix your newly discovered Self, that means—live your Light! To do that, you must get courageous—feel the rage of the heart—and let go of the layers you have put between you and life.

If during your Miracle-Mindedness work, you've unearthed an artist—by all means paint! If you've discovered a poet or a writer within yourself, write!—just for the sake of writing—with no care at all as to what other people may think. Who cares what they think! This is your time to prove to yourself that you can live fully and *freely from your heart.*

Next (and you only have permission to practice this facet of the work once you've owned and expressed your amazing, Self-discovered, and Soul-embracing talents first), you extend your Soul-Full Self and your talents to others, as a gift to them, always remembering—YOU are the gift! Your outer wrapping is only the smallest part of what you have to offer—all of the "real goods" are on the inside! Realizing this puts you firmly on the road to living a truly transformed, authentic life.

So here is your assignment. One of the most powerful gifts we can give to any other person is to hold a strong belief in their potential. The only greater gift is to first hold an unwavering belief in ourselves that allows us to transcend the limiting beliefs associated with the thought, "I am a body," and then demonstrate our own unbounded nature and Self-love on a daily basis. Take a few moments to connect with your Soul and from this standpoint discern what you believe about how you look, what weight you feel is optimum, how much you need to eat, and what types of foods bring you the deepest satisfaction and connection to life. Write down your insights if you like. Then vow to act on them—aligning your beliefs with your actions. Be a living breathing example of Self-Mastery, then others will respect you and easily believe your input and opinion as you encourage them to be the best person they can be.

"Living life fully is between you and you!"

~ Maureen Whitehouse

CHAPTER THIRTY-EIGHT

Feed Another

"The poor are hungry not only for food; they are hungry to be recognized as human beings. They are hungry for dignity and to be treated as we are treated. They are hungry for our love."
~ Mother Teresa

AS I WAS DOGGEDLY PLODDING along my Spiritual path, I came across Marianne Williamson's best-selling book, *Return to Love*. In it, she very lucidly explains the principles of the profound Spiritual work, *A Course in Miracles*, which many years later I would begin teaching myself. At that time, however, many of its principles baffled me, so I greatly appreciated her clarity. One insight Marianne imparted that particularly grabbed me was that if you find yourself upset about things that seem "wrong" to you, such as world hunger, then do something about it. But to that comment she added an intriguing twist—she said, don't do it for the others; do it for yourself. That is where you need healing of your perception most.

I took this advice quite literally and applied it to an area of my life that I felt needed healing—my relationship with food. As a model and commercial actress, I had spent so much time with the affluent and "beautiful people" and was fortunate to live a very abundant life. Yet deep inside of myself, I felt it was obscene that so many others were apparently just getting by in our abundant world. It made me feel guilty—something that *A Course in Miracles* points out is a humanly-made emotion and definitely not from God. So I became determined to find God in this situation.

Not long after this, I had an "aha moment" about how to do something. I spoke to the principal at my daughter's elementary school about setting up a partnership between the school and a local homeless shelter that had a soup kitchen and food pantry. We started out small, just gathering food for Thanksgiving baskets. But even this usually amounted to two or three van-loads of provisions. The effort grew over time to include sponsorships and clothing drives as well. But what I loved most about the experience was that the children got to deliver the food directly to the shelter with me and the other volunteers. Their faces would light up at being chosen to help, and the love and respect that they felt for themselves as they unloaded boxes was palpable. They felt connected. While driving the van on the way back to school afterwards, I loved looking in the rearview mirror to see the children chatting animatedly, or more often just sitting, smiling ear-to-ear, reveling in the glow of the experience. And needless to say, my heart healed as I felt I could genuinely feel great gratitude for the Souls who offered us this opportunity for involvement.

The basis of the miraculous is that we are all one, and the only thing that separates us is time and space. It's important for those of us who are seemingly "more fortunate" or "advanced" in life to remember that that's just what's seen on the level of form. Those "unfortunate" who are physically distressed may, in fact, be a bit further along the evolutionary path of the Soul than those who are apparently more fortunate. Notice how helping them actually helps *you* transcend labels and limiting beliefs.

You'll know that you've really begun to recognize a greater sense of connectedness to all beings when you have the inclination to close any gap that exists between yourself and others. If you are "well-off", you'll want to help another get a leg up on the ladder of life.

If you find that you're experiencing unsettling circumstances around food—like the inability to exercise your willpower when you pass a fast food restaurant or see a gooey, sugar-and-fat-laden dessert—it will always help for you to create a new appreciation for eating. And that appreciation can be one that doesn't rely on your taste-buds or the feeling of a full stomach. By deciding to feed another, you can acquire a reverence for the connecting virtue of food that goes much deeper.

There are a plethora of opportunities out there to do some hands-on volunteer work in food pantries, shelters, churches, nursing homes, children's hospitals and hospices. Next time you see a homeless person, ask them if they would like something to eat. If they say yes, give them food instead of money. Doing so will easily connect you with them—and your Truest Self.

MAKING FRIENDS OF STRANGERS

Around the same time that I was coordinating the food-pantry deliveries, I had an early morning appointment one day in downtown Boston. I was still modeling then, and had an interview for a possible job. After circling the area in search of a parking space, I happened to find a perfect spot just one block away from my destination.

I was relieved that I found the parking space sooner than I had expected, and even more so when I reached for the quarter roll I usually keep in the ashtray only to find the tray empty. I took the one quarter I had and put it in the meter, and then turned to walk down the street to a nearby coffee shop to get a cup of tea and the needed change. I immediately noticed a homeless couple just a few feet away from me "camped out" in the enclave of a church.

It was a rather brisk morning, and so a few minutes later as I ordered my tea, my mind wandered back to the man and woman hunkering under their blankets. I decided to order two more teas and two nice warm croissants. Then I handed the tea and croissants to the pair as I headed back to my car.

As I did this, it dawned on me that I would be gone for about two and a half hours, and the maximum time allowed on the meter was only two hours. It seemed completely logical to me that these folks could feed the meter for me.

I turned back to the two of them and said, "Hey, could you do me a favor?" With surprised looks on their faces, both of them immediately said, "Sure." The man then actually turned to look behind him to see if I could possibly be talking to someone else! Smiling, I told them my dilemma and gave them two quarters, asking them to feed my meter when the time was up.

Then I left, confident that I could breathe easy and take my time. However, when I got more than halfway down the block, I realized I forgot to put any of the other quarters I'd just procured at the coffee shop into the meter. I ran back to do just that.

I got back to my car almost a full 10 minutes later. As I passed the couple in the enclave, they were still talking about me and I heard the woman say, "She really trusts us. I'm surprised that she trusts us."

It wasn't until I heard them say those words that I realized that I did trust them. I hadn't even thought twice about them not being able to do this task for me. I simply saw them as I see all people now—as miraculous and, at the core of their true essence, Perfect.

And the way I saw the situation through miraculous perception was that I was put on that street at that particular time because the Powers That Be knew I wouldn't buy into the picture of two hapless, degenerate people. My Soul knew I would rise to the occasion and claim my True essence—as one who can unearth the Spirit of "Christ" and Perfection in others. This is something we can all do—*if we so choose.*

After my appointment, I went back to the coffee shop for a couple of hot soups and rolls for "my friends." They were just packing up their things, probably all of their earthly belongings, when I got back to the church entryway. The man said they had to go now, but they had waited for me and put the quarters in the meter just like I'd asked. Both of them were literally beaming at me. When I handed them the soup, the woman looked me directly in the eyes—something I have a feeling they didn't get the chance to do to strangers all that often—and said, "Thank you for being so nice and God bless you." I sincerely replied, "And the same to you."

In this situation, I knew with all of my heart that much more had been taught and learned and exchanged in this "chance encounter" than our separate selves would ever be able to grasp—but that the Oneness of our hearts fully felt. Turning away, I saw that the car parked directly behind me had a parking ticket on the windshield. I thought, Oh my, had that driver only known!

Put in its proper perspective, food can be seen for what it is first and fore-most—a vehicle for connecting to the Divine source within us and a way to empower ourselves and others and give and receive Love.

"Happiness is not perfected until it is shared."

~ Jane Porter

SOMETHING TO CHEW ON

Composer Gustav Mahler once said, "To take responsibility is to keep the ability to respond." Seen in this light, it's easy to realize why feeding another is an effortless way to cultivate the ability to be with someone else and in the present moment—thus feeding your own Soul. Think about how you have given through the gift of food. Can you do more?

SOUL-FULL EXERCISE #38

The next time you find yourself discouraged or despondent about any facet of your life, realize that in that moment you are in denial of the power that lies within you. Begin to see such feelings not as a reason to introvert but as a call to extend yourself from a deeper place within you. That way, you can expand your world rather than contracting into an enticing pity party centered on "poor me" thoughts that come from the ego. Self-pity will never allow you to feel power-full or to know your true nature as a force for change. After taking control of the direction of your thinking, do something for another that you would want done for yourself if you happened to be in their shoes. *We are one.*

CHAPTER THIRTY-NINE

Let Us Break Bread Together

"We should look for someone to eat and drink with, before looking for something to eat and drink."

~ Epicurus

I'VE FOUND THAT one way to insure you're eating from a position of emotional fullness is to share the experience with those you love.

It wasn't too long ago that most families gathered around the table each and every night to enjoy dinner together, with members of the extended family joining them on weekends. Mealtime created an opportunity for joining and deepening communion with one another. Opening the mouth not only brought the nourishment of the food, but also communication with one another—a mix that is deeply satisfying.

Today it's not unusual for family members to be scattered at all three meal-times, with parents working, traveling on business trips, or attending to otherwise important obligations, and children participating in school activities, team sports, or hobbies. Often people settle for eating alone or with the TV, a newspaper, or a book. This means a good deal of the *love-ly* experience of eating is often missed. What so many of us don't realize is that it's *greatly missed.*

MY MOST FULFILLING MEAL EVER

I've never felt as full—physically, mentally, vitally, emotionally and Spiritually—as the day I enjoyed my life's most satisfying meal, a meal in which we literally supped on love.

I had been Spiritual journeying in India with one of my most favorite people in the whole world, a person very well accomplished at the arts of appreciation and of being in the moment. Together we enjoyed many profound and Synchronistic experiences. On our way back to the States, we stopped in Europe where we met up with his sister.

One morning, the three of us traveled up the coast of Italy from Assisi to the small coastal town of Cinque Terre. The name Cinque Terre means *five fingers*, describing the way the land's five mountainous peninsulas jut out dramatically slicing into the ocean below. As we roamed in and out of the various shops on one of the fingers, appreciating the local artisans' goods, the three of us lost track of time. It was already peak mealtime when we realized that all of us were famished. However, we unanimously decided not to settle for just any restaurant for lunch, although most of the eateries were full due to the hour. We agreed that above all else, the place had to have *a view*.

We stopped at one tiny little picturesque spot and perused the lunch menu. Before we knew it, the owner swept us up and seated us at a table inside, since all of the tables outside were full. He assured us that it was too late to find anywhere else to eat. We were disappointed, since the tables outside were on a veranda overlooking the ocean. However, we'd made an unstated pact to be led by the moment so we went with the flow.

Once seated, we noticed that we were in front of a large floor-to-ceiling window, with its shutters closed. So we asked if it were possible to open the shutters. The owner replied by enthusiastically flinging the shutters apart to reveal the most breathtaking view. We were perched on the edge of a cliff overlooking the sea, with multi-colored homes built into the mountainsides all around us, and scattered fishing vessels below.

We were the only ones seated inside. It was a tiny place, and we could hear nearly every sound of the lively bustle taking place in the kitchen as the meals were prepared. When it came time to order, the sounds of the kitchen helped us realize the folly of trying to discern for ourselves what to eat. We asked the owner, who was now doubling as our waiter, to bring us his favorite meal. "Bravo," the man said, eyes twinkling with delight as he swept away the menus.

While waiting for the first course, we drank in every bit of the experience along with the suggested glass of house wine. All three of us simultaneously realized that we were at the beginning of a utopian experience. After the food arrived, our eyes met as we tasted our first bite, and all of us nearly burst out laughing with our mouths full. It was beyond description, almost painfully delicious, and we tried to contain our mile-wide smiles in order to chew. All we could murmur between forkfuls was "Mmmmmm." The sights, the sounds, the smells, the feelings, the tastes were all wonderful. Our every sense was being tickled to life.

What were we eating? The "house special," of course—Sardines in Tomato Sauce! This dish made our experience even more delightful—since we each ate mostly all vegetarian at the time, and it could easily have been considered "breaking the rules." But as we chewed each delectable morsel, we threw all care to the wind—quite literally—out the window it went carried on the peels of our bellyful laughter.

Our delight only intensified during the meal as one-by-one the rest of the members of the owner's family, who had been working in the kitchen, emerged to sit at the only other table inside the restaurant to eat their lunch together as well. This is something which we were told that they always did at the end of the busy mealtime. They thoroughly enjoyed one another's company and were evidently loving their meal—and each other—as well.

The owner would pop up from his seat from time to time to ask us how we were, as if that were necessary. The three of us stated the obvious when we replied in unrehearsed unison, "This is the best meal I have ever eaten!" and then burst out laughing again. Smiling, he replied, "People always say that." His response only made us laugh all the more, since we knew it was true. Although we'd had just one glass of wine, all of us felt completely drunk on the ecstasy of the moment.

We left the restaurant after finishing our meal with a bellyful of solace unlike any I have ever known before or since. That was the Fall, after I'd

"My idea of heaven is a great big baked potato and someone to share it with."

~ Oprah Winfrey

spent a good part of the Summer writing this book. Many times, I'd asked for guidance from the Divine to make this book as helpful as possible and to show me if I'd left out anything that was vitally important for others to realize. I know that meal was God's way of answering my request. Eating can be a way of filling our every sense with Divine delight. We just have to come to the table fully surrendered to the moment by opening our minds, our hearts and our bellies to Soul-Fullness in order to know that.

SOMETHING TO CHEW ON

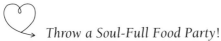

Next time you share a meal with those you love, see it as an unsurpassable opportunity to receive not only the food but also nourishment from the relationships. Choice moments can fill you up for an entire lifetime.

SOUL-FULL EXERCISE #39

Throw a Soul-Full Food Party!

Have a party with a mindful theme. This can be an intimate gathering or a full-blown bash. Prepare, or have everyone bring, wonderful foods made with organic, sustainable ingredients. Then after the guests have all arrived and the table is laden with goodies, share "grace" and gratitude with them in whatever way you feel is most authentic and Soul-Full for you. Let them know that they are a very important part of your life—then fully enjoy the feast and each other!

Food as a Healer

"The wise man should consider that health is the greatest of human blessings. Let food be your medicine."
~ Hippocrates, The Father of Medicine (460—377 BC)

SINCE ANCIENT TIMES, the medical profession has been enamored with food. Long before Hippocrates proclaimed food to have curative effects, healers were writing food remedies for common diseases on stone tablets. Papyrus prescriptions dating back to 4000 BC list foods as therapeutic. And it's widely known that Oriental cultures have long regarded food as an important aspect of medicine. In fact, the tendency for the medical profession to separate food and healing is a fairly recent phenomenon. But it appears that this is one that may be relatively short-lived.

Now there is a reemergence of healing-food advocates, particularly among the alternative-health community. But that's not the only place where questions are being asked and answered with regard to the inherent curative and preventive powers in foods. Research is happening all over the world in mainstream labs, medical centers and academic institutions. In addition, due to heightened public awareness and interest in less-invasive and alternative medical therapies world-wide, many governments are beginning to join the search for disease antidotes in the diet in a big way.

REFLECTIONS IN NATURE

In his book *Medicine Throughout Antiquity*, medical historian Benjamin Lee Gordon, MD, writes about an ancient text called the Doctrine of Signatures. He notes: "This doctrine was probably the earliest therapeutic system in the history of medicine." Gordon adds that translations of medical texts from the 7th century BC show that physician-priests referred to the Doctrine to find remedies in Assyro-Babylonian times.

The Doctrine states that for every part of our human body there is a corresponding part in nature. Just as is so typical in the world of Spirit, the macrocosm and microcosm are inseparable and always reflective of one another in the physical world. But the trick is… how do we find these mirroring aspects of nature?

Indigenous tribes had their "medicine man or woman" to do this for them—special tribal members who were known for being tapped into the Soul of creation and so could feel "the pulses" of the earth every bit as well as the pulses of a human beings. These wise-ones found—often at opposites ends of the earth simultaneously—that the cure resembled the malady in shape, color or structure. Dr. Gordon writes, "To make the search easier, the Creator stamped all objects medically beneficial to mankind."

Most homeopathic remedies make use of this concept, using an extremely diluted solution of the very substance that would typically cause a symptom in larger doses. For example, Silicea is a remedy made from silicone (a mineral) which is also used in the electronics industry to make silicone chips. Silicone is chosen because it is particularly inert. Silicea, the homeopathic remedy, is for people with no mental or physical energy who prefer inertia to action. It has a strengthening influence, allowing the person to feel physically and emotionally stronger, and better able to "move into" life with enthusiasm and confidence. In traditional Oriental Medicine, ginseng root—which resembles the human form—became known as a "whole-body tonic," and it was used as a general cure-all and to promote virility and longevity. Years ago, the philosopher Herbert Spencer wrote that the perfect correspondence always prevails in nature and that one thing is always balanced by another.

There's one catch to using the Doctrine's premise—chemical derivatives of foods and plants are not as powerful as the original plant extracts or whole food itself. If you isolate an apparent beneficial chemical or property from a plant, it may even have an opposite effect when administered and cause an elevation of the symptoms you hoped to alleviate. For instance, the extract from the plant belladonna, which reduces fever when administered in a precise way, could actually cause a fever if administered in too high a dose. It is apparent that nature has an innate intelligence that is best utilized when respected. Just as you can't mix up a whole bunch of nutrients found in an apple and viola! have a real apple, some foods cure best when eaten whole.

A PIECE OR THE WHOLE ENCHILADA?

Hold a piece of fruit or a vegetable and realize that each food is made up of 10,000 or more elements. If you become mindful of this, even for just a few moments, it's not difficult to see that nature is exquisite!

Each food holds an intricate and vast universe within itself. Why then focus on individual nutrients at the expense of the whole?

Given the vitamin fads and crazes that abound today, could it be doing us more harm than good to rely on supplements to take the place of eating a conscious, whole, well-balanced diet rich in a variety of life-giving and supporting foods? So many people have resorted to "eating on the run" and popping a few vitamins "to keep healthy and fit" when the (Divine) point was never to make the dysfunctional symptoms of separation from Soul more comfortable.

Looking at nutrition this way, disease can be a very useful prod to pull us out of an acceptance of fragmentation and separation and get us back on track honoring the essential call of our Soul, from within, to live as one with the whole.

Do you feel fit or fat? That may sound like a logical question to the millions of people who equate an optimal weight with fitness. However, what if instead of seeing "fit" as solely a physical attribute, you considered fitness to be a symptom of inner well-being—an inner state that just so happens to manifest physically?

Soul-Fullness fitness and health means that you're connected with a deeper sense of Self, which is your Eternal Being. This Self doesn't get sick, nor does it tire. When you sleep at night, this Self blithely creates—unencumbered by the shackles of your mind and body—in the dream world. The Art of Soul-Full Living is the art of allowing the veil between that free-Spirited dream state and your living, waking "reality" to slowly dissolve. The fact is that life is here *for you.*

So what does sickness and disease mean to one who realizes that? It means simply that there is a far greater experience of life available to you—you just have to **wake up** to it.

ACKNOWLEDGING THE WAKE-UP CALL

Sometimes illness can serve to be a powerful wake-up call that there is far too much *dis-ease* in our lives. A Soul-Full approach is the *ease-full* approach to eating and to life. By connecting you to all of life, this approach helps you to tap the flow of energy that can stimulate the body's natural ability to rejuvenate and heal.

When viewed objectively (a perspective that's not all that common due to the fear that typically surrounds illness), disease is actually the body's self-defense effort. Therefore, it is not a negative condition to be avoided, combated, and suppressed at all costs, but can trigger a positive constructive process aimed at healing and restoring the body back to its natural healthful state. Seen this way, disease can be viewed as a very helpful signal that something is amiss in our bodies—often because something is amiss in our lives. If we pay attention to these signals and act to make corrections directed at the causes and not the symptoms, then diseases can actually be seen as extremely beneficial aids to us on all levels.

It's important not to rush to cover up or treat symptoms before we take the time to look at what we may be consuming in our lives—on all levels—that could have initiated the illness. This evaluation process can call attention to an unbalanced condition in our lives and lead to powerful healing that takes place in ways far beyond that which we are now allowing into our experience. Part of the changes triggering the healing can take place in our diet.

ANN WIGMORE AND HER LEGACY

Sometimes necessary changes call for helpers or guides to lead the way. The Hippocrates Health Institute is a wholeness center in South Florida where the primary healing modality is organically grown, enzyme-rich vegetarian food. It is their experience that this dietary approach, complemented by positive thinking, is an extremely effective path to optimum health. I personally know many people who've spent time at Hippocrates in order to heal themselves of such diseases as cancer, arteriosclerosis, severe allergies and irritable bowel syndrome. The results of choosing this alternative path to healing have been nothing short of miraculous for them.

The foundation for the Hippocrates Health Institute began four decades ago, when visionary and humanitarian Ann Wigmore created a concept for healing based on the Hippocratic wisdom of "Let food be your medicine." Together with another kindred Soul, Viktoras Kulvinskas, she established a comprehensive institute in Boston, Massachusetts that taught people to draw the power to transform the quality of their lives from within their vast inner resources. Wigmore's passion for healing was no doubt fueled as she watched her grandmother treat wounded soldiers with grasses during World War I. She came to the United States while still a child and, in the 1950s, called on those memories of her grandmother when treating personal health problems.

Wigmore would go on to start a revolution in the world of nutrition that has continued to grow to this day. To many, her name is synonymous with the history of a health movement that has pushed alternative health-care measures into the forefront of the US and world consciousness. Her efforts—and the efforts of others like her—are largely responsible for cultivating an awareness that's sparked the modern research that has firmly

"By healing you learn of wholeness, and by learning of wholeness you learn to remember God."

~ A Course in Miracles

established the links between certain foods and health risks. Now we are seeing more research into the link between particular foods and health benefits.

Meanwhile, the fact is that people from all walks of life have opted to choose food as their healer when faced with a choice between the conventional and holistic approaches. Many, many of these same individuals can tell stories of substantial and even full recovery from illness. What was once considered miraculous is today becoming more commonplace.

"Seeing illness as misfortune, especially one that is undeserved, may obstruct the system. Coming to see illness as a gift that allows you to grow may unlock it."

~ Andrew Weil, MD

EXAMPLES OF HEALING FOODS

To give you some tangible examples, I've listed some food-remedies below that you may find valuable. Look in health food stores for the more unusual items I've mentioned. Also, find other remedies in the books listed in the resources section at the end of this chapter.

- **Burns**—Use fresh aloe vera gel both internally and externally. Eat raw aloe vera gel, raw manuka honey, avocados, olives, olive oil, spirulina and parsley.

- **Common cold**—Drink fresh water with the juice of one lemon, 1 Tbsp. of raw honey, and a thumb-sized amount of grated ginger added. This recipe can also be warmed and drunk as a "tea." Also, figs are excellent mucus dissolvers.

- **Constipation**—Eat lots of high-fiber, chlorophyll-rich foods such as green vegetables and add whole flax seeds, ground flax seeds, or flax oil to your diet.

- **Depression**—Throughout the day, eat lots of mildly-sweet fruits, such as berries, to keep your blood-sugar level high.

- **Eyesight**—Increase the amount of raw foods in your diet. The raw foods most often associated with improving eyesight are all berries, most especially blueberries and goji berries (a Himalayan berry found at health food stores), plus lychees, grapes, tumeric, blue-green algae, spirulina and dark green vegetables. Stop eating cooked fats, primarily animal fats.

- **Headache**—The ancient Romans and Greeks used fennel to treat migrane headaches. It thins the blood and so lessens the pressure on the blood vessels as the blood flows more freely.

- **Muscle Soreness**—Muscle soreness often results from the accumulation of too much lactic acid and uric acid in the body's tissues. To counteract acid build-up, drink alkaline green juices made from green vegetables, and eat spirulina and hemp seed.

- **PMS** (Pre-Menstrual Syndrome)—When women menstruate, they detoxify so this is a great time to get in sync with the body's natural rhythms. If you suffer from PMS each month, try cutting back on food or stop eating altogether during your menses. Do this by fasting on green juices for one to three days. When you resume eating, eat a diet of raw, live food while you continue to menstruate. Incorporate seaweeds into your regular diet as they are especially abundant in minerals and iron.

- **Skin problems**—For beautiful skin, eat plenty of foods rich in silicon—such as lettuces, okra, cucumber and radishes—and sulfur—which include aloe vera, cruciferous vegetables (broccoli and cauliflower), onion, garlic, red bell peppers, and hot peppers. Also of great benefit are the "good fats" found in coconut meat and coconut oil, as well as hempseed, borage and flax seed oil. All cooked fats should be avoided.

- **Ulcers**—Cabbage, which is high in the amino acid glutamine, is beneficial in healing ulcers. For best results, drink it juiced, mixed with other juices such as cucumber, celery or apple. Or eat it raw in salads.

GIVE YOURSELF TIME FOR HEALING

Something interesting happens when you step into alignment with your Soul, and make powerful healing life changes from the inside-out. Unlike with the typical "slash and burn" medical approach (that can appear to be an "instantaneous fix"), the effects of healing are typically very subtle at first, and often not at all apparent to the naked eye. That's because the most vital, central organs heal and transform first, and then next the bones and musculature, and finally the outer perimeter of the body is the last to heal. Also, food choices have a cumulative effect on the body. Just as it took you some time to feel the ill-affects of your detrimental lifestyle choices, so too does it take time to heal.

SOMETHING TO CHEW ON

Bernie S. Siegel, MD, once said, "Diseases can be our Spiritual flat tires—disruptions in our lives that seem to be disastrous at the time, but end by redirecting our lives in a meaningful way."

SOUL-FULL EXERCISE #40

Consider the adage "You are what you eat" in a deeper way. When you consume food, it literally becomes you. If you're eating only what is grown with love, prepared with love, and served with love, your body's cells will be swimming in love—the most powerful healing energy on the planet. If you have been plagued by repetitive, ill-health of any kind, consider what and how you've been eating. Also, make it a practice to trace any health challenges (effects) when they arise, no matter if they be acute symptoms or long-standing addictions, back to their source (or true cause). On a blank piece of paper, or in your journal, ask, "What is the true cause of this health challenge?" Then wait in stillness until you hear the answer that your Soul, your Inner Wisdom, has been waiting patiently to relate to you. Record your answer, but don't stop there! Follow through and make the necessary dietary and lifestyle changes—all the while listening to the promptings of your Soul.

In addition, are you finding that you're feeling "vitamin deficient"? Instead of popping a few supplements, slow down, relax, breathe and reconnect by eating a whole, fresh organic apple. Then when you're finished, plant the apple seeds, or save them until you find a time when you can. Reconnect with life. Become one with the whole. That's the cure for every dis-ease.

"We should consider every day lost on which we have not danced at least once."

~ Friedrich Nietzsche

RESOURCES

The Complete Guide to Health and Nutrition by Gary Null

Healing with Whole Foods by Paul Pitchford

Eat More, Weigh Less by Dean Ornish, MD

Hippocrates Live Food Program by Ann Wigmore

The Food Pharmacy by Jean Carper

Food—Your Miracle Medicine by Jean Carper

Super Foods by Steven Pratt, MD and Kathy Mathews

Food and Healing by Annemarie Colbin

Foods that Heal by Bernard Jensen

The Cancer Prevention Diet by Mishio Kushi

Encyclopedia of Natural Medicine by Joseph Pizzorno and Michael Murray, ND

Healing Foods by Michael Murray, ND, Joseph Pizzorno, ND
    and Lara Pizzorno, MA, LMT

Hippocrates Health Institute

www.hippocratesinst.com

Bon Appétit!

"As soon as you trust yourself, you will know how to live."
~ Johann Wolfgang von Goethe

OK. NOW, LET'S STEP BACK, take a big deep breath, and take a wider view of things for a moment.

You are a Soul. You came to Earth to remember that, and to wake up from the unsatisfying dream of limitation and separation. Your time here began when you breathed your first breath. You will leave with your last. In between those breaths everything you do is left up to you and your free will.

But here's a word of advice. No matter what it is that you choose to do, you will not, and cannot, be truly happy if you are out of step with the Divine and unconscious of your own inherent goodness. By focusing on your connection to the deeper Soul of life, you naturally fall into step—without effort, strife or strain.

FEEDING YOUR SOUL, IMPACTING THE WORLD

"One of
the very nicest
things about life is
the way we must
regularly stop
whatever it is we
are doing and
devote our
attention
to eating."

~ Luciano Pavarotti

We are now entering into a new era on earth. One in which humanity is beginning to wake up from the separating dream of selfishness. We are just beginning to realize that both heaven and hell have always existed—not "somewhere out there"—but within every one of us and right here on this earth. It's up to each one of us to choose whether it's heaven or hell that we manifest and experience in our lives.

This planet is currently being faced with many challenges—terrorism, global warming, pollution, starvation, disease, homelessness, natural disasters and weapons of destruction in the hands of fearful and power-hungry leaders, to name but a few. To me these events all have a human and not a Divine origin. Take a deep breath and a small step back into your Soul, and you will see that it is our incessant movement and unceasing hunger that keeps so many people experiencing themselves in the "wrong place at the wrong time"—which is hell by the way—grabbing for all of the alluring things that promise an ever-evasive brand of happiness. That is what keeps this ball of confusion in motion. But at the same time, our frenetic energies are impacting everything; that is how powerful we are. So it's now time for each of us to use the powers we all possess **consciously**—since we are the dreamers of the dream. We can make life a blissful experience, or a nightmare. *Only we humans can stop the inhumanity!*

The wounds of this world are gaping now—far too big for Band-Aids and far too evident to ignore. But that's alright because now we can see more clearly that change is necessary. We can learn from our mistakes and reclaim our power on an individual and collective level. We can begin to be gentle with one another, consume responsibly in harmony with the laws of love, and come together to co-create a new earth—*with Soul.*

The way is now being paved by many for an experience here on earth that is greater than anything that has come before. If you've been moved in any way—either inwardly, or to action—by anything that you've read in this book, then you are the living, breathing proof that the new reality is upon us. You are the evidence that we can all learn to change our minds and open our hearts, and as Mahatma Ghandi said, "*Be the change we wish to see in the world.*"

What we are experiencing is a Divine wake-up call. It's time *now* to stop being so blindly selfish, to stop creating and consuming so many products that absolutely do not contribute to our well-being or survival, which even harm and endanger our lives. When you begin to see the entire world on your plate each and every time you eat—when you see how your choices impact you and the world—you automatically align with a deeper truth and commit to living it. Love yourself and everything you consume and then pass this awareness on, one blessed plate-full at a time, to another. What an example! That is truly the way to change your thoughts about the world.

And keep the other lifestyle practices in mind; stop buying products that harm or endanger lives. Carefully review what it is that you support with your dollars, your energy, and your time. Be congruent with your beliefs, words and actions, and vow to support only those services that bless the family of humanity and help build a kinder, better and safer world. And always remember that *all we need is one **fully** loving person to heal this world*. YOU are the one person who can make a difference when you raise up your voice in conviction and become a living example of the power of love to others. Just start where you are today, with something as simple as the next meal you eat, or your next trip to the grocery store. No truly impactful revolution begins on a grandiose scale, but with one person's simple willingness to show up and lovingly and authentically live the life that unfolds before them. That is the opportunity available to you *right now*.

A RECAP

Now, as one last gentle reminder, here is a list of some of the most powerful and effective ways discussed in this book to eat Soul-Fully:

1. **First and foremost—Eat with love, what is grown with love, prepared with love, and served with love**—always remembering *you are a Soul!*

2. Know that an underlying principle in all your food choices is to seek quality that you can feel on a Soul level.

3. Choose sustainable, organically grown, hormone-free, free-range, locally grown foods whenever possible. This connects you with your true compassionate Soul.

4. Prepare food with presence, realizing that the main ingredient to add is love.

5. Bless your food and feel gratitude for all that brings abundance to your life.

6. Eat a rainbow assortment of fruits and vegetables with a full spectrum of pigments—recognizing that eating this way fills us up with beauty and Light, affecting not only our body, but our mind and Spirit as well.

7. Eat to regulate your blood-sugar level—avoiding The "7 Energy Stealers," for a well-balanced, centered and peaceful persona.

8. Do not over-consume meat and other animal foods.

9. Eat the "good fats."

10. Eat in moderation, remembering that "less is more" and allowing the Light-within to shine bright.

11. Keep salt intake low and potassium intake high. Potassium—essential to life and health—also helps the body's cells conduct energy more effectively. Potassium is found in fresh fruits and vegetables.

12. Do a periodic fast or cleanse—to "Lighten up."

13. Drink sufficient water every day. It will help increase the flow in your life.

14. Breathe deeply!—remembering it is one of the most powerful ways to connect with the Soul.

15. Finally, *be still…* and know you are One with God.

"I am not a body. I am free.
For I am still as God created me."
~ *A Course in Miracles*

THE LOVE SCALE OF "FOODS"

I also felt it important to include the quick-reference chart on the following page to remind you which foods (and elements) will keep you most healthy, balanced and Soul-Full. The foods that contain the most love, radiance, rejuvenation and positive energy begin at the top of the chart, and those with the least love and positive energy are listed at the bottom. This chart was adapted from the "Karma Chart," found in David Wolfe's book, *The Sunfood Diet Success System.*

More than any chart or anything else for that matter, there is, however, one universal truth to follow. *By paying attention to your body, through caring self-observation and by remaining centered on your Soul, it is possible to discern how your individual needs can best be met, throughout all the seasons of your life.* A low protein, low fat or entirely raw food diet is not a goal or even an ideal to achieve. But what's important to learn is how to glean from your body's innate wisdom all that you need to know about yourself. Then lift that up even higher to align with the Light of your Soul.

Study the information in this book, sit with it, grow with it, and play with it in order to determine what has particular relevance for you. Then, most importantly, vow to yourself that you will eat what helps you to maximize your energy flow, connects you to your Soul, and promotes the greatest experience of vitality that you can give to yourself.

A key to living a vibrant, free and joyous life is to remember that anything you eat with judgment, guilt or fear will bind you to the imprisoning limitations of body-identification. Conversely, anything you eat with love further aligns you with your liberating Divine nature—your Soul.

EAT WITH SOUL

Highest Love	Sunlight
Soul-Full	Fresh air
(Alkaline)	Water
	Mother's milk
	Fatty fruits (avocado, durian, olives)
	Sweet fruits (melons, berries, bananas, papaya, mango)
	Non-sweet fruits (bell pepper, cucumber, tomato)
	Raw plant foods prepared with love
	Greens (picked by the leaf with root remaining in ground to regenerate)
	Seaweeds
	Onion and garlic bulb (root-ball viable)
	Milk given freely from free-range animals
Neutral	Edible flowers
	Greens picked by killing the plant
	Onion and garlic bulb (root-ball killed)
	Hybrid seeds (rice, wheat, legumes)
	Coconut
	Tree nuts
	Seeds
	Hybrid roots (carrots, beets, potatoes)
	Eggs, insects, fish
Fear	Milk taken from enslaved animals
Soul-Less	Animal muscle, organ fat and blood (most especially
(Acidic)	inhumanely caged and feed-lot raised)

Note: Your intention to align with your Soul is the number one requisite to Soul-Full Eating. Therefore all blessed food, eaten with love—no matter what the food is—is Soul Food!

GOOD-BYE FOR NOW

We've come a long way together in this delicious journey and I thank you from the bottom of my heart for joining me.

At this point, you've gotten all of the basics to connecting with your Soul through eating. But there's one last ingredient that only you can add to this experience—*yourself*. Come to this feast called life with *all* of yourself. If you choose to talk, walk, sing, laugh, dance *and eat* with all of your being, you will always, always feel full.

The next time you pick up a forkful of your favorite food, do it with Soul— with every inch of your Being. Raise it to the heavens treating it like a toast at a madcap New Year's Eve party. Fill this act with fervor, let it feed your heart's delight and open you to the infinite possibility that this one bite can be your doorway to the Divine.

To Life!

May blessings abound for you as you
eat your way into your heavenly home!

Amen.

At This Feast

I don't want to be the only one here
Telling all the secrets—

Filling up all the bowls at this feast
Taking all the laughs.

I would like you
To start putting things on the table
That can also feed the Soul
The way I do.

That way
We can invite

A hell of a lot more
Friends.

~ Hafiz, 14th century Persian mystic poet

"Life is the sum of all your choices."

~ ALBERT CAMUS

ADDITIONAL RESOURCES

ETHICAL AND SUSTAINABLE FOOD SOURCES

Whole Foods

www.wholefoodsmarket.com

Wild Oats

www.wildoats.com

Trader Joe's

www.traderjoes.com

ORGANIC

You can find a vast and wonderful array of organic products at health/natural-food stores, food coops, and some regular supermarkets. Here are websites to check out if you'd like even more information about where to find organic items.

The Organic Consumers Association

www.organicconsumer.org

The Rodale Institute (the "Granddaddy" of the organic movement)

www.rodaleinstitute.org

Green People

www.greenpeople.org

Fair Trade

These sites give information about fair-traded foods:

The Fair Trade Federation

www.fairtradefederation.org

The Fair Trade Labeling Organizations International

www.fairtrade.net

Transfair USA

www.transfairusa.org

Compassionate Eating
(Loving Animals and the Environment)

To find out more about how to get started eating Vegan—the surefire way to be certain you are not harming animals—here are some excellent websites:

People for the Ethical Treatment of Animals

www.VegCooking.com and www.GoVeg.com

Vegan Outreach

Offers delicious recipes and great advice at:

www.veganoutreach.org

Compassion Over Killing

More recipes and good advice:

www.TryVeg.com

The Physician's Committee for Responsible Medicine

Find vegetarian starter kits as well as recipes and advice at:

www.pcrm.org

Index

Also Available from Axiom Audio Productions
by Maureen Whitehouse

- **Miracle Manifesting**, 2 CD Set, 90 minutes, $17.00

- **How to Be in Love All of the Time**, 2 CD Set. 90 minutes, $17.00

- **The Soul at Work**, 4 CD Set (includes meditation CD), approx. 120 minutes, $37.00

- **The Path of the Soul**, 4 CD Set , approx. 180 minutes, $37.00

- **Conscious Couples**, 4 CD Set, approx. 180 minutes, $37.00

- **Conscious Parenting**, 4 CD Set, approx. 180 minutes, $37.00

Order online at *www.experienceaxiom.com* or call 1-800-611-6165.

Email Mini Courses

- **The E3 Transformational Triad**, 90 day Email Mini-Course, $87.00

- **30 Days to Miracle Mindedness**, $37.00

- **30 Days to Miracle Matrixing**, $37.00

- **30 Days to Miracle Mastery**, $37.00

- **The Soul at Work**, 27 Day Email Mini-Course, $37.00

Exclusively available online at *www.experienceaxiom.com*.

Soul-Full Supplements
Proprietary blends

- **Green Food Formula**

- **Vegetarian Enzymes**

- **Probiotics**

- **Plant Minerals**

Exclusively available online at *www.soul-fulleating.com*.

"Wherever you go,
go with all of your heart (and Soul)."

~ Confucius (and Maureen)

Notes

Notes

Notes

Notes

Notes

Notes

Notes

Notes